Evidence-Based Practice in Suicidology: A Source Book

Evidence-Based Practice in Suicidology: A Source Book

Maurizio Pompili
Roberto Tatarelli
(Editors)

HOGREFE

Library of Congress Cataloging in Publication

is available via the Library of Congress Marc Database under the
LC Control Number 2010925398

Library and Archives Canada Cataloguing in Publication

Evidence-based practice in suicidology : a source book / Maurizio Pompili,
Roberto Tatarelli, editors.

Includes bibliographical references and index.
ISBN 978-0-88937-383-9

1. Suicide–Prevention. 2. Suicide. I. Pompili, Maurizio. II. Tatarelli, Roberto.

RC569.E95 2010   616.85'8445   C2010-902136-3

PUBLISHING OFFICES
USA: Hogrefe Publishing, 875 Massachusetts Avenue, 7th Floor, Cambridge, MA 02139
Phone (866) 823-4726, Fax (617) 354-6875; E-mail customerservice@hogrefe-publishing.com
EUROPE: Hogrefe Publishing, Rohnsweg 25, 37085 Göttingen, Germany
Phone +49 551 49609-0, Fax +49 551 49609-88, E-mail publishing@hogrefe.com

SALES & DISTRIBUTION
USA: Hogrefe Publishing, Customer Services Department, 30 Amberwood Parkway,
Ashland, OH 44805
Phone (800) 228-3749, Fax (419) 281-6883, E-mail customerservice@hogrefe.com
EUROPE: Hogrefe Publishing, Rohnsweg 25, 37085 Göttingen, Germany
Phone +49 551 49609-0, Fax +49 551 49609-88, E-mail publishing@hogrefe.com

OTHER OFFICES
CANADA: Hogrefe Publishing, 660 Eglinton Ave. East, Suite 119-514, Toronto, Ontario M4G 2K2
SWITZERLAND: Hogrefe Publishing, Länggass-Strasse 76, CH-3000 Bern 9

Hogrefe Publishing
Incorporated and registered in the Commonwealth of Massachusetts, USA, and in Göttingen, Lower Saxony, Germany

Printed and bound in the USA
ISBN 978-0-88937-383-9

Table of Contents

Foreword

The most widely cited definition of evidence-based medicine is:

> . . . the conscientious, explicit, and judicious use of current best evidence in making decisions about the care of individual patients. The practice of evidence based medicine means integrating individual clinical expertise with the best available external clinical evidence from systematic research. By individual clinical expertise we mean the proficiency and judgement that individual clinicians acquire through clinical experience and clinical practice.

The term "evidence," in English, means the type of knowledge derived from research, and although the term does not translate particularly well into Italian, French, or German, the term "evidence-based decision-making" has stuck and has become popular. The propositions made by professionals can be divided into those that are based on research evidence, evidence-based propositions, and those that are based on experience or opinion or on values. The former are not morally superior to the latter, but are less personal and less subjective, and there is fairly general agreement that decisions for both individuals and for populations or groups of patients should be based on research evidence.

"Evidence-based" is a term, of course, which includes not only the word "evidence" but also the word "based," and decisions that are based on evidence do need to take into account the particular needs of the individual patient or group of patients, as shown in the diagram below:

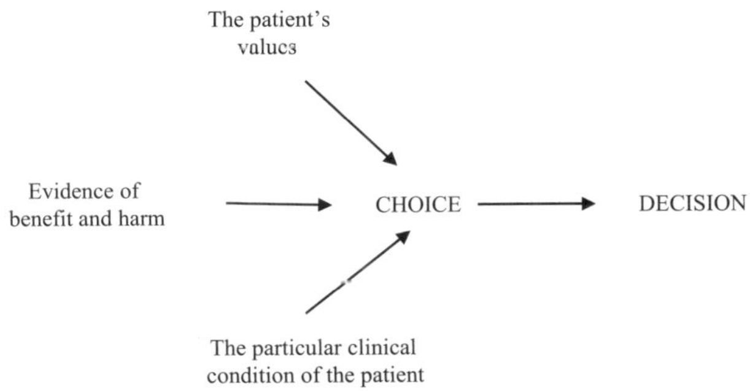

Relating the evidence to the individual's clinical condition, their other diagnoses, or risk factors, for example, sometimes called personalized medicine, requires the skills of a clinician. Even then values have to be taken into account, and not all clinicians or policy-makers are equally adept at managing values.

Evidence-based decision-making is most difficult when the evidence is scanty and when the values are strong, and in the prevention of suicide both these criteria hold true. Nevertheless, for both individuals and for populations it is essential that an evidence-based approach be taken. When resources are scarce, the best use has to be made of those resources. It is also important for those who are skilled in the management of evidence to appreciate that evidence-based decision-making is evidence-based, and that values may drive a decision more than evidence. If public values demand that something be done, then the values may be deemed more important than the evidence if the evidence is that the type of action being proposed is ineffective.

In a democracy, values are more important than evidence. To the policy-maker, the official, the presentation of evidence is a core responsibility. If the decision goes against them, then they have to consider whether they can accept this value-based decision or whether they should resign.

In both the prevention of suicide in the individual and in the population, evidence and values need to be brought together; what is required then is good judgment, and that is sometimes even scarcer than good evidence.

Sir Muir Gray
NHS National Knowledge Service
Summertown Pavilion
Middle Way
Oxford OX2 7LG
UK
Tel.: +44 7770 970 997
E-mail: muir.gray@medknok.net

The Framework

Evidence-Based Practice in Suicidology

What We Need and What We Need to Know

Maurizio Pompili[1,2]

[1]Department of Neurosciences, Mental Health and Sensory Functions, Suicide Prevention Center, Sant'Andrea Hospital, Sapienza University of Rome, Italy
[2]McLean Hospital, Harvard Medical School, Boston, MA, USA

Suicide prevention has become a national imperative in most countries worldwide, and a huge amount of resources has been invested to reduce the tragic loss of human lives that we witness each day. Despite great efforts in suicide prevention, the reduction of suicide rates does not parallel the ever-increasing investments both in economic and in human resources terms.

One of the most important obstacles in the prevention of suicide is the lack of solid evidence-based practices for delivering a sound intervention. Yet, suicidology proposes many interventions that have turned out to be effective. To some extent, in the health care domain, many practices are believed to be more or less a matter of one's own intuition, as if suicide prevention were a kind of art that some people may be able to master better.

Can we talk of "the art" of suicide prevention? Yes and no. The former because you must be really close to certain aspects of human suffering to deal with suicidal individuals and the latter because we must rely on shared principles that derive from evidence. With Hippocrates, medicine became a science and he was the one who stated "Where there is love for mankind, there is the love for the art of healing," David Sackett – one of evidence-based medicine's best proponents – once famously said that, when it comes to medicine, "Art kills" (Zuger, 1997). Whenever suicide prevention is based on our own intuition, we run the risk of not providing the best available care for an individual and, even worse, run the risk of losing that individual by suicide. In fact, relying on our scheme of reasoning or learned behavior may turn out to be extremely dangerous when dealing with suicidal subjects.

Prevention must be based on the most sound and best evidence available. Suicide prevention must begin with identifying prevention strategies, followed by conducting research to determine if these strategies work. Whenever we believe that we have an effective strategy, we should explore the impact and cost of that strategy in a community setting and then work for improving the strategy and its delivery.

The term *evidence-based programs* generally refers to interventions that have been evaluated and found to produce the desired results – in this case, reductions in suicidal behaviors or risk. The term *evidence-based prevention* can refer to those programs and also to effective *processes* for developing prevention programs, such as assessing local needs and assets, basing program content on up-to-date research and theory, tailoring programs to specific target audiences, designing multiple program components to work synergistically, and conducting evaluations. Choosing evidence-based *programs* and using effective *processes* are both important for effective prevention.

Recently, Berman (2008) raised the issue stating that we need scientific evidence "or at least a strong, logical argument based on the premise 'it is more likely than not ....' " He challenged the audience by asking for credible responses worthy of consideration for the following issues:

1. Is there evidence that suicide prevention public awareness programs or strategies save lives? (If not, why do organizations continue to spend limited available monies on these?)
2. Is there evidence that universal prevention programs are more cost effective and efficacious than indicated prevention programs? (If not, why are these so much more often put into effect?)
3. Is there evidence that the level of activity of suicidal thoughts (vague or passive ideation compared to detailed or active ideation) is directly related to suicidal behavior; that is, is there evidence that the more active and detailed the ideation, the greater risk of behavior (suicide attempt or death) and/or the more vague or passive the ideation the less risk behavior?
4. Is there evidence, other than anecdotal, to support the idea that giving away the prized possessions should be considered a warning sign (acute risk factor) for suicide? (If not, why is this so frequently mentioned as a warning by so many organizations educating the public about suicide's warning signs?)

Rodgers, Sudak, Silverman, and Litts (2007) reported that expert-based review systems rely primarily on the experience of experts to determine what is evidence-based. These systems are used by experts to evaluate program effectiveness. While some prevention fields could boast of multiple registries of evidence-based programs and formidable arrays of published studies summarized in quantitative reviews, suicide prevention has relatively little to show in the way of evidence-based programs. Little is known about the effectiveness of many of these programs. The Suicide Prevention Action Network USA (SPAN USA Inc., 2001) reported that the "The single greatest obstacle to the effective prevention of suicide is the lack of evaluation research" (p. 19).

Pouliot and De Leo (2006) stated that:

> The current emphasis on psychiatric disorders in published research needs to be balanced by a better study of the socioenvironmental contributors to suicide, particularly by stimulating the attention on conceiving and adopting standardized instruments and/or structured interviews that may favor the appropriate weighting of these variables. Efforts in this direction promote a truly ecological approach for understanding suicide and assist in the development of better preventive strategies.

In describing a practice as evidence-based, we mean that a body of research evidence supports the practice's effectiveness. According to the Institute of Medicine:

> Effectiveness refers to the care that is based on the use of systematically acquired evidence to determine whether an intervention produces better outcome than alternatives – including the alternative of doing nothing.

Expert-based review systems rely primarily on the experience of experts to determine what is evidence-based. Such systems are used by experts to evaluate program effectiveness.

According to Sackett, Rosenberg, Gray, Haynes, and Richardson (1996):

> Evidence-based medicine is the conscientious, explicit, and judicious use of current best evidence in making decisions about the care of individual patients. The practice of evidence-based medicine means integrating individual clinical expertise with the best available external clinical evidence from systematic research. By individual clinical expertise we mean the proficiency and judgment that individual clinicians acquire through clinical experience and clinical practice.

By best available external clinical evidence we mean clinically relevant research, often from the basic sciences of medicine, but especially from patient-centered clinical research, to the accuracy and precision of diagnostic tests (including the clinical examination), the power of prognostic markers, and the efficacy and safety of therapeutic, rehabilitative, and preventive regimens. Without clinical expertise, practice risks becoming tyrannized by evidence, for even excellent external evidence may be inapplicable to or inappropriate for an individual patient.

The best external clinical evidence can be obtained only if a hierarchy of evidence is taken into account. This hierarchy is usually provided as follows, the evidence at the top of the list being the most reliable:

- Systematic reviews and meta-analyses (discussion of validity and confidence intervals)
- Randomized controlled trials (discussion of validity, magnitude, and clinical significance of results)
- Cohort studies
- Case-control studies
- Cross-sectional surveys
- Case reports.

Evidence-based medicine is not restricted to randomized trials and meta-analyses. It involves tracking down the best external evidence with which to answer our clinical questions. To consider an evidence-based approach, we should rely on the four-step approach:

- Formulate a clinical question
- Search for relevant information
- Evaluate the evidence for validity and usefulness
- Apply the evidence to the particular clinical situation/individual patient.

Last but not the least the evidence-based professional should filter the evidence, that is he or she should perform a critical appraisal of what is found.

The Example of the Suicide Prevention Resource Center

The US Suicide Prevention Resource Center (SPRC) (www.sprc.org) promotes the implementation of the National Strategy for Suicide Prevention and enhances the nation's mental health infrastructure by providing states, government agencies, private organizations, colleges and universities, and suicide survivor and mental health consumer groups with access to the science and experience that can support their efforts to develop programs, implement interventions, and promote policies to prevent suicide.

The organization has established *the Best Practices Registry (BPR) for Suicide Prevention* whose purpose is to identify, review, and disseminate information about best practices that address specific objectives of the *National Strategy for Suicide Prevention*. The registry has three sections: Section I: Evidence-Based Programs; Section II: Expert and Consensus Statements; and Section III: Adherence to Standards. The three sections are not intended to represent "levels" of effectiveness, but rather include different types of programs and practices reviewed according to specific criteria for that section. BPR listings include only materials submitted and reviewed according to the designated criteria and do not represent a comprehensive inventory of all suicide prevention initiatives.

Section I: Evidence-Based Programs

This section contains interventions that have undergone rigorous evaluation and have demonstrated positive outcomes. Section I includes listings from two sources: (1) interventions reviewed and rated by Substance Abuse and Mental Health Services Administration's (SAMHSA's) National Registry of Evidence-Based Programs and Practices, and (2) programs reviewed as part of the SPRC/American Foundation for Suicide Prevention Evidence-Based Practices Project.

Section II: Expert and Consensus Statements

This section lists statements that summarize the current knowledge in the field and provide "best practice" recommendations to guide program and policy development.

Section III: Adherence to Standards

This section contains suicide prevention programs and practices, including awareness materials, educational and training programs, protocols, and policies, that have been implemented in specific settings (as opposed to Section II statements that offer general guidance to the field). These programs address specific objectives of the *National Strategy for Suicide Prevention* and their content has been reviewed for accuracy, likelihood of meeting objectives, and adherence to program design standards. Being listed in this section means that the program content meets the stated criteria; inclusion does not mean that the practice has been proven effective through evaluation (those programs are listed in Section I). While this section does not include treatments, it does contain practices that support treatment such as case-finding, compliance, and aftercare.

The BPR is designed to support program planners in creating effective suicide prevention programs. This section explains briefly how the BPR fits into the concept of evidence-based prevention and provides suggestions for using the BPR as part of a data-driven planning process.

Principles of Suicide Prevention Effectiveness

According to Suicide Prevention Action Network USA (SPAN USA Inc., 2001), the following principles should be taken into account when designing prevention actions:

- Prevention programs should be designed to enhance protective factors. They should also work toward reversing or reducing known risk factors. Risk for negative health outcomes can be reduced or eliminated for some or all of a population.
- Prevention programs should be long term, with repeat interventions to reinforce the original prevention goals.
- Family-focused prevention efforts may have a greater impact than strategies that focus only on individuals.
- Community programs that include media campaigns and policy changes are more effective when individual and family interventions accompany them.
- Community programs need to strengthen norms that support help-seeking behavior in all settings, including family, work, school, and community.
- Prevention programming should be adapted to address the specific nature of the problem in the local community or population group.
- The higher the level of risk of the target population, the more intensive the prevention effort must be and the earlier it must begin.
- Prevention programs should be age-specific, developmentally appropriate, and culturally sensitive.
- Prevention programs should be implemented with no or minimal differences from how they were designed and tested.

Toward a Definition of Suicidology

Suicidology can be defined as the scientific study of suicide and suicide prevention. The term (and the concept) was first used by Shneidman (1964) and has since then been used in a number of ways such as to describe a new training scheme (Fellowship in

Suicidology, 1967); as part of a new journal (Bulletin of Suicidology, 1967); and to label a new association (The American Association of Suicidology, 1968). Suicidology is unlike other behavioral sciences in that it has usually included not just the study of suicide but also its prevention, in other words it incorporates appropriate clinical interventions to prevent suicide, a feature not always taken into consideration in the many contributions towards understanding suicide. The focus of suicidology is not necessarily completed suicide but above all the treatment of suicidal individuals. Suicides die with their unique life histories and dealing with pooled data or statistics would appear inappropriate for understanding the human misery of these individuals. Maris, Berman, and Silverman (2000) stated that:

> While suicidologists give lip service to the multidisciplinary study of suicide, in actual fact most of us have very narrow and specialized domain assumption – usually those related to our professional training and subdisciplinary paradigms.

It is perhaps received wisdom in suicidology that suicidal individuals are experiencing unbearable psychological pain or suffering and that suicide may be, at least in part, an attempt to escape from this suffering.

As reported by Maris and colleagues (2000), the building blocks of a systematic theory of suicide include definition, basic concepts (lethality, motive, suicidal career, etc.), hypothesis, models, and research results. Regardless of such items, some concepts are so basic to suicide that they can be thought of as the commonalities of suicide. Shneidman (1985) listed some practical measures for helping highly suicidal persons:

1. Stimulus (unbearable pain): reduce the pain
2. Stressor (frustrated needs): fill the frustrated needs
3. Purpose (to seek a solution): provide a different answer
4. Goal (cessation of consciousness): indicate alternatives
5. Emotion (hopelessness-helplessness): give transfusion of hope
6. Internal attitude (ambivalence): play for time
7. Cognitive state (constriction): increase the options
8. Interpersonal act (communication of intention): listen to the cry, involve others
9. Action (egression): block the exit
10. Consistency (with lifelong patterns): invoke previous positive pattern of successful coping.

The 1950s: Los Angeles Suicide Prevention Center

This book was in the final stages of preparation when Edwin Shneidman passed away. He was no doubt the person who fathered suicidology and who gave me some insight for this book during our long and regular chats on the telephone. The discipline was born under the star of searching for evidence related to suicide. Shneidman's search for evidence was a breakthrough in understanding suicide. He proposed the first experiment in the field and this was an effort to understand it scientifically.

As in most important developments in science, serendipity played a big role. It was not a particular interest in the topic that first moved Shneidman to get involved with suicide research, but rather his normal duties. In the last period of his life, he recalled the following event in 1949:

> I was 31 and a clinical psychologist at Brentwood Veterans Administration Neuropsychiatric Hospital, and the superintendent asked me to prepare letters for his signature to two new widows whose husbands had recently committed suicide. On my own I went to the county coroner's office to find relevant background material and discovered a vault with hundreds of suicide notes. My contribution was to recognize their enormous potential, behavioral science potential. My further contributions were not to read them (so as to remain blind) and to invent, on the spot, a new genre of document, namely the elicited suicide note from non-suicidal persons so as to be able to compare genuine suicide notes in a real double-blind experiment. The day I went to the Coroner's office was somewhat an epiphany of my life. I then called Norman Farberow, who had recently completed a dissertation on suicidal patients using my Make a Picture Story test. Norman and I blindly analyzed each genuine and simulated suicide note. We published the results in a paper entitled "Clues to Suicide" (Shneidman & Farberow, 1956) and the following year we published another short paper entitled "Some comparisons between genuine and simulated suicide notes" (Shneidman & Farberow, 1957). In 1957 we co-edited *Clues to Suicide* (Shneidman & Farberow, 1957). That was the birth of Suicidology.

Obviously, only a few decades later, the new discipline became known as a major field of science.

Psychological Autopsy Studies

During the development of suicidology, psychological autopsy became a major tool to understand suicide. This procedure introduced the psychological element into the study of suicide. Hitherto, suicide was studied anecdotally, statistically, sociologically but hardly psychologically. The psychological autopsy develops relevant information where the mode of death is unclear. Obviously one can write a biography without knowing the chief character directly, but by depending on people who knew the decedent as the informants. The psychological autopsy method involves a retrospective investigation of the deceased person and uses psychological information gathered from personal documents; police, medical, and coroner records; and interviews with family members, friends, coworkers, school associates, and health care providers to clarify equivocal deaths. The aim of the procedure is to achieve a clear picture of the personality preceding the event. Much credit for the success of the psychological autopsy belongs to Dr. Theodore Curphey, the Los Angeles coroner, who recognized the real benefits of that procedure. Shneidman had prophetically used the term for the first time in a book on Thematic Test Analysis, stating something that was going to become relevant afterwards (Shneidman, 1951):

> . . . To present a study in which the emphasis is on the prediction of behavior rather than the validation of the technique; i.e., to hold a "psychological autopsy" on one case (p. 4)... Dr. James G. Miller has indicated rather succinctly that "Diagnosis is irrelevant and unproductive unless it is also prediction at the same time." He has also, in the same context, pointed out the need for clinico-pathologic conferences in psychology similar in function

> to those held in medicine. This book, then, is a sort of "psychological autopsy," wherein the postmortem is performed not on the patient but on the test interpretations. This is made possible by the availability of the clinical and psychiatric data... (p. 6).

The Problem With Psychological Autopsy Studies

Over the past decades, psychological autopsies have provided important elements for understanding suicide. Most of the data that come from psychological autopsy studies support the idea that individuals who die by suicide were suffering from a psychiatric disorder. Studies labeled as psychological autopsies report little information on the psychology of the deceased.

The assumption derived from psychological autopsy studies that the vast majority of individuals who die by suicide suffered from a mental disorder at the time of their death has, however, several biases. First, scholars worldwide use the term psychological autopsy for any retrospective investigation and such studies lack the comprehensive data gathering obtained from interviewing key persons. It is rather easy to classify a subject as depressed when in fact he or she was understandably sad for what was a mess in his or her life. Most of the data obtained from psychological autopsy studies are derived from a forensic environment, physicians, or death registries and much less often from family members or friends who could make sense of the depressive features that are distinguishable from clinical depression. Suicide is a problem of the human condition or, as Shneidman points out, "it is a dissatisfaction of the status quo."

Pouliot and De Leo (2006) have highlighted many issues related to psychological autopsies, concluding that the medical model often fails to provide sufficient evidence that a disorder could lead to suicide. In most psychological studies conducted so far, suicide is almost exclusively researched under single paradigmatic umbrella of medicine. Pouliot and De Leo proposed that, according to the medical model, suicide is the consequence of biologically based alterations of the brain, where psychiatric symptoms are expressions of the disease caused by the alterations. Data reported by Cavanagh, Carson, Sharpe, and Lawrie (2003) support the notion that between 88% and 95% of suicides were suffering from a psychiatric disorder. These data contrast with evidence from prospective case studies which show that, at 10 to 20-year follow-up, the risk of suicide in adolescents suffering from major depression is 7.7% (Weissman et al., 1999), 3.4% for alcoholics (Murphy & Wetzel, 1990), and 3.8% in depressed patients (Gladstone et al., 2001).

As a psychiatrist, my model for depicting suicide refers to the two distinct dimensions that often overlap: the one comprising psychiatric disorders and the other referring to suicidality. When substantial overlapping exists, there is a major risk of suicide as the patient is "attacked" in two ways. However, suicide can occur with no psychiatric disorder when profound distress and psychological pain become unbearable and when suicide is seen as the perfect solution. In suicidal individuals, psychological pain affects the very core of their human condition and threatens life, which cannot be accepted in its present condition. This is precisely the aspect that characterizes suicide deaths and is absent in vast majority of psychiatric patients. A psychiatric disorder alone is, therefore, not sufficient for precipitating suicide. There must be the suicidality dimension that carries some variant of negative emotions, such as heightened inimicality (acting against the individual's best interest); exacerbation of perturbation (refers to how disturbed the individual is); increased constriction of intellectual focus; tunneling or narrowing of the mind's content (dichotomous thinking); and the idea of cessation – the idea the insight that it is possible to stop consciousness and put an end to suffering (Pompili, in press).

In other words, the motives for suicide can be traced in the variables surrounding the individual viewed as a unique human being whose personality contains the real reasons for wishing suicide (Figure 1).

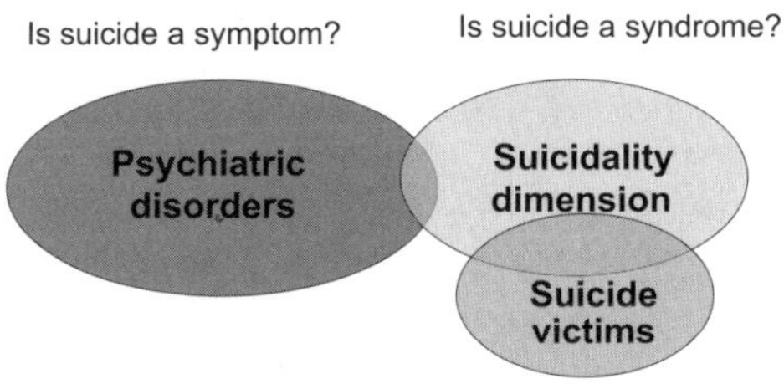

Figure 1. Suicide is better understood as the result of variables traceable in the suicidality dimension. This dimension generally includes: heightened inimicality (acting against the individual's best interest); exacerbation of perturbation (refers to how disturbed the individual is); increased constriction of intellectual focus and tunneling or narrowing of the mind's content (dichotomous thinking); the idea of cessation (the insight that it is possible to stop consciousness and put an end to suffering).

In medicine and psychology, the term syndrome refers to a group of several clinically recognizable features, signs (as observed by a physician), symptoms (as reported by the patient), phenomena, or characteristics that often occur together, so that the presence of one feature alerts the physician to the presence of the others. In suicidology, we have many features that are associated with suicide risk, but no single factor has been demonstrated to be necessary or sufficient to cause suicide.

Choron (1972) cites Gaupp's work (1910) as the milestone for understanding suicide from the biopsychological point of view; that is, there are forces that do not rise to the consciousness of individuals and thus cannot constitute motives, and forces that are related to race, age, sex, work, and social status. This perspective has been challenged by psychiatry that relates individuals who die by suicide to abnormal mental states. Ringel (1953) considered suicide as "the conclusion of a pathological psychic development." Weisman (1971) wondered whether suicide was a disease and proposed that "Suicide is neither a moral dilemma nor a mental disease but a form of life-threatening behavior resembling a declaration of war of a petition for bankruptcy." There is "suicidal sickness," but no evidence of an organic "disease" to explain it. However, the concept of "disease" is a cultural abstraction that excludes other dimensions of sickness, such as conflict and crisis.

Esquirol (1838) said that suicide was a symptom of insanity and, therefore, those who commit suicide are psychiatrically disturbed. Esquirol developed the perspective that suicide is a psychiatric problem and wrote:

> All that I have said up to now, the facts which I have reported, proves that suicide presents all the characteristics of insanity of which it is but a symptom; that there is no point for a unique source of suicide, since one observes it in the most contradictory circumstances, and because it is symptomatic or secondary, be it in acute delirium, or chronic, besides, the autopsy of suicides made so far did not throw much light on the subject of pathological changes (p. 639).

Considering suicide risk as a symptom impairs the opportunity to fully investigate and understand this aspect. If a patient has fever or headache, and if this ailment were thought to be part of pneumonia or cancer, clinicians would treat the disease as a whole rather than each symptom separately.

This phenomenological approach promises to aid our understanding of suicide, helping us understand rather than explain the behavior. Jaspers' (1959) assumption that we can explain a phenomena without understanding it at all is of particular interest here. Jaspers separated the study of subjective phenomena as experienced by the patients from the study of other psychological data. He introduced the difference between explanation and understanding and focused on the latter. Jaspers distinguished two types of psychiatric entities: developments that we can come to understand and processes that can be explained, even though they are not understandable. For instance, reactive depression is understood insofar as we can put ourselves in the place of the sufferer; most often, this is also true for suicidal behavior. On the other hand, we owe our emphasis to Kraepelin (1921) on documenting the longitudinal course of psychiatric disorders. As for suicide, he stated that: "The patients, therefore, often try to starve themselves, to hang themselves, to cut their arteries, they beg that they may be burned, buried alive, driven out into the woods and there allowed to die"; however, he did not emphasize on what was happening in their tormented mind, a feature often neglected when only DSM-Kraepelinian diagnostic criteria are taken into account.

The lack of association between suicide and psychiatric disorders has been dealt with in various studies (e.g., De Leo, 2004), and scholars have come to believe that alternative solutions must be found because the vast majority of depressed, schizophrenic, alcoholic, or organically psychotic patients do not commit or even attempt suicide (Leenaars, 2004; Lester, 1987, 1989). Hopelessness as a psychological construct has been reported to be a more important mediator of suicide risk than depression. Studies involving the Beck Hopelessness Scale (Beck, Weissman, Lester, & Trexler, 1974) found that the extent of negative attitudes about the future (pessimism) was a better predictor of suicidal intent than depression (Beck & Steer, 1988). This indicates that it is not necessarily important how you feel right now, for example, being depressed, but it is important to trust whether the future would bring changes in your condition. This is particularly true for suicidal individuals experiencing the uniqueness of their suffering that, for them, has no escape and no future solution. It was suggested that:

> The interest in classifying populations of suicidal patients by their psychiatric diagnoses is being supplemented by an interest in understanding what makes a minority of patients within any given diagnostic category suicidal while the majority are not suicidal (Hendin, 1986).

These observations are reinforced by the response of patients to psychiatric treatment. For instance, Ahrens and Müller-Oerlinghausen (2001) investigated a group of high-risk patients with recurrent affective disorders (n = 167) who had made one or more suicide attempts before the start of lithium prophylaxis within a collaborative project. According to their recurrence-related response to long-term lithium prophylaxis, patients were classified into three groups: excellent (n = 45), moderate (n = 81), and poor responders (n = 41). Only depressive episodes leading to hospitalization were considered. With regard to suicidal behavior in this select group of high-risk patients, there was a significant decrease in the rate of suicide attempts as compared to the prelithium figures. This was the case not only in those patients with excellent treatment outcome, but also in those patients with moderate or even poor response to lithium prophylaxis, suggesting an effect on the suicidal dimension independent of the effect on psychiatric symptoms.

A similar finding emerges from a study by Prudic and Sackeim (1999) using electroconvulsive therapy (ECT). They found that ECT responders and nonresponders showed a large decrease in scores on the suicide item of the Hamilton Rating Scale for Depression, and this decrease was greater than the average improvement on other items.

Moreover, recent studies on the role of antidepressants in reducing suicide risk have failed to provide strong evidence with regard to their possible role in increasing or decreasing suicide risk. Pooling trials of antidepressants (including both tricyclics and SSRI versus placebo) might have yielded a nonsignificant result that was not in favor of one or the other (Baldessarini et al., 2006; Baldessarini, Pompili, & Tondo, 2006).

A psychological autopsy helps clarify an equivocal death by interviewing people who knew the deceased individual (spouse, grown-up children, neighbors, employers, or physicians) and by analyzing his or her clinical records.

The psychological autopsy focuses on what is usually the missing element: The *intention* of the deceased in relation to his or her own death

- Time interval between death and interviews
- Interviewers
- Biases related to informants
- Control groups.

The current emphasis on psychiatric disorders in published research needs to be balanced by a better study of the socioenvironmental contributors to suicide, particularly by focusing attention on conceiving and adopting standardized instruments and/or structured interviews that may favor the appropriate weighting of these variables. Efforts in this direction will promote a truly ecological approach for understanding suicide and will assist in the development of better preventive strategies (Pouliot & De Leo, 2006).

A Discourse to Reconcile the Evidence-Based Practice and the Real World

Suicide prevention was considered in the real world as a mission for rescuing suicidal individuals during crisis or period of great distress. The first example of this is the Lemberg Volunteer Rescue Society (1893–1906) that may be considered the earliest organization devoted to suicide prevention. In 1906, The Salvation Army opened an Anti-Suicide Bureau in London and, during the same year, a religious-based organization, named National Save-A-life League was founded in New York City. In 1947, a professionally staffed center focusing on the prevention of suicide was established at the Neuropsychiatric Clinic of the University of Vienna. In 1953, Rev. Chad Varah began offering help to suicidal persons out of a Central London Church and then established The Samaritans, "to befriend the suicidal and despairing." *He believed suicidal people needed a way of being in touch with someone to whom they could talk at any time of day or night that was right for them.*

In remembering what was noticed in his suicidal individuals, he stated that:

> Often individuals who seemed desperate when they called for an appointment to see him declined his offer for therapy after spending hours in his waiting room. He observed that while they were waiting they discussed their problems with the "ordinary" volunteers who were making appointment and serving tea and were helped as much as they would been from seeing a professional therapist (Mishara, 2008).

In psychology and psychiatry, *phenomenology* is used to refer to subjective experiences or their study. The experiencing subject can be considered to be the person or self, for purposes of convenience. Scholars worldwide have puzzled over what makes a person suicidal and what individuals who die by suicide have in their minds. Most often, the focus is not on the motives for suicide nor on the phenomenology of this rare act, but it is rather on what is found from small cohorts of suicidal individuals. Each day, dozens of papers on suicide are added to the enormous literature related to this topic.

One abiding feature of "experiences" is that, in principle, they are not directly observable by any external observer. For example, we might ask, "Is my experience of redness the same as yours?" While it is difficult to answer such a question in a concrete manner, the concept of intersubjectivity is often used as a mechanism for understanding how human beings are able to empathize with one another's experiences, and indeed to engage in a meaningful communication about them. The phenomenology of suicide addresses an important epistemological question on poor communication between people and how to bridge the gap in communication of human suffering. Many studies analyzing the incidence of psychiatric disorder in suicides employ after-the-fact diagnosis and are often criticized for their lack of objectivity. The main argument is that a decision of the psychiatrist is biased *if he believes that suicidal people must be mentally ill.* This bias is indirectly confirmed by statistics: "the highest estimate of mental illness when a sample had been diagnosed before suicide was 22 percent. Afterward the highest estimate was 90 percent" (Temoche, Pugh, & Macmahon, 1964).

The use of after-the-fact diagnosis may lead to a kind of tautology. In simple words, "We say, in essence, 'All people who attempt suicide are mentally ill.' If someone asks, 'How do you know they are mentally ill?', the implied answer is, 'Because only mentally ill persons would try to commit suicide.' " Since killing oneself is against nature, no normal person would commit such an act; therefore, those who commit suicide are considered mentally ill, BUT why do the vast majority of mentally disordered people even if faced by the same dramatic situations encountered by suicides not actually kill themselves.

According to Bertolote et al.'s estimation in 2003, the number of patients in published works that specifically studied the psychiatric diagnosis of people who died by suicide was relatively small (*n* = 15,629). Of the 15,629 cases of suicide with information on psychiatric diagnosis, slightly over 50% (*n* = 8,205 cases) originated from genuine studies on the general population. The remainder of the cases included subjects who were previously admitted to psychiatric hospitals, where the details of their diagnoses were found in the medical charts (Bertolote, Fleischmann, De Leo, & Wasserman, 2003). The association of suicide and mental disorders has been widely discussed and documented, leaving out the key role of the management of mental disorders in the prevention of suicide.

Bertolote, Fleischmann, De Leo, and Wasserman (2004) calculated that, if we apply the depression treatment effectiveness of 52% on average, indicated in the World Health Report 2001 (World Health Organization, 2001), instead of an idealistic but unattainable 100%, and supposed that an average of 50% of people with depression were correctly identified and treated, the impact on suicide rates would be about 7.8%. On a global basis, this would reduce the suicide rates from a world average of 15.1 per 100,000 to 13.9 per 100,000 (Bertolote et al., 2003). Considering alcohol-related disorders, with an average effectiveness of 30% (World Health Organization, 2001) and 50% of identification and treatment, the reduction expected would be about 2.6%, thus reducing the global suicide rate from 15.1 per 100,000 to 14.6 per 100,000. Similar results can be obtained for schizophrenia, the third disorder most frequently associated with suicide (14.1%) and applying the same type of calculations, with an average effectiveness of 78% (World Health Organization, 2001) and 80% of identification and treatment, one would have an impact of 8.9%, thus reducing global suicide rates from 15.1 per 100,000 to 13.7 per 100,000.

Examples of Evidence-Based Educational Programs for Reducing Suicide

Risk of Suicide and Related Adverse Outcomes After Exposure to a Suicide Prevention Program in the US Air Force: Cohort Study

A multilayered intervention was targeted at reducing the risk factors and enhancing the factors that are considered protective. The intervention consisted of removing the stigma of seeking help for a mental health or psychosocial problem, enhancing the understanding of mental health, and changing policies and social norms. Relative risk reductions (the prevented fraction) for suicide and other outcomes were hypothesized to be sensitive to broadly-based *community prevention efforts* (family violence, accidental death, and homicide). Additional outcomes not exclusively associated with suicide were included because of the comprehensiveness of the program.

Implementation of the results of the program was associated with a sustained decline in the rate of suicide and other adverse outcomes. A 33% relative risk reduction was observed for suicide after the intervention; reductions for other outcomes ranged from 18% to 54% (Knox, Litts, Talcott, Feig, & Caine, 2003). After the implementation of a broadly-based, community-level suicide prevention program in the US Air Force, there were fewer suicides. The ongoing program also reduced the rates of other adverse outcomes that shared similar underlying risk factors (Figures 2 and 3).

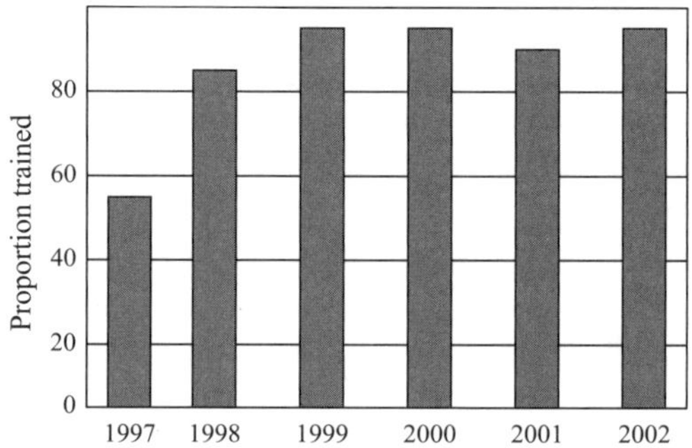

Figure 2. Proportion of Air Force personnel trained in suicide prevention (1997–2002).

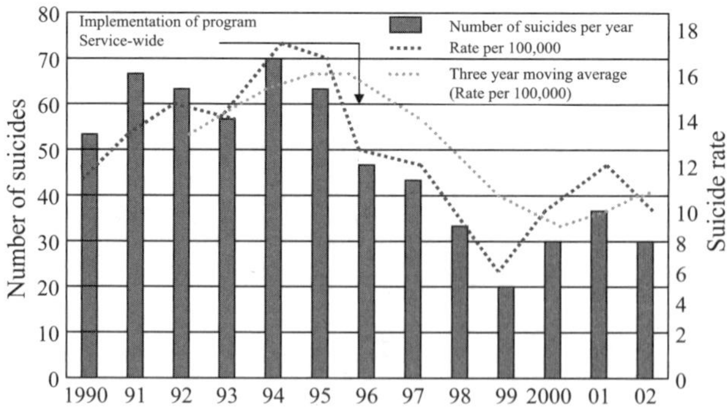

Figure 3. Number of suicides, suicide rates, and 3-year moving average for rates of suicide, US Air Force, 1990–2002.

PROSPECT (Prevention of Suicide in Primary Care Elderly: Collaborative Trial) aims at preventing suicide among older primary care patients by reducing suicidal ideation and depression (Alexopoulos et al., 2005). Implementation of the program relies on educating primary care physicians to recognize the symptoms and apply a clinical algorithm based on depression treatment guidelines for older patients from the American Psychiatric Association, the Agency for Healthcare Research and Quality, and the Texas Department of Mental Health. In a randomized controlled trial, unadjusted rates of suicidal ideation decreased 12.9% among patients receiving PROSPECT (29.4–16.5%), compared with a 3.0% decrease (20.1–17.1%) among patients receiving treatment as usual (p = .01).

Suicide prevention should, therefore, be targeted to identifiable key areas of difficulty. The first approach is to provide proper education on suicide prevention to all professionals involved in health care. Being able to recognize the warning signs for suicide should be a first goal for any suicide prevention campaign. An example of this is the program in Gotland, Sweden, where successful suicide prevention was achieved through the education of primary care doctors (Rutz, 2001; Rutz, von Knorring, Pihlgre, Rihmer, & Walinder, 1995; Rutz, von Knorring, & Walinder, 1992; Rutz, von Knorring, Walinder, & Wistedt, 1990).

Brief Psychological Intervention After Deliberate Self-Poisoning

This intervention provides four sessions of psychotherapy for adults who deliberately poisoned themselves. According to Guthrie et al. (2001), "This therapy entails identifying and helping to resolve interpersonal difficulties which cause or exacerbate psychological stress" (p. 1). The intervention is delivered by nurse therapists at the patient's home. Four, 50-minute sessions are offered over the course of a month. During each session, therapists assessed the risk of suicide and communicated with the patient's general practitioner.

A randomized two-group design was used by evaluators to determine the intervention effectiveness. One hundred nineteen patients who deliberately poisoned themselves were assigned either to a psychotherapy (intervention) group or to a treatment-as-usual (control) group. Psychotherapy group members demonstrated statistically significant less suicidal ideation and depression compared to the treatment-as-usual group members. In addition, at the 6-month follow-up, it was found that only 9% of psychotherapy group members had harmed themselves again compared with 28% of treatment-as-usual group members.

Suicidal behavior ranges from ideation, to nonfatal attempts, to completions, all of which have their own different subtypes and levels of seriousness or lethality. It is important to decide whether we are trying to assess an individual's suicide risk or a population's suicide risk, and over what time frame (this weekend, in several weeks, this year, or over a lifetime) (Maris, 2002). Women attempt suicide more than men do, and one of the most obvious reasons attributed to this factor is that they choose different methods for suicide. Men are more likely to use firearms and hanging, whereas women are more likely to use poisons and medication. The methods used by men are more lethal than those used by women and, therefore, women are more easily saved when treated in an emergency department. However, as Lester (1984) pointed out, within any one method for suicide, men are still more likely to die than women; therefore, differences in the choice of method cannot be the sole explanation for sex differences in the outcome of suicidal actions.

In the 1960s, Stengel (1964) stated that people completing suicide and people unsuccessfully attempting suicide constituted two different groups only because the age and sex distributions were so different. Suicide is more common among elderly people and among men, whereas younger people and women predominate among those who make nonfatal attempts. Beautrais (2001) also concluded that attempted and completed suicides are two overlapping populations that share common psychiatric diagnosis and historical feature but are distinguished by gender (males are more likely to kill themselves) and patterning of psychiatric disorder (attempters were more likely than those dying by suicide to have a current diagnosis of anxiety disorder and to be socially isolated). Arguing that the two groups also differ in their intent and motives, Kreitman, Philip, Greer, and Bagley (1969) proposed the term parasuicide to replace the label "attempted suicide," thereby stressing that the differences between those completing and those attempting suicide are not simply a question of the outcome of the self-destructive act (Bille-Brahe et al., 1995). More recently, the terms self-injurious behavior and self-poisoning (depending on which method is used to injure the self) have become more common.

A World Health Organization Working Group (Working Group on Preventive Practices in Suicide and Attempted Suicide, 1986) defined attempted suicide as follows: Attempted suicide (parasuicide) is an act with a nonfatal outcome, in which an individual deliberately initiates a nonhabitual behavior that, without intervention from others, will cause self-harm, or deliberately ingests a substance in excess of the prescribed or generally recognized therapeutic dose, and which is aimed at realizing changes that the subject desired via the actual or expected physical consequences. The definition of attempted suicide includes acts interrupted by others before the actual self-harm occurs (e.g., a person removed from a railway track before the train arrives), but excludes, as is the case of completed suicide, self-harmful acts by people who do not understand the meaning or consequences of their act (e.g., because of developmental disability or severe mental illness).

Nonfatal suicidal behavior has often been considered to be a manipulative act. In 1961, Farberow and Shneidman's book, entitled The Cry for Help, noted the desire of attempted suicides to get attention from others. Lester (1987) has in fact stressed that, even if the suicidal act results in punishment, the person may still find it rewarding, especially if a previous attempt was ignored by others. Sifneos (1966) studied a group of attempted suicides and found that the manipulative aspect of the behavior was a common feature in the sample. The majority of his patients were satisfied with the results of their manipulative behavior and were not motivated to receive psychotherapy. Anxiety was lacking in these patients, and they appeared apathetic and fatalistic. They were more introspective and self-centered, had few but rather intense relationships, had difficulty expressing their emotions, and had exaggerated expectations for themselves.

The Trouble With Nomenclature

One problem faced when studying nonlethal suicidal behavior is the lack of consensus on the terms that should be used to refer to these types of behaviors (O'Carroll et al., 1996). Self-injurious behavior exists on a continuum from actions without conscious intent to die, to actions with lethal intent that do not result in death (suicide attempts), to intentional, self-inflicted death (completed suicide). Often it is difficult to identify a person's intent to die, and so it is difficult to differentiate attempted suicide from self-injurious behavior in which there is no intent to die. The label "attempted suicide" should be used only in the case of those individuals who wish to die and who survive by chance; that is, they are rescued and taken to an emergency department, the lethality of the gesture being high. A more precise classification of suicide attempts would be one that included lethality as well as a measure of the intent to kill oneself. Then we would be able to distinguish between a superficial cut made by an individual who wished to solve an interpersonal conflict and a firearm shot in the head of an individual who survived thanks to a complicated neurosurgical operation. Presently, both individuals are labeled as suicide attempters by some researchers.

A major clarification of the nomenclature in suicidology was suggested by O'Carroll et al. (O'Carroll et al., 1996; Silverman, Berman, Sanddal, O'Carroll, & Joiner, 2007a, 2007b), but researchers continue to use rival nomenclatures, and it is not unusual to encounter researchers using inappropriate terms for describing suicidal individuals.

Attempted suicide should be distinguished from suicidal gestures. A suicidal gesture occurs when a person, for example, swallows some aspirins or increases by three- to four-fold the dosage of benzodiazepines that he or she takes regularly each day. Although there is a small chance of dying in this manner, these are low-lethality methods for attempting suicide. These individuals may be psychologically distressed, but they are not planning to die. They should, however, be taken seriously and receive psychiatric treatment (Lester, 1989).

According to the revised nomenclature (Silverman et al., 2007a, 2007b), a suicide attempt is now defined as self-inflicted, potentially injurious behavior with a nonfatal outcome for which there is evidence (either explicit or implicit) of intent to die. A suicide attempt may result in no injuries, injuries, or death. If there is some degree of suicidal intent, then it is labeled suicide attempt, type I (no injury), or suicide attempt, type II (with injury), regardless of the degree of injury or the lethality of method. It is, therefore, considered an act with intent to die, and is distinguished from self-harm or self-injurious behavior.

Self-reports of suicide attempts also have limited validity due to inconsistent definition and problem with recall bias (Kjoller, Norlev, & Davidsen, 2004). Freeman, Wilson, Thigpen, and McGee (1974) reported that most of the people included in their study of the intention to kill oneself after self-injurious behavior called their suicidal behavior a suicide attempt when in fact their intention to die was minimal. In the CDC's Youth Risk Behavior Survey (Centers for Disease Control and Prevention, 2005), only one in three adolescents who reported a suicide attempt required any medical attention. Meehan, Lamb, Saltzman, and O'Carroll (1992) reported that, for every ten self-reported attempts, only one led to hospitalization. This indicates that the term is used to describe other forms of distress or self-injury. We share O'Carroll et al.'s (1996) opinion who stated that "Because the term 'attempted suicide' potentially means so many different things, it runs, the risk of meaning almost nothing at all" (p. 238).

Suicide attempts and other acts of self-harm that result in nonfatal injuries take a heavy toll on the health of younger persons. In 2002, an estimated 124,409 visits to US emergency departments were made after attempted suicides or other self-harm incidents by persons aged 10–24 years (Centers for Disease Control and Prevention, 2004). The CDC analyzed self-report data from the 2001 nationally representative sample of high school students in the US and found that students who reported attempting suicide during the preceding 12 months were nearly four times more likely to report fighting than those who reported not attempting suicide. The observed association between suicide attempts and fighting suggests that violence prevention programs directed at reducing both suicide and fighting are appropriate for younger persons. Although mechanisms linking suicidal behavior and interpersonal violence are unclear, characteristics such as aggressiveness, impulsivity, substance abuse, depression, and hopelessness appear to increase the risk for both suicidal and violent behaviors (Plutchik, 1995; Pompili et al., 2007; Trezza & Popp, 2000).

Hospitals should handle suicides more effectively. Specifically, immediate acceptance of the patient and treatment should be the first duty of hospitals. Occasionally, hospitals in some countries do not accept patients with suicidal ideation or after an attempted suicide, an unacceptable policy. Some of the common reasons for refusing registration and admission include a nonaccepting attitude on the part of the hospital staff, considering suicide emergencies as increasing the workload, thinking that suicidal patients are merely seeking attention, and medicolegal fears (such as lawsuits). The unsympathetic attitude of some hospital staff discourages people from seeking help. Publicity should be provided about first-aid measures and the location of emergency help centers, especially for handling poisoning and burn injuries. Many common household first-aid practices could, in fact, be dangerous, and there should be no delay in taking the affected person to a hospital.

This section has reviewed some of the issues concerning attempted suicide and provided a selective review of the topic. Nevertheless, even a comprehensive analysis of this ambiguous behavior would find it difficult to draw definitive conclusions. Despite common usage of the term, attempted suicide may be confused with other self-harm behaviors. The term "attempted suicide" should be used only when there is clear intention to die but, for some reason, the individual is rescued. Even among genuine suicide attempters, the lethality of the action should be taken into account. Lethality, that is the probability that death will occur (or the medical seriousness of the injury), may help classify suicide attempters and plan effective treatments. An attempted suicide is also a cry for help, but we should bear in mind that focusing on this aspect of suicide attempt could result in undertreatment of these individuals. Clinicians should assess the suicidal intent and lethality of attempted suicides and provide clear treatment plans for them. Their behavior carries a high probability of repetition, and attempted suicide is a major risk factor for subsequent completed suicide.

Meehan et al. (1992) stressed the need to assess suicide attempts better through precise protocols in the emergency room aimed at describing what really happened, determining if hospitalization was needed, and above all assessing whether the injuries were intended to cause death. A partnership between medical staff working in the emergency department and mental health professionals would be of great help in the assessment of suicide attempts (Pompili, Girardi, Ruberto, Kotzalidis, & Tatarelli, 2005).

Conclusion

Know Yourself for Suicide Prevention: Combining Evidence-Based Practice With Personal Experience When Facing Suicidal Individuals

The saying "Know thyself" may refer by extension to the ideal of understanding human behavior, morals, and thought, because ultimately to understand oneself is to understand other humans as well. The Ancient Greek aphorism "Know yourself" was inscribed in the pronaos (forecourt) of the Temple of Apollo at Delphi. Many clinicians perform a careful assessment of suicide risk in these patients and assume that suitable treatments will resolve the suicidal risk. They rarely investigate suicidality in-depth in their patients. There are myths and resistances that impair a proper understanding of suicidal people.

Most of the studies have evaluated short-term risk factors for suicidal behavior, such as current suicidal ideation and recent suicide attempts (particularly in the context of severe major depressive episode), the major precursors and the most powerful predictors of attempted and completed suicide. There is the need to reconcile this with the fact that suicide might be better understood as phenomenon centered in the individual. In other words, the motives for suicide can be traced in the variables surrounding the individual viewed as a unique human being whose personality contains the real reasons for wishing suicide.

Suicide prevention programs have been implemented *before* appropriate assessments are completed, so gaps may exist in knowledge about the efficacy, effectiveness, safety, or economic impact of specific prevention strategies. Without evaluation of programs, we do not know if the program benefits or harms the people we are trying to help. The focus should be on what patients feel rather than on how they can be categorized. Many unfortunate patients may quickly take their lives because they cannot wait for relief. Most desperate patients, enraged patients, or intensely anxious patients show what they feel in their faces, body movements, and demeanor.

References

Ahrens, B., & Muller-Oerlinghausen, B. (2001). Does lithium exert an independent antisuicidal effect? *Pharmacopsychiatry, 34*(4), 132–136.

Alexopoulos, G. S., Katz, I. R., Bruce, M. L., Heo, M., Ten Have, T., Raue, P., et al. (2005). Remission in depressed geriatric primary care patients: A report from the PROSPECT study. *The American Journal of Psychiatry, 162*(4), 718–724.

Baldessarini, R. J., Guzzetta, F., Hennen, J., Pompili, M., Soldani, F., Tondo, L., et al. (2006). *Effects of psychotropic drug treatments on suicide risk.* Paper presented at the ACNP 2006 Annual Meeting.

Baldessarini, R. J., Pompili, M., & Tondo, L. (2006). Suicidal risk in antidepressant drug trials. *Archives of General Psychiatry, 63*(3), 246–248.

Beautrais, A. L. (2001). Suicides and serious suicide attempts: Two populations or one? *Psychological Medicine, 31*(5), 837–845.

Beck, A. T., & Steer, R. A. (1988). *Beck hopelessness scale – Manual.* San Antonio: Harcourt Brace Javanovich.

Beck, A. T., Weissman, A., Lester, D., & Trexler, L. (1974). The measurement of pessimism: The hopelessness scale. *Journal of Consulting and Clinical Psychology, 42*(6), 861–865.

Berman, A. L. (2008). Twenty questions, maybe more ... message from the executive director. *Newslink, 35*, 6.

Bertolote, J. M., Fleischmann, A., De Leo, D., & Wasserman, D. (2003). Suicide and mental disorders: Do we know enough? *British Journal of Psychiatry, 183*, 382–383.

Bertolote, J. M., Fleischmann, A., De Leo, D., & Wasserman, D. (2004). Psychiatric diagnoses and suicide: Revisiting the evidence. *Crisis, 25*(4), 147–155.

Bille-Brahe, U., Schmidtke, A., Kerkhof, A. J., De Leo, D., Lonnqvist, J., Platt, S., et al. (1995). Background and introduction to the WHO/EURO Multicentre Study on Parasuicide. *Crisis, 16*(2), 72–78, 84.

Cavanagh, J. T., Carson, A. J., Sharpe, M., & Lawrie, S. M. (2003). Psychological autopsy studies of suicide: A systematic review. *Psychological Medicine, 33*(3), 395–405.

Centers for Disease Control and Prevention. (2004). *Morbidity and mortality weekly report* (No. 53\22). Centers for Disease Control and Prevention.

Centers for Disease Control Prevention. (2005). *Youth risk behavior surveillance system.* Centers for Disease Control and Prevention.

Choron, J. (1972). *Suicide.* New York: Charles Scribner's Sons.

De Leo, D. (2004). Suicide prevention is far more than a psychiatric business. *World Psychiatry, 3*(3), 155–156.

Esquirol, J.-E. (1838). *Des maladies mentales considérées sous le rapport médical, hygiénique et médico-légal* [On mental disorders, considered in the medical, public health, and legal medicine report]. (Vol. 1). Paris: J.-B. Baillière et fils.

Freeman, D. J., Wilson, K., Thigpen, J. D., & McGee, R. K. (1974). Assessing intention to die in self-injury behavior. In C. Neuringer (Ed.), *Psychological assessment of suicide risk* (pp. 18–42). Springfield: Charles C. Thomas.

Gaupp, R. (1910). *Über den Selbstmord. Zweite vermehrte Auflage* [On suicide. 2nd, enlarged ed]. München: Verlag der Ärztlichen Rundschau.

Gladstone, G. L., Mitchell, P. B., Parker, G., Wilhelm, K., Austin, M. P., & Eyers, K. (2001). Indicators of suicide over 10 years in a specialist mood disorders unit sample. *Journal of Clinical Psychiatry, 62*(12), 945–951.

Guthrie, E., Kapur, N., Mackway-Jones, K., Chew-Graham, C., Moorey, J., Mendel, E., et al. (2001). Randomised controlled trial of brief psychological intervention after deliberate self poisoning. *British Medical Journal, 323*(7305), 135–138.

Hendin, H. (1986). Suicide: A review of new directions in research. *Hospital & Community Psychiatry, 37*(2), 148–154.

Jaspers, K. (1959). *General psychopathology.* Baltimore: The John Hopkins University Press.

Kjoller, M., Norlev, J., & Davidsen, M. (2004). *Recall bias and suicidal behavior in a six year follow-up study.* Paper presented at the 10th European Symposium on Suicide and Suicidal Behaviour, Copenhagen, Denmark.

Knox, K. L., Litts, D. A., Talcott, G. W., Feig, J. C., & Caine, E. D. (2003). Risk of suicide and related adverse outcomes after exposure to a suicide prevention programme in the US Air Force: Cohort study. *British Medical Journal (Clinical Research ed.), 327*(7428), 1376.

Kraepelin, E. (1921). *Manic-depressive insanity and paranoia* (R. M. Barclay, Trans.). Edinburgh: E&S Livingstone.

Kreitman, N., Philip, A. E., Greer, S., & Bagley, C. R. (1969). Parasuicide. *British Journal of Psychiatry, 115*(523), 746–747.

Leenaars, A. (2004). *Psychotherapy with suicidal people*. Chichester: Wiley.

Lester, D. (1984). Suicide. In C. S. Widon (Ed.), *Sex roles and psychopathology* (pp. 145–156). New York: Plenum.

Lester, D. (1987). *Suicide as a learned behavior*. Springfield: Thomas.

Lester, D. (1989). *Questions and answers about suicide*. Philadelphia: The Charles Press.

Maris, R. W. (2002). Suicide. *Lancet, 360*(9329), 319–326.

Maris, R. W., Berman, A. L., & Silverman, M. M. (2000). *Comprehensive textbook of suicidology*. New York: The Guildford Press.

Meehan, P. J., Lamb, J. A., Saltzman, L. E., & O'Carroll, P. W. (1992). Attempted suicide among young adults: Progress toward a meaningful estimate of prevalence. *American Journal of Psychiatry, 149*(1), 41–44.

Mishara, B. L. (2008, February). The passing of two telephone helpline pioneers. In *IASP News Bulletin*.

Murphy, G. E., & Wetzel, R. D. (1990). The lifetime risk of suicide in alcoholism. *Archives of General Psychiatry, 47*(4), 383–392.

O'Carroll, P. W., Berman, A. L., Maris, R. W., Moscicki, E. K., Tanney, B. L., & Silverman, M. M. (1996). Beyond the Tower of Babel: A nomenclature for suicidology. *Suicide & Life-Threatening Behavior, 26*(3), 237–252.

Plutchik, R. (1995). Outward and inward directed aggressiveness: The interaction between violence and suicidality. *Pharmacopsychiatry, 28*(Suppl. 2), 47–57.

Pompili, M. (in press). Exploring the phenomenology of suicide. *Suicide & Life-Threatening Behavior*.

Pompili, M., Girardi, P., Ruberto, A., Kotzalidis, G. D., & Tatarelli, R. (2005). Emergency staff reactions to suicidal and self-harming patients. *European Journal of Emergency Medicine, 12*(4), 169–178.

Pompili, M., Innamorati, M., Lester, D., Brunetti, S., Tatarelli, R., & Girardi, P. (2007). Gender effects among undergraduates relating to suicide risk, impulsivity, aggression and self-efficacy. *Personality and Individual Differences, 43*, 2047–2056.

Pouliot, L., & De Leo, D. (2006). Critical issues in psychological autopsy studies. *Suicide & Life-Threatening Behavior, 36*(5), 491–510.

Prudic, J., & Sackeim, H. A. (1999). Electroconvulsive therapy and suicide risk. *Journal of Clinical Psychiatry, 60*(Suppl. 2), 104–110, discussion 106–111.

Ringel, E. (1953). *Der Selbstmord, Abschluß einer krankhaften psychischen Entwichlung. Eine Untersuchung an 745 geretteten Selbstmördern* [Suicide, completion of a morbid psychological development. A research on 745 rescued suicides]. Vienna, Düsseldorf: Maudrich.

Rodgers, P. L., Sudak, H. S., Silverman, M. M., & Litts, D. A. (2007). Evidence-based practices project for suicide prevention. *Suicide & Life-Threatening Behavior, 37*(2), 154–164.

Rutz, W. (2001). Preventing suicide and premature death by education and treatment. *Journal of Affective Disorders, 62*(1–2), 123–129.

Rutz, W., von Knorring, L., Pihlgren, H., Rihmer, Z., & Walinder, J. (1995). Prevention of male suicides: Lessons from Gotland study. *Lancet, 345*(8948), 524.

Rutz, W., von Knorring, L., & Walinder, J. (1992). Long-term effects of an educational program for general practitioners given by the Swedish Committee for the Prevention and Treatment of Depression. *Acta Psychiatrica Scandinavica, 85*(1), 83–88.

Rutz, W., von Knorring, L., Walinder, J., & Wistedt, B. (1990). Effect of an educational program for general practitioners on Gotland on the pattern of prescription of psychotropic drugs. *Acta Psychiatrica Scandinavica, 82*(6), 399–403.

Sackett, D. L., Rosenberg, W. M., Gray, J. A., Haynes, R. B., & Richardson, W. S. (1996). Evidence based medicine: What it is and what it isn't? *British Medical Journal, 312*(7023), 71–72.

Shneidman, E. S. (1951). *Thematic test analysis*. New York: Grune and Stratton.

Shneidman, E. S. (1964). Grand old man in suicidology. A review of Louis Dublin's Suicide: A sociological study. *Contemporary Psychology, 9*, 370–371.

Shneidman, E. S. (1985). *Definition of suicide*. Northvale: Aronson.

Shneidman, E. S., & Farberow, N. L. (1956). Clues to suicide. *Public Health Reports, 71*(2), 109–114.

Shneidman, E. S., & Farberow, N. L. (1957). Some comparisons between genuine and simulated suicide notes in terms of Mowrer's concepts of discomfort and relief. *Journal of General Psychology, 56*, 251–256.

Sifneos, P. E. (1966). Manipulative suicide. *Psychiatric Quarterly, 40*(3), 525–537.

Silverman, M. M., Berman, A. L., Sanddal, N. D., O'Carroll, P. W., & Joiner, T. E. (2007a). Rebuilding the tower of Babel: A revised nomenclature for the study of suicide and suicidal behaviors. Part 1: Background, rationale, and methodology. *Suicide & Life-Threatening Behavior, 37*(3), 248–263.

Silverman, M. M., Berman, A. L., Sanddal, N. D., O'Carroll, P. W., & Joiner, T. E. (2007b). Rebuilding the Tower of Babel: A revised nomenclature for the study of suicide and suicidal behaviors. Part 2: Suicide-related ideations, communications, and behaviors. *Suicide & Life-Threatening Behavior, 37*(3), 264–277.

SPAN USA Inc. (2001). *Suicide prevention: Prevention effectiveness and evaluation*. Atlanta: SPAN USA.

Stengel, E. (1964). *Suicide and attempted suicide*. London: Penguin Books.

Temoche, A., Pugh, T. F., & Macmahon, B. (1964). Suicide rates among current and former mental institution patients. *Journal of Nervous and Mental Disease, 138*(2), 124–130.

Trezza, G. R., & Popp, S. M. (2000). The substance user at risk of harm to self or others: Assessment and treatment issues. *Journal of Clinical Psychology, 56*(9), 1193–1205.

Weisman, A. D. (1971). Is suicide a disease? *Life Threatening Behavior, 1*(4), 219–231.

Weissman, M. M., Wolk, S., Goldstein, R. B., Moreau, D., Adams, P., Greenwald, S., et al. (1999). Depressed adolescents grown up. *Journal of the American Medical Association, 281*(18), 1707–1713.

Working Group on Preventive Practices in Suicide and Attempted Suicide. (1986). (No. ICP/PSF 017(S)). Copenhagen: WHO Regional Office for Europe.

World Health Organization. (2001). *World health report 2001: Mental health: New understanding, new hope*. Geneva: World Health Organization.

Zuger, A. (1997, December 16). A new way of doctoring: By the book. *New York Times,* p. B11.

About the Author

Maurizio Pompili, MD, PhD, is Professor of both Suicidology and Epidemiological Psychiatry at Sapienza University of Rome where he received his MD degree, training in psychiatry (both summa cum laude), and doctoral degree in Neurosciences. He is also part of the Community at McLean Hospital – Harvard Medical School, USA. He is the recipient of the American Association of Suicidology's 2008 Shneidman Award for "Outstanding early career contribution to suicidology." He has published more than 200 papers on suicide including original research articles, book chapters, and editorials.

He edited and co-edited several national and international books including the latest *Suicide in the Words of Suicidologists* and *Suicide: A Global Perspective*. He provided validation studies for psychometric instruments to assess suicide risk and he is the Italian National Representative to the International Association for Suicide Prevention (IASP).

Maurizio Pompili
Department of Psychiatry
Sant'Andrea Hospital
Via di Grottarossa 1035
00189 Rome
Italy
Tel.: +390633775675
E-mail: mpompili@mclean.harvard.edu

Evidence-Based Medicine in Mental Health

General Principles

Delia Cimpean and Robert E. Drake

Dartmouth Medical School, Dartmouth Psychiatric Research Center, Lebanon, NH, USA

Historically, as medicine replaced religious and folk treatments, the standard method of determining effectiveness of treatments was based on the capacity of individual doctors to observe and draw conclusions from experience with small numbers of patients. Even with the best observers, the results of these case series were subject to bias and confounding variables, arising from having patients with dissimilar conditions, from confusing effects of treatment with the natural history of the disease, from using surrogate outcomes, or from patient and provider expectations.

The impressions of individual clinicians have proved notoriously inaccurate in judging the effectiveness of treatments. The medical literature is replete with examples of ineffective or harmful treatments that enjoyed great popularity, sometimes for centuries, before they were replaced by effective treatments. In mental health, long-term hospitalization, megavitamins, and psychosurgery were eventually proved to be harmful or ineffective by careful research. At the same time, scientific research has developed and confirmed the effectiveness of numerous mental health interventions, including medications, psychotherapies, social therapies, and rehabilitation approaches, most of which are still underutilized today.

We have adopted the term "patient" throughout the chapter for clarity, recognizing that there is inconsistency among writers, with the term patient being replaced gradually with other terms, such as "user," "client," or "consumer," to represent the shift from traditional paternalistic approaches to shared participation in the medical decision-making process.

Three Approaches to Evidence-Based Medicine

The specific term "evidence-based medicine" was introduced in 1990 to refer to a systematic approach to helping practitioners apply scientific evidence to decision-making at the point of contact with a specific patient (Drake & Goldman, 2003; Guyatt & Rennie, 2002). As the philosophy, major tenets, and techniques of the movement have evolved, evidence-based medicine has strongly influenced the practices offered in health care programs, individual health care decision-making, and the oversight of medical and public health systems. These three aspects of evidence-based medicine are in many ways separate but equally important. (a) Evidence-based practices refer to general approaches to health care that have been validated multiple times and that should be widely available (Institute of Medicine (US), Committee on Quality of Health Care in America, 2001; Woolf, DiGuiseppi, Atkins, & Kamerow, 1996). For example, people with serious mental illnesses should have access to systematic medication management, assertive community treatment, and supported employment in any clinic. (b) Within any of these practices or other practices, clinicians and their patients should make individual decisions regarding care based on evidence-based techniques, which combine research evidence, patient's preferences, and clinician judgment (Sackett, 1995), and which we describe in detail below. (c) Finally, current quality assurance techniques require that overall performance and outcomes of programs, clinicians, and clients be monitored through evidence-based management (Sederer, 2009). For example, electronic medical records can be used, at the level of clinician, program, or clinic, to determine if patients who meet specific criteria (such as the presence of depression) are receiving appropriate interventions (such as screening for suicidal thoughts and behaviors).

Each of these three approaches assumes the fundamental principles of evidence-based medicine: accepting basic health care values, recognizing the importance of science, recognizing the complexity of scientific evidence, balancing science with patient's values and preferences, and the criticality of clinician expertise (Drake, 2005).

Basic Health Care Values

The philosophy and ethics of health care recognize several basic values (Backlar & Cutler, 2002; Beauchamp & Childress, 2001). Chief among them are autonomy, beneficence, avoiding maleficence, and justice. Patients and their families should be treated with respect. Patients have rights to autonomy, choice, and self-determination in relation to their bodies and health care decisions. Health care practitioners should be truthful and share information. They should try to help and avoid harming the patient. Quality health care should be provided equally to everyone.

Evidence-based medicine fully endorses these and other basic health care values. A patient who seeks treatment for depression, for example, has a right to receive full information about the illness, to understand the available treatments and their expected outcomes and potential side effects, and to make an informed choice and give consent regarding treatment. The individual's rights may be contravened only in specific circumstances, such as when he or she presents an immediate life-threatening risk to self or others.

Knowing the scientific evidence and sharing it in a collaborative way with the patient shows respect. Without knowing the evidence, practitioners cannot be certain that they are avoiding harm and doing their best to help. Without understanding the evidence, patients cannot be truly informed and thus cannot make informed decisions about their health care.

While these beliefs and values are consistent with patient-centered care in the rest of medicine, in the mental health field they have been identified by a variety of different terms, such as social inclusion, community integration, empowerment, and recovery, which counter long-standing attempts to segregate and institutionalize people with psychiatric disabilities.

Scientific Evidence

During the 20th century, the scientific study of disease and treatment became the keystone of modern health care (Le Fanu, 1999). The scientific method is in fact what separates modern medicine from folk remedies, religious cures, and various other approaches to health not supported by evidence. Scientific approaches to understanding illness, such as epidemiologic methods and randomized controlled trials of interventions, have solved hundreds of medical problems, saved millions of lives, separated numerous effective treatments from an even greater number of ineffective or harmful treatments, and helped society to save billions of dollars. The scientific method is valued because it offers the most reliable, efficient, and unbiased approach to establishing the causes of illness and the effectiveness of treatments. Common sense, logic, history, and research argue against other approaches, such as relying on authorities, traditions, religious ideas, or the anecdotal experience of individual clinicians (Sagan, 1995).

The Complexity of Evidence

Critics of evidence-based medicine point out that researchers often disagree about the scientific evidence, that the scientific evidence is often limited to specific types of patients or settings, and that there is no strong research evidence (e.g., randomized controlled trials) to inform many common clinical decisions. All of these arguments are valid. In fact, one of the major assumptions of evidence-based medicine is that the scientific evidence has many limits and must be used judiciously (Guyatt & Evidence-Based Medicine Working Group, 2008). Evidence-based medicine assumes that there is always a hierarchy of evidence. Some clinical decisions can be guided by high-level, more reliable, and more extensive evidence than others.

There are essentially always limitations on the quality of the evidence in general, and on the applicability of the evidence to specific patients and situations. Complex psychosocial treatments are constantly evolving, and randomized controlled trials are rare. In many cases, the existing randomized trials are totally unhelpful because they address an intervention that is no longer used. Obviously, randomized controlled trials of discarded interventions are less helpful than quasi-experimental studies of current interventions. Sometimes only quasi-experimental studies are available, so these constitute the best available evidence. Sometimes observational studies allow extremely strong inferences (e.g., hip replacement surgery for debilitating osteoarthritis was so dramatically effective that it was never tested in controlled trials), and randomized controlled trials are unnecessary (Guyatt et al., 2008). Further, much of the evidence regarding harmful effects of treatments comes from large observational studies.

In the typical clinical situation, the available evidence, even if strong, does not match a specific patient perfectly. For example, several randomized clinical trials show the effectiveness of a particular intervention, but the specific patient might differ from the average patient in those trials because she has North-African background, is over age 75, or has diabetes. How do the clinician and patient use the evidence in this situation? This is where clinical experience and understanding the effects of co-occurring illnesses, treatments, and other factors are critical.

Patient's Preferences

Evidence-based medicine assumes that scientific evidence is only one important component of decision-making (Haynes, Devereaux, & Guyatt, 2002). A second involves including the patient's values, goals, preferences, and participation in shared decision-making. A third is the sum of local circumstances: the availability of hospitals, specialists, programs, insurance, supports, and other resources that affect health care decisions. All of these must be considered to make optimal decisions.

Patient's preferences, local conditions, or societal decisions about resources often override the scientific evidence, especially in situations where the evidence is weak (Wennberg, Fisher, & Skinner, 2002). Consider a few examples. One patient understands the evidence that electroconvulsive treatment (ECT) is the most effective treatment for depression but decides to decline ECT. Unless competence to make the decision is at issue, or the depression is so severe that the safety of the patient is at stake, the patient's preference always overrides the scientific evidence. An elderly patient with Alzheimer's disease develops pneumonia, and antibiotic therapy clearly would be effective for his condition. But before developing severe dementia, this patient expressed a strong preference for rejecting medical treatments to prolong his life. His physician therefore prescribes pain medications to prevent suffering but not antibiotics to treat the pneumonia. A third patient has panic disorder, for which cognitive-behavioral therapy (CBT) is clearly an effective treatment. However, in the local mental health center, there are no CBT-trained psychotherapists available. The patient's physician therefore recommends medications to treat the panic disorder rather than CBT until the patient can travel to a large medical center for a course of this psychotherapy.

The focus on patient's preferences assumes that patients have access to accurate and understandable scientific information. As the medical field advocates for patient's preferences and shared decision-making (Charles, Gafni, & Whealen, 1999), it is clear that truly informed choice requires access to accurate information (O'Connor et al., 2003). Otherwise, patients make choices that are based on the opinions of their social contacts, the biases of vested interest groups (e.g., marketing), or the individual knowledge and opinions of their local health care providers. With access to accurate information, patients make choices that are highly differentiated. That is, their treatment choices often differ from what their providers might recommend, from what their peers choose, and from what they would choose in the absence of such information (Wennberg et al., 2002). Nevertheless, informed patient choice, which is termed shared decision-making in medicine, often leads to better outcomes, not just higher satisfaction and adherence to treatment but improved biomedical outcomes. Standards are rapidly developing for how information should be synthesized and presented to patients in an unbiased fashion, but this is an area that needs further research (Gigerenzer, Gaissmaier, Kurz-Milcke, Schwartz, & Woloshin, 2007).

The emphasis on accurate information and shared decision-making implies a fundamental shift away from the traditional model of medical authority in which the physician decides what the best treatment is and tells the patient what to do. Shared decision-making means that the provider shares information about reasonable and available treatments and their likely effects, both benefits and side effects, based on scientific information, and engages the patient in a process that involves the patient taking as much responsibility as he or she is able and willing to take in terms of understanding the treatments and outcomes, making informed choices, and learning to manage his or her illness.

Evidence-based medicine prescribes attention to patient preferences for outcomes as well as treatments. For example, a patient may value avoiding medication side effects more than eliminating symptoms. This emphasis in medicine is totally congruent with what has been termed the philosophy of recovery in mental health. Recovery implies attention to functioning and quality of life, rather than just symptom control (Onken, Craig, Ridgway, Ralph, & Cook, 2007). Practices that are identified as evidence-based in mental health typically have patient preferences built in at several points of decision-making because choice corresponds with better patient outcomes (Bond & Salyers, 2004).

Clinical Judgment

Working with the patient to understand the scientific evidence, to adjust the evidence to the particular characteristics of the patient and his or her circumstances, to incorporate the patient's preferences and decisions, and to include the specifics of local factors requires a great deal of clinical judgment (Haynes et al., 2002). In fact, as the scientific evidence proliferates, as demands for patient-centered care increase, and as health care organizations constrain time and decisions, the need for clinical expertise has expanded dramatically. More than ever before, correct diagnosis and prescribing are related to improved outcomes. More than ever before, patients are demanding information and a role in health care decision-making. And more than ever before, attempts to control health care costs are impinging on health care decision-making. How can all of these pressures be managed at the point of contact between practitioner and patient?

The simple answer is that there is no substitute for clinical expertise. The clinician must first understand the individual patient and his or her illness. If the diagnosis were incorrect or if the clinician misunderstood the individual patient's preferences, scientific evidence would not help. For example, clinical skills are needed to identify the fact that a client who has survived a recent heart attack and who does not participate in the cardiac rehabilitation program prescribed may have actually developed major depression that needs urgent diagnosis and treatment as it is associated with increased mortality postmyocardial infarction (Shiotani et al., 2002; Strik, Lousberg, Cheriex, & Honig, 2004; Ziegelstein et al., 2000). Similarly, prescribing an evidence-based medication that causes sexual side effects to a patient who finds these side effects intolerable is unlikely to be effective. A clinician who fails to make the correct diagnosis or to elicit information about the side effect's importance to the patient will not have helped the patient.

Second, the better the clinician understands the scientific evidence, the better he or she could determine how it applies to a specific patient. Because of the rapidity of medical developments, keeping up with evidence-based practice is exceedingly difficult. The clinician must master information technology and be able to find and understand information rapidly. Consider, for example, the situation of a patient with a serious liver infection called hepatitis C complicated by depression. The randomized controlled trials of treatments for hepatitis C infection have shown efficacy but have excluded patients with depression. Should the clinician recommend the treatment? In most cases, there will be additional evidence (usually weaker evidence) regarding potential interactions between the treatment and the comorbid condition. In other cases, the clinician must use knowledge of these other conditions and good judgment to discuss with the patient whether the treatment will be tolerated and effective in these specific circumstances.

Third, the clinician must also understand the local health care situation accurately. The elderly patient who already has regular support from family and a visiting nurse, for example, may have a different capacity to monitor side effects and take medicines accurately than a similar patient without local supports. What if there is no family and no opportunity for a visiting nurse? Clinical judgment is required to put all of the pertinent factors together.

Current Approaches to Evidence-Based Mental Health Treatment

Evidence-Based Practices

Evidence-based practices are health care interventions that are shown to be effective by consistent scientific evidence, generally several controlled trials (Institute of Medicine (US), Committee on Quality of Health Care in America, 2001). The evidence-based practices movement advocates that when there are competing interventions available, patients should be given accurate information about alternative interventions and outcomes, and those interventions that are supported most strongly by scientific evidence should be among the choices available to patients (Drake, Rosenberg, Teague, Bartels, & Torrey, 2003).

Current evidence-based treatments for severe mental illnesses, such as depression, bipolar disorder, and schizophrenia, are as effective as current treatments for most other chronic medical illnesses. Despite extensive evidence regarding effective psychosocial and pharmacological treatments for mental illness, which have been summarized as evidence-based practices, research shows that these interventions are not available routinely to patients seeking mental health treatment (Lehman & Steinwachs, 1998; Mojtabai, 2009). In the 1990s, only 20–30% of people with persistent depression and anxiety in the United States were using appropriate counseling and/or medication (Young, Klap, Shoai, & Wells, 2008), and there was variation in using appropriate ECT (Weissman et al., 1988). Among people with severe mental illness, only 15% received minimally adequate treatment (Wang, Demler, & Kessler, 2002). Still, evidence-based practices are typically unavailable or ignored in favor of intuition and clinical experience. The "science-to-practice gap" refers to the discrepancy between what we know works and what we actually offer in routine mental health settings. Policy-makers, administrators, clinicians, advocates, insurers, and researchers generally agree that the gap between science and practice must be closed; mental health programs and practitioners have an obligation to provide the most effective treatments to patients and their family members via evidence-based practices.

Efforts to identify evidence-based practices have been led by groups such as the American Psychological Association (Chambless & Ollendick, 2001), The British Medical Journal Publishing Group (www.group.bmj.com), The Cochrane Collaborative (www.cochrane.org), The National (US) Evidence-Based Practices Project (Drake et al., 2001), The Schizophrenia Patient Outcome Research Team (PORT) (Lehman & Steinwachs, 1998), and Texas Medication Algorithm Project (TMAP) (Miller et al., 1999) that have assembled teams to review and synthesize the evidence regarding treatment of mental illness. Some of these groups have also incorporated additional elements of systems engineering such as patient education and systematic assessments to facilitate the implementation of identified evidence-based practices. Efforts to implement effective interventions have been at most modestly successful when based on passive diffusion of research findings, clinical guidelines, or even on quality improvement processes (Drake, 2009). The attempts at complete systems reengineering, with multiple components aimed at activating patients, complex electronic medical records, and decision support, based on the widely implemented model of chronic care in medical illness, have been effective in various settings and populations, including with mental illness (Coleman, Mattke, Perrault, & Wagner, 2009). These models need fundamental organizational support. For example, in serious mental illness, if work is the patient's goal, supported employment interventions should be available. Implementing such a practice in an outpatient mental health setting requires training of the staff who will deliver the intervention, ongoing supervision, and data feedback. In suicide prevention, evidence-based practices such as systematic screening for depression of populations at risk followed by referral to clinical evaluation would similarly require organizational support, and mechanisms need to be in place to train and supervise the providers of the intervention in the required skills, as well as ongoing data feedback to ascertain the fidelity and the outcomes of the implementation.

Evidence-Based Decision-Making

The current definition of evidence-based medicine emphasizes the fact that the scientific evidence is not the only component of evidence-based medicine. Rather, evidence-based medicine means practicing medicine based on scientific evidence, complemented with clinical experience as it applies to the clients' unique set of concerns, values and preferences (Sackett, Rosenberg, Gray, Haynes, & Richardson, 1996). Clinical experience and training are needed to understand the diagnosis and the treatments, to know the local health care system, and to evaluate the scientific evidence. One common misconception regarding evidence-based practice in the mental health field is that it prescribes a standard, rigid approach for all patients, thereby eliminating patient choice and preferences. Along with many patient advocacy groups, the evidence-based practices movement supports the maximization of patient choice and self-determination (Bond & Salyers, 2004). A treatment with the strongest evidence may not be the optimal treatment for a particular individual, who may have specific risk factors that preclude the treatment, for whom the treatment may not be available or affordable in a given situation, or who may have a different preference.

Evidence-Based Program Management

In efforts to implement evidence-based practices, proven interventions need to be adapted to local circumstances. As the success of implementation may highly depend on the actual adherence to the practice implemented, programs of implementing evidence-based practices need to have built-in ways to evaluate the quality of the implementation. Fidelity scales have been developed for some evidence-based practices (Bond, Drake, & Becker, 2008).

Information technology facilitates patient-clinician communication and use of evidence-based decision supports. Importantly, it also creates the capacity to monitor quality of care at the level of patient, clinician, program, clinic, agency, or system (Freedman, 2003). Several approaches have been developed for management (Sederer, 2009). For example, software for medication monitoring can identify instances of potential adverse medication interactions, proscribed practices, or medications likely to worsen health status at the point of prescription. Data can also be used to review overall patterns of practice post hoc. Utilization review, performance monitoring, and standards of care are among the terms used to describe these activities.

Consider the possibilities for preventing suicide. Electronic medical records in any mental health or addiction clinic could not only guide clinicians to follow evidence-based guidelines for assessment and treatment but could also provide feedback to supervisors, team leaders, and quality assurance directors regarding the numbers of patients who screen positive for suicide risk, who receive a full suicide assessment, who receive treatments consistent with their assessments, and who are followed up according to established guidelines. Thus, patients who are considered at risk but who are not receiving evidence-based care could be identified immediately by managers for review. At higher administrative levels, such as a county or provincial mental health authority, programs could be monitored for rates of appropriate suicide assessment, treatment, and follow-up. Educational interventions could thereby target specific clinicians or clinics that are not meeting the standards of care.

Sources of Research Evidence/Hierarchy of Evidence

The highest quality for making a decision about an individual patient is actually the *N* of 1 randomized controlled trial, in which the patient switches from active treatment to placebo several times under double-blind conditions (Guyatt & Evidence-Based Medicine Working Group, 2008). In most clinical situations, this approach is not feasible, so the highest standard becomes the systematic review of randomized controlled trials. As we move down the hierarchy, the criteria involve designs with less control that allow less certainty of inference (e.g., quasi-experimental studies, followed by systematic observational studies, followed by unsystematic clinical observations), fewer studies, and less external validity (or generalizability) (Drake, Latimer, Leff, McHugo, & Burns, 2004).

a. *Systematic reviews and meta-analyses*. The gold standard of evidence is represented by meta-analyses (results across studies are combined using statistical methods) and systematic reviews (results are presented descriptively). Systematic reviews are focused on a single question rather than a diagnosis. For example, a review might focus on the following question: "What is the effectiveness of exercise for people with depression?" The question is searched systematically and comprehensively, ideally in published and unpublished databases, to avoid publication bias. There are predetermined inclusion and exclusion criteria for the studies identified in the search, to avoid selection bias, and an adequate assessment of the quality of the studies included. The quality of the review is high if the quality of the studies included is high. The results are pooled and often expressed as risk ratios for each study, within a 95% confidence interval. The result range is clinically significant if the confidence interval does not contain the null value and is more precise if the confidence intervals are narrow. The importance of the results can be better appreciated if the results are clearly displayed (typically using Forest plots).
b. *Randomized controlled trials*. The most internally valid scientific experiments are randomized controlled trials. In this design, the researchers attempt to control

variables that may influence a particular outcome to maximize the chance that differences in outcome are attributable to the treatments. Typically, clinical interventions are designed to work for people with specific problems, and often, only individuals with one condition, or mental illness, will be included in a study. Research participants (patients in this case) agree to participate in the study and subject themselves to the risks of experimental research. Participants are randomized to two or more groups, usually intervention and control groups. A successful randomization ensures that the distribution of the participants and thus of other predictable and unpredictable individual characteristics that may influence outcome is similar between the groups. Ideally, participants, intervention providers, and evaluators are blinded to the treatment condition to avoid bias derived from treatment expectations. Great care is exercised to make sure that all the participants in all groups are treated the same in other regards, with the exception of the intervention delivered. All participants need to be accounted for at the end of the study. This means that researchers need to know the participants who stopped the intervention prematurely and, as much as possible, understand why that happened. The intent-to-treat analysis includes all participants who started the intervention, regardless of whether they have stayed enough in the study to finish it, or not. In such an analysis, the participant who dropped out at some point would have the last recorded observation included in the analysis (even if the last one is the same as the first one recorded!). This analysis is also called "last observation carried forward" and is a conservative way of expressing results. Presumably, the participants who did not complete the intervention would show less improvement, decreasing the expectation for overall improvement from the treatment. On the other hand, this approach may be closer to what happens in real settings, as a number of patients would not complete the intervention in real settings either.

Recently, there has been increased emphasis on the ways of reporting results that are more intuitive and applicable to the clinical practice. Number needed to treat (NNT) is easy to calculate and shows the number of participants who had the outcome of interest specifically due to the intervention. Eight elderly patients with depression need to be treated with selective serotonin-reuptake inhibitors for one patient to show significant clinical improvement that would not have happened if treated with placebo alone (Wilson, Mottram, Sivanranthan, & Nightingale, 2001). Knowing the NNT for different interventions that have the same outcome for the same disorder can help the clinician and the patient choose between interventions. Effect size is another measure of the magnitude of treatment based on the differences between continuous variables. A rule of thumb states that effect sizes are small at around 0.2, medium at around 0.5, and large at 0.8 (Cohen, 1969). In general, in psychiatry, effect sizes are either small or medium. For example, the effect size for antidepressants used in the treatment of depression in the elderly is around 0.6, and the effect size of psychotherapy in the same category of population is around 1 (Pinquart, Duberstein, & Lyness, 2006).

c. *Cohort studies*. These studies include two groups (cohorts) of patients, one which receives the exposure of interest and one which does not. Cohort studies follow participants forward for the outcomes of interest. For example, two cohorts of adult participants, with and without depression, had their body mass index assessed prospectively for 10 years to understand whether people with depression are more likely to become obese (Patten et al., 2009).
d. *Case-control studies*. These studies identify patients who have the outcome of interest (cases) as well as similar patients without the same outcome (controls) and assess retrospectively whether they had the exposure of interest. For example, suicidal and nonsuicidal elderly depressed participants were compared on prior tests of executive function, attention, and memory (Dombrovski et al., 2008).
e. *Cross-sectional surveys*. These studies assess a defined population at a single point in time, with exposure and outcomes determined simultaneously. For example, numerous cross-sectional studies have assessed the mental health of populations that were exposed to recent disasters.
f. *Case series reports*. These studies describe a series of patients with the outcomes of interest. No control group is involved.
g. *Qualitative studies*. Qualitative studies assess a small number of patients in depth, often to understand how patient's experience and value different treatments, experiences, or outcomes.

Efficacy Versus Effectiveness

In the hierarchy of evidence, the design of the study is meant to maximize the internal validity of the research. However, internally valid studies are difficult to generalize to populations and settings outside the clinical trial. While validity requires inclusion of a homogeneous population in the trial, often treatment populations in clinical settings are heterogeneous, and have multiple comorbidities including medical, mental health, and substance abuse problems. Administering a controlled intervention in the trial is essential to attribute outcomes to the intervention, but in clinical settings, often the intervention cannot achieve the same degree of standardization. A trial with high internal validity, therefore, demonstrates the efficacy of an intervention, but the findings are difficult to generalize to real clinical settings. The effectiveness of a practice, on the other hand, is determined by its ability to produce a positive effect in a real-world setting with real-world populations. Ideally mental health practices are both efficacious and effective (McHugo et al., 2006).

A number of new approaches have been employed recently to bridge the gap between efficacy and effectiveness. Practical clinical trials compare clinically relevant interventions (as opposed to comparing the experimental intervention and control), include participants recruited from a variety of practice settings, and collect a range of health outcomes (Tunis, Stryer, & Clancy, 2003). Innovative research designs have utilized methods such as equipoise stratified design (STAR-D) (Rush, Fava, & Wisniewski, 2004), outcomes-based re-randomization schemes (CATIE) (Stroup et al., 2003), and other methods that help answer clinically relevant questions and help interpret and generalize meaningful outcomes to real practice settings.

Optimizing and Improving Practice

Many common clinical situations do not have answers anchored in evidence. New evidence-based practices need to be developed to respond to common clinical questions. Efficacy trials are performed in isolated controlled conditions with homogeneous populations, unlike real practice. Future research focused predominantly on effectiveness trials is more likely to produce evidence that is relevant to real practice. As patient-centered medicine develops further, interventions should address outcomes that correspond to patients' goals. Qualitative work in this area has repeatedly identified the fact that patients' goals for treatment are often related to independence, relationships, employment, and other areas of meaningful behavior, such as parenting, rather than to control of various aspects of illness.

Implementing an evidence-based practice includes promoting behavioral change in providers. While availability of guidelines has not been shown to change behaviors, predisposing strategies, enabling and reinforcing, learning through active participation, and mandated outcomes help change a practice (Torrey, Finnerty, Evans, & Wyzik, 2003). Information technology is an essential component of system change. As electronic medical records systems become widespread, they will provide reminders and alerts to providers, education and self-management instruction to patients, regular monitoring of clinical and patient-significant outcomes to all parties, and data for program monitoring (Drake, 2009).

In evidence-based decision-making, the four-step approach to evidence-based decision-making directs practitioners to (1) formulate a clinical question, (2) search for relevant information, (3) evaluate the evidence for validity and usefulness, and (4) apply the evidence to the particular clinical situation/individual patient (Hatala & Guyatt, 2002). Formulating the clinical question involves transforming the data obtained from a complex client-provider encounter into a clinical question that is searchable using electronic interfaces. Appropriate databases for searches may be the fast-growing Cochrane Database of Systematic Reviews for meta-analyses, Evidence-based Mental Health or the ACP Journal Club for appraised articles, or Medline, accessed through PubMed, Google scholar, or other interfaces. The appraisal of evidence for validity involves applying known validity criteria for each type of evidence, and unbiased organizations increasingly perform this function. Clinical significance is also critical: for example, does a one-point statistically significant change on a depression scale mean improvement in depression? Applying the evidence to the individual clinical situation in the context of the patient's values and preferences is the last step, fundamental to appropriate use of the evidence. This includes a way of communicating results to patients to facilitate understanding and decision-making. For example, results are more intuitive if expressed in absolute risks or numbers needed to treat (or to harm), rather than in relative risks (Taylor & Chang, 2008).

Here again, the clinical skills of the provider are needed to clarify the clinical question, understand the relevance of the evidence for a particular patient, and communicate the results to the patient. These are all fundamental steps of the process of making shared clinical decisions based on evidence.

Implementing evidence-based medicine in real practices has been only modestly helped by issuing guidelines and using quality improvement methods (Shojania & Grimshaw, 2005). Instead, the transformation of the system of care, with the help of health information technology, electronic medical records, learning communities, web-based training, and shared decision-making, is better suited to drive the adoption of these practices and methods.

In general medicine, the chronic care model, which is the most widely implemented model of care, includes six different components (Wagner et al., 2001). Clinical information systems allow practices to keep patient registries to identify and select for intervention certain populations at risk, also to integrate electronic assessments, treatment planning, services, outcomes, and algorithms. Other components of this program include providing decision support that incorporates evidence-based guidelines into registries, flowcharts, and assessments to clinical teams. This model was shown to improve outcomes across diseases such as diabetes, asthma, cardiovascular disease and depression (Coleman et al., 2009). In reviews, such interventions are more successful when they incorporate multiple rather than single methods (Coleman, Austin, Brach, & Wagner, 2009). No one component produces the same outcomes by itself. A fundamental issue in program management is obtaining outcome data for feedback on the fidelity of implementation of the evidence-based practice and outcomes. Health information technology enables these processes.

Potential Problems, Costs, and Resources

Evidence-based practices require system changes that can be costly to implement and maintain. Further, the gains may only be appreciated much later. In many countries, including the US, financing is poorly aligned with the evidence base (Goldman et al., 2001). The availability of information technology, which is essential to implementation and program management, is still uneven in the US and elsewhere. Existing evidence-based practices do not address all patient and clinical needs, and do not generalize to all cultures. Stakeholders express concerns that due to limited finances, implementation of evidence-based practices would limit the resources for implementation of other favored services, which may be helpful even though they do not yet have evidence (Essock et al., 2003). Clinicians often lack skills and the time necessary to acquire new skills. Many clinicians express the concern that abiding by strict guidelines might de-emphasize the clinician-patient relationship and clinical judgment.

Logic suggests several answers to concerns. Ineffective services are often even more expensive, especially in terms of human suffering, than evidence-based practices. Evidence-based practices are themselves patient-centered, which is part of the reason that they are effective. Ethically, patients should have an evidence-based practice offered as an available choice. Providers of course need to use clinical judgment to best apply the evidence to the unique patient. For policy-makers, supporting implementation of evidence-based practices is choosing to support outcomes that patients desire.

Further Reading

1. Sackett et al. (1996) Evidence-based medicine: what it is and what isn't. This editorial published in the *British Medical Journal* defines evidence-based medicine as a patient-centered integration of individual clinical expertise with the best available external clinical evidence from systematic research.
2. Drake et al. (2003) Fundamental principles of evidence-based medicine applied to mental health care. The fundamental principles of evidence-based medicine: using the best available evidence, individualizing the evidence, attending to patient's preferences, and expanding clinical expertise, have important implications for the adoption of evidence-based practices and evidence-based policy decisions in mental health care.
3. Gigerenzer et al. (2007) Helping doctors and patients make sense of health statistics. Statistics may be misleading to patients and doctors. The authors recommend using frequency statements instead of single-event probabilities, absolute risks instead of relative risks, mortality rates instead of survival rates, and natural frequencies instead of conditional probabilities to improve transparency of risk communication.
4. Drake (2009) Implementing evidence-based practices for people with schizophrenia. Implementation literature specific to schizophrenia, including medication practices, psychosocial interventions, information technology, and state- and federal-level interventions, has changed gradually from passive diffusion to system re-engineering, following the pattern outlined by the chronic care model in general health care.
5. McHugo et al. (2006) Enhancing validity in co-occurring disorders treatment research. Adoption of evidence-based interventions in routine practice settings requires focus on external and ecological validity, and change in research focus from efficacy studies to more credible and valid effectiveness studies.

References

Backlar, P., & Cutler, D. L. (2002). *Ethics in community mental health care*. New York: Plenum.

Beauchamp, T. L., & Childress, J. F. (2001). *Principles of biomedical ethics*. New York, NY: Oxford University Press.

Bond, G. R., Drake, R. E., & Becker, D. R. (2008). An update on randomized controlled trials of evidence-based supported employment. *Psychiatric Rehabilitation Journal, 31*(4), 280–290.

Bond, G. R., & Salyers, M. P. (2004). Prediction of outcome from the Dartmouth assertive community treatment fidelity scale. *CNS Spectrums, 9*(12), 937–942.

Chambless, D. L., & Ollendick, T. H. (2001). Empirically supported psychological interventions: Controversies and evidence. *Annual Review Psychology, 52*, 685–716.

Charles, C., Gafni, A., & Whealan, T. (1999). Decision-making in the physician-patient encounter: Revisiting the shared treatment decision-making model. *Social Science & Medicine, 49*(5), 651–661.

Cohen, J. (1969). *Statistical power analysis for the behavioral sciences*. New York: Academic Press.

Coleman, K., Austin, B. T., Brach, C., & Wagner, E. H. (2009). Evidence on the Chronic Care Model in the new millennium. *Health Affairs (Millwood), 28*(1), 75–85.

Coleman, K., Mattke, S., Perrault, P. J., & Wagner, E. H. (2009). Untangling practice redesign from disease management: How do we best care for the chronically ill? *Annual Review of Public Health, 30*, 385–408.

Dombrovski A. Y., Cyranowski J. M., Mulsant B. H., Houck P. R., Buysse D. J., Andreescu C., et al. (2008). Which symptoms predict recurrence of depression in women treated with maintenance interpersonal psychotherapy? *Depression and Anxiety, 25*(12), 1060–1066.

Drake, R. (2005). The principles of evidence-based mental health treatment. In R. E. Drake, M. R. Merrens, & D. W. Lynde (Eds.), *Evidence-based mental health practice: A textbook* (pp. 45–65). New York: W.W. Norton.

Drake, R. E., Essock, S., & Bond, G. R. (2009). Implementing evidence-based practices for people with schizophrenia. *Schizophrenia Bulletin, 35*, 704–713.

Drake, R. E., & Goldman, H. H. (2003). *Evidence-based practices in mental health care*. Arlington, VA: American Psychiatric Association.

Drake, R. E., Goldman, H. H., Leff, H. S., Lehman, A. F., Dixon, L., Mueser, K. T., et al. (2001). Implementing evidence-based practices in routine mental health service settings. *Psychiatric Services, 52*(2), 179–182.

Drake, R. E., Latimer, E. A., Leff, H. S., McHugo, G. J., & Burns, B. J. (2004). What is evidence? *Child & Adolescent Psychiatric Clinics of North America, 13*(4), 717–728.

Drake, R. E., Rosenberg, S. D., Teague, G. B., Bartels, S. J., & Torrey, W. C. (2003). Fundamental principles of evidence-based medicine applied to mental health care. *Psychiatric Clinics of North America, 26*(4), 811–820, vii.

Essock, S. M., Goldman, H. H., Van, T. L., Anthony, W. A., Appell, C. R., Bond, G. R., et al. (2003). Evidence-based practices: Setting the context and responding to concerns. *Psychiatric Clinics of North America, 26*(4), 919–938, ix.

Freedman, J. (2003). The role of information technology in evidenced-based practice. *Psychiatric Clinics of North America, 26*(4), 833–850, vii–viii.

Gigerenzer, G., Gaissmaier, W., Kurz-Milcke, E., Schwartz, L., & Woloshin, S. (2007). Helping doctors and patients make sense of health statistics. *Psychological Science in the Public Interest, 8*(2), 53–96.

Goldman, H. H., Ganju, V., Drake, R. E., Gorman, P., Hogan, M., Hyde, P. S., et al. (2001). Policy implications for implementing evidence-based practices. *Psychiatric Services, 52*(12), 1591–1597.

Guyatt, G. & Evidence-Based Medicine Working Group. (2008). *Users' guides to the medical literature: A manual for evidence-based clinical practice.* New York: McGraw-Hill Medical.

Guyatt G., Haynes B., Jaeschke R., Meade M. O., Wilson M., Montori V., et al. (2008). The philosophy of evidence-based medicine. In G. Guyatt et al. (Eds.), *Users' guides to the medical literature: essentials of evidence-based clinical practice* (2nd ed., pp. 9–16). New York: McGraw-Hill Medical.

Guyatt, G., & Rennie, D. (Eds.). (2002). *Users' guides to the medical literature: A manual for evidence-based clinical practice.* Chicago, IL: American Medical Association.

Hatala, R., & Guyatt, G. (2002). Evaluating the teaching of evidence-based medicine. *Journal of the American Medical Association, 288*(9), 1110–1112.

Haynes, R. B., Devereaux, P. J., & Guyatt, G. H. (2002). Clinical expertise in the era of evidence-based medicine and patient choice. *ACP Journal Club, 136*(2), A11–A14.

Institute of Medicine (US), Committee on Quality of Health Care in America. (2001). *Crossing the quality chasm: A new health system for the 21st century.* Washington, DC: National Academy Press.

Le Fanu, J. (1999). *The rise and fall of modern medicine.* London: Little, Brown.

Lehman, A. F. & D. M. Steinwachs. (1998). Patterns of usual care for schizophrenia: Initial results from the schizophrenia patient outcomes research team (PORT) client survey. *Schizophrenia Bulletin 24*(1): 11–20; discussion 20–32.

McHugo, G. J., Drake, R. E., Brunette, M. F., Xie, H, Essock, S. M., & Green, A. I. (2006). Enhancing validity in co-occurring disorders treatment research. *Schizophrenia Bulletin, 32*(4), 655–665.

Miller, A. L., Chiles, J. A., Chiles, J. K., Crismon, M. L., Rush, A. J., & Shon, S. P. (1999). The Texas medication algorithm project (TMAP) schizophrenia algorithms. *Journal of Clinics Psychiatry, 60*(10), 649–657.

Mojtabai, R. (2009). Unmet need for treatment of major depression in the United States. *Psychiatric Services, 60*(3), 297–305.

O'Connor, A. M., Stacey, D., Rovner, D., Holmes-Rovner, M., Tetroe, J., Llewellyn-Thomas, H., et al. (2003). Decision aids for people facing health treatment or screening decisions. *Cochrane Database of Systematic Reviews(2)*, CD001431.

Onken, S. J., Craig, C. M., Ridgway, P., Ralph, R. O., & Cook, J. A. (2007). An analysis of the definitions and elements of recovery: A review of the literature. *Psychiatric Rehabilitation Journal, 31*(1), 9–22.

Patten, S. B., Williams, J. V., Lavorato, D. H., Brown, L., Mc Laren, L., & Eliasziw, M. (2009). Major depression, antidepressant medication and the risk of obesity. *Psychotherapy and Psychosomatics, 78*(3), 182–186.

Pinquart, M., Duberstein, P. R., & Lyness, J. M. (2006). Treatments for later-life depressive conditions: A meta-analytic comparison of pharmacotherapy and psychotherapy. *American Journal of Psychiatry, 163*(9), 1493–1501.

Rush, A. J., Fava, M., & Wisniewski, S. R. (2004). Sequenced treatment alternatives to relieve depression (STAR*D): Rationale and design. *Control Clinical Trials, 25*(1), 119–142.

Sackett, D. (1995). Evidence-based medicine. *Lancet, 346*(8983), 1171.

Sackett, D. L., Rosenberg, W. M., Gray, J. A., Haynes, R. B., & Richardson, W. S. (1996). Evidence based medicine: What it is and what it isn't. *British Medical Journal, 312*(7023), 71–72.

Sagan, C. (1995). *The demon-haunted world: Science as a candle in the dark.* New York: Random House/Ballantine Books.

Sederer, L. I. (2009). Science to practice: Making what we know what we actually do. *Schizophrenia Bulletin, 35*, 714–718.

Shiotani, I., Sato, H., Kinjo, K., Nakatani, D., Mizuno, H., Ohnishi, Y., et al. (2002). Depressive symptoms predict 12-month prognosis in elderly patients with acute myocardial infarction. *Journal of Cardiovascular Risk, 9*(3), 153–160.

Shojania, K. G., & Grimshaw, J. M. (2005). Evidence-based quality improvement: The state of the science. *Health Affairs (Millwood), 24*(1), 138–150.

Strik, J. J., Lousberg, R., Cheriex, E. C., & Honig, A. (2004). One year cumulative incidence of depression following myocardial infarction and impact on cardiac outcome. *Journal of Psychosomatic Research, 56*(1), 59–66.

Stroup, T. S., McEvoy, J. P., Swartz, M. S., Byerly, M. J., Glick, I. D., Canive, J. M., et al. (2003). The National Institute of Mental Health Clinical Antipsychotic Trials of Intervention Effectiveness (CATIE) project: Schizophrenia trial design and protocol development. *Schizophrenia Bulletin, 29*(1), 15–31.

Taylor, C. B, & Chang, V. Y. (2008). Issues in the dissemination of cognitive-behavior therapy. *Nordic Journal of Psychiatry, 62*, 37–44.

Torrey, W. C., Finnerty, M., Evans, A., & Wyzik, P. (2003). Strategies for leading the implementation of evidence-based practices. *Psychiatric Clinics of North America, 26*(4), 883–897, viii–ix.

Tunis, S. R., Stryer, D. B., & Clancy, C. M. (2003). Practical clinical trials: Increasing the value of clinical research for decision making in clinical and health policy. *Journal of the American Medical Association, 290*(12), 1624–32.

Wagner, E. H., Austin, B. T., Davis, C., Hindmarsh, M., Schaefer, J., & Bonomi, A. (2001). Improving chronic illness care: Translating evidence into action. *Health Affairs (Project Hope), 20*(6), 64–78.

Wang, P. S., Demler, O., & Kessler, R. C. (2002). Adequacy of treatment for serious mental illness in the United States. *American Journal Public Health, 92*(1), 92–98.

Weissman, M. M., Leaf, P. J., Tischler, G. L., Blazer, D. G., Karno, M., Bruce, M. L., et al. (1988). Affective disorders in five United States communities. *Psychological Medicine, 18*(1), 141–153.

Wennberg, J. E., Fisher, E. S., & Skinner, J. S. (2002). Geography and the debate over Medicare reform. *Health Affairs (Millwood)* (Suppl. Web Exclusives), W96–W114.

Wilson, K., Mottram, P., Sivanranthan, A., & Nightingale, A. (2001). Antidepressant versus placebo for depressed elderly. *Cochrane Database of Systematic Reviews(2)*, CD000561.

Woolf, S. H., DiGuiseppi, C. G., Atkins, D., & Kamerow, D. B. (1996). Developing evidence based clinical practice guidelines: Lessons learned by the US preventive services task force. *Annual Review of Public Health, 17*, 511–538.

Young, A. S., Klap, R., Shoai, R., & Wells, K. B. (2008). Persistent depression and anxiety in the United States: Prevalence and quality of care. *Psychiatric Services, 59*(12), 1391–1398.

Ziegelstein, R. C., Fauerbach, J. A., Stevens, S. S., Romanelli, J., Richter, D. P., & Bush, D. E. (2000) Patients with depression are less likely to follow recommendations to reduce cardiac risk during recovery from a myocardial infarction. *Archives of Internal Medicine, 160*(12), 1818–1823.

About the Authors

Delia Cimpean, MD, is Assistant Professor of Medicine and Psychiatry at Dartmouth Medical School.

Robert E. Drake, MD, PhD, is Professor of Psychiatry and Community and Family Medicine at Dartmouth Medical School and Director of the Dartmouth Psychiatric Research Center.

Robert E. Drake
Dartmouth Psychiatric Research Center
Rivermill Commercial Center
85 Mechanic St., Suite B4-1
Lebanon, NH 03766
USA
Tel.: +1 603 448 0263
E-mail: Robert.E.Drake@Dartmouth.edu

Improving Suicide Risk Assessment With Evidence-Based Psychiatry

Robert I. Simon

Georgetown University School of Medicine, Washington, DC, USA

Suicide risk assessment is a core competency that psychiatrists are expected to acquire (Scheiber, Kramer, & Adamowski, 2003). The purpose of suicide risk assessment is to identify treatable and modifiable risk and protective factors that inform the patient's treatment and safety management requirements. Evidence-based psychiatry can enhance suicide risk assessment by diminishing reliance on lore, tradition, and unaided clinical impression. Acceptance of expert opinion solely based upon respect for authority is giving way to evidence-based medicine.

Patients at risk for suicide often confront the psychiatrist with life-threatening emergencies. Most clinicians rely on the clinical interview and certain valued questions and observations to assess suicide risk (Sullivan & Bongar, 2006). The psychiatrist, unlike the general physician, does not have laboratory tests and sophisticated diagnostic instruments available to assess the suicidal patient. In evaluating an emergency cardiac patient, the clinician can order a number of diagnostic tests and procedures, for example, EKG, serial enzymes, imaging, and catheterization. The psychiatrist's diagnostic instrument is systematic suicide risk assessment that is informed by evidence-based psychiatry. No suicide risk assessment *method* has been empirically tested for reliability and validity (Simon, 2006). The standard of care encompasses a range of reasoned approaches to suicide risk assessment. Utilizing evidence-based psychiatry is best practice. It is not, however, a standard of care requirement. Moreover, the law does not require the mental health professional to provide ideal, best practice, or even good patient care. The clinician's legal duty is to provide adequate patient care.

Sackett et al. (1996) defined evidence-based medicine as: "The conscientious, explicit, and judicious use of current best evidence in making decisions about the care of individual patients." The method of evidence-based psychiatry is described by Gray (2004). The preferred study designs for determining harm (risk) are cohort and case-control studies. Online evidence-based psychiatric information sources include: National Electronic Library for Mental Health (comprehensive sources); Evidence-Based Mental Health (structured abstracts); Cochrane Database of Systematic Reviews (systematic reviews); and PubMed (original articles).

Evidence-Based Suicide Risk and Protective Factors: Some Examples

In Table 1, examples of evidence-based suicide risk factors are arranged according to the hierarchy of supporting evidence. The hierarchy of supporting evidence for studies of harm (risk) include: systematic reviews (meta-analysis), the highest level of evidence, followed by cohort studies (prospective or retrospective) and case-control studies (retrospective) (Gray, 2004). In a retrospective cohort study, a historical cohort is identified through the existing records for outcomes of interest at initiation of the study. Dependence on existing records, however, raises questions of data quality (Gray, 2004). Nonevidence-based suicide risk factors are based upon case reports, case series, and lastly, clinical opinion and clinical consensus. Clinical opinion and clinical consensus are important in suicide risk assessment, if buttressed by evidence-based studies. The extensive literature on suicide contains many well-designed studies on suicide risk factors that go beyond the scope of this chapter.

Systematic Reviews (Meta-Analysis)

Psychiatric Diagnosis

Harris and Barraclough (1997), in a systematic review (meta-analysis), abstracted 249 reports from the medical literature on the mortality of mental disorders. They compared the numbers of suicides in individuals with mental disorders with those expected in the general population. The standardized mortality ratio (SMR) is a measure of the relative risk of suicide for a particular disorder compared with the expected rate in the general population (SMR of 1). The SMR was calculated for each disorder by dividing observed mortality by expected mortality (see Table 2).

The highest relative risk for suicide was associated with eating disorders. The SMR for eating disorders was significantly higher than those for major affective disorders and substance abuse disorder. Virtually all psychiatric disorders, except for mental retardation, are associated with an increased risk of suicide. The importance of making an accurate psychiatric diagnosis, one of the most important indicators of risk for suicide, is essential for a competent suicide risk assessment (Simon, 2004).

Physical Illness

Physical illness, especially in the elderly, is associated with suicide risk. Quan et al. (2002), in a systematic review (meta-analysis), found that the psychiatrically ill elderly with any of the illnesses such as cancer, prostatic disorder (excluding prostatic cancer), and chronic pulmonary disease were more likely to complete suicide than those without the illness.

Table 1. Suicide risk and protective factors: Examples of evidence-based studies

Suicide risk factors

Systematic reviews (meta-analysis)

- Psychiatric diagnosis (Harris & Barraclough, 1997; Kessler, Borges, & Walters, 1999)
- Physical illness (Harris & Barraclough, 1997; Quan, Arboleda-Florez, Fick, Stuart, & Love, 2002)

Cohort studies

- Deliberate self-harm (Cooper et al., 2005)
- Anxiety (Fawcett et al., 1990)
- Child abuse (Brown et al., 1999; Dube et al., 2005)

Case-control studies

- Violent threats: Impulsivity and aggression (Conner et al., 2001; Dumais et al., 2005; Mann et al., 2008)
- Melancholia (Grunebaum, Galfalvy, Oquendo, Burke, & Mann, 2004)
- Comorbidity (Beautrais et al., 1996; Hawton, Houston, Haw, Townsend, & Harris, 2003)

Suicide protective factors

Case-control studies

- Protective factors (Malone et al., 2000)
- Religious affiliation (Dervic et al., 2004)
- Reason for living inventory (Linehan, Goodstein, Nielsen, & Chiles, 1983)

Harris and Barraclough (1997), identified, by statistical overview, a number of specific medical illnesses that were associated with increased suicide risk: HIV/AIDS, malignant neoplasms as a group, head and neck cancers, Huntington's chorea, multiple sclerosis, peptic ulcer, renal disease, and spinal cord injury and systemic lupus erythematosus. Recognizing specific medical conditions that are associated with increased risk of suicide aids the clinician's suicide risk assessment.

Cohort Studies

Deliberate Self-Harm

In a prospective cohort study of 7,968 deliberate self-harm (DSH) patients, Cooper et al. (2005) found an approximate 30-fold increase in risk of suicide compared with the general population during a 4-year follow up period. Suicide rates were highest within the first 6 months after the initial self-harm. The authors underscored the importance of early intervention following self-harm. Female patients were at high risk for suicide.

Hawton and Zahl (2003) conducted a follow-up study of 11,583 patients who presented to a hospital between 1978 and 1997. The authors found a significant and persistent

Table 2. Mental and physical disorders and mortality

Disorder	SMR*
Eating disorders	23.14
Major depression	20.35
Sedative abuse	20.34
Mixed drug abuse	19.23
Bipolar disorder	15.05
Opioid abuse	14.00
Dysthymia	12.12
Obsessive-compulsive disorder	11.54
Panic disorder	10.00
Schizophrenia	8.45
Personality disorders	7.08
AIDS	6.58
Alcohol abuse	5.86
Epilepsy	5.11
Child and adolescent disorders	4.73
Cannabis abuse	3.85
Spinal cord injury	3.82
Neuroses	3.72
Brain injury	3.50
Huntington's chorea	2.90
Multiple sclerosis	2.36
Malignant neoplasma	1.80
Mental retardation	0.88

*Standardized mortality ratio (SMR) is calculated by dividing observed mortality by expected mortality. Adapted from Harris and Barraclough (1997).

risk of suicide. In this study, the risk was far higher in men than in women. In both genders, suicide increased markedly with age at initial presentation.

Anxiety

Fawcett et al. (1990) identified short-term suicide risk factors derived from a 10-year prospective study of 954 patients with major affective disorders that were statistically significant for suicide within 1 year of assessment. The risk factors included panic attacks, psychic anxiety, loss of pleasure and interest, moderate alcohol abuse, diminished concentration, global insomnia, and depressive turmoil (agitation). Clinical interventions directed at treating the anxiety-related symptoms in patients with major affective disorders can rapidly diminish suicide risk (Fawcett, 2001).

Child Abuse

Dube et al. (2005) conducted a retrospective cohort study of 17,337 adult Health Maintenance Organization members from 1995 to 1997. Compared to individuals reporting no sexual abuse, a history of suicide was more than twice as likely among both men and women who experienced childhood sexual abuse. Brown et al. (1999) studied a cohort of 776 randomly selected children from a mean age of 5 years to adulthood over a 17-year period. Adolescents and young adults with a history of childhood abuse were three times more likely to become depressed or suicidal than individuals without such a history. Childhood sexual abuse effects were the largest and most independent of associated factors. The risk of repeated suicide attempts was eight times greater in the case of individuals with a history of sexual abuse.

The nature and extent of childhood sexual abuse is associated with the severity of suicide risk. Fergusson, Horwood, and Lynsky (1996) followed a birth cohort of 1,019 males and females from birth to age 18. There was a consistent relationship between the extent of childhood sexual abuse and the risk of a psychiatric disorder. Individuals reporting intercourse were at the highest risk for psychiatric disorders and suicidal behaviors. An essential part of the psychiatric examination and systematic risk assessment is inquiry about childhood abuse.

Case-Control Studies

Violent Threats: Impulsivity and Aggression

Violent threats or behavior toward others is a suicide risk factor. Clinicians more commonly encounter patients who threaten violence against themselves. Violence, however, has a vector. It can be directed at oneself, at others, or both, as in murder-suicide. Conner et al. (2001), in a case-control study, found that violent behavior in the last year of life was a significant risk factor for suicide. The relationship was especially strong in individuals with no history of alcohol abuse, in younger individuals, and in women. In the study, 753 suicide victims were compared with 2,115 accident victims. Violent behavior distinguished suicide victims from accident victims. The findings were not attributable to alcohol abuse disorders alone.

Dumais et al. (2005), using a case-control design, found that higher levels of impulsivity and aggression were associated with suicide. One hundred four male suicide completers who died during an episode of major depression were compared to 74 living depressed male subjects. Current (6-month prevalence) alcohol abuse/dependence and current drug abuse/dependence disorders increased the risk of suicide in individuals with major depression. Impulsive and aggressive behaviors underlied these risk factors. Mann et al. (2008), in a retrospective study of 408 patients with mood, schizophrenia spectrum, or personality disorders who externally directed aggression, distinguished past suicide attempters from non-attempters. The risk of future suicide attempts was also increased in the aggression group.

Melancholia

Do melancholic features associated with Major Depressive Disorder confer a higher risk of suicide attempts than in nonmelancholic major depression? Grunebaum, Galfalvy, Oquendo, Burke, and Mann (2004), in a case-control study, compared suicide attempts in 377 melancholic with those in nonmelancholic patients. Melancholia was associated with more serious past suicide attempts and the increased probability of suicide attempts during follow-up. While major depression is associated with a high risk of suicide, melancholia is a less commonly recognized feature of major depression that may further increase the risk of suicide attempts or completions.

Comorbidity

Psychiatric patients often present with more than one psychiatric disorder. For example, a bipolar patient may be diagnosed with borderline personality disorder and substance abuse. Beautrais et al. (1996) found that individuals who made serious suicide attempts had high rates of comorbid mental disorders. Three hundred two consecutive individuals who made serious suicide attempts were compared with 1,028 randomly selected subjects. The risk of suicide increased with increasing comorbidity: Subjects with two or more disorders were at 89.7 times increased risk for suicide than those with no psychiatric disorder. Comorbidity is an independent suicide risk factor.

Employing a case-control design, Hawton et al. (2003) assessed 111 patients who attempted suicide (72 females and 39 males). They found that more patients with comorbid disorders had made previous attempts and repeated attempts during the follow-up period. Comorbidity of Axis I disorders and personality disorders was present in 44% of patients. In a national population survey of 5,877 respondents conducted between 1990 and 1992, Kessler et al. (1999) discovered that a dose-response relationship existed between the number of comorbid psychiatric disorders and suicide attempts.

Protective Factors: Reasons for Living

Malone et al. (2000) assessed 84 patients with a DSM-IIIR diagnosis of major depression. Of the 84 patients, 45 had attempted suicide and 39 had not. The depressed patients who had not attempted suicide expressed more responsibility toward family, more fear of social disapproval, more moral objections to suicide, greater coping and survival skills, and more fear of suicide than the depressed patients who had attempted suicide. The authors concluded that the assessment of reasons for living should be part of the assessment of patients at risk for suicide.

The Linehan Reasons for Living Inventory (Linehan et al., 1983) assesses the strength of a patient's commitment not to die. The inventory is a 48-item self-report measure that takes about 10 minutes to administer. A 72-item version is also available. Internal consistency is high. The inventory's test-retest reliability is moderately high for 3 weeks. The inventory is sensitive to improvements in depression, hopelessness, and in suicidal patients with borderline personality disorder receiving treatment.

How important are religious beliefs for preventing suicide? Dervic et al. (2004) assessed 371 depressed inpatients for religious affiliation. Patients without a religious affiliation had significantly more suicide attempts and more first-degree relatives who completed suicide than patients with religious affiliations. Unaffiliated patients were younger, less often married, fewer had children. They also had less contact with family members. Patients with no religious affiliation had fewer reasons for living, especially moral objections to suicide. There was no difference in subjective and objective depression, hopelessness, or stressful life events. The authors concluded that greater moral objection to suicide and lower aggression level in religiously affiliated patients may act as protective factors against suicide attempts.

Religious beliefs may not necessarily be a protective factor against suicide. In some patients, religious beliefs can be challenged by severe mental illness. For example, a bipolar patient stated hopelessly that "God has forsaken me." A devout, severely depressed patient hurled "blasphemous" insults at God. In a twist, where religion became a facilitating risk factor, a suicidal patient stated, "God will forgive me if I kill myself." Severe mental illness can overcome a patient's protective factors.

Clinical Experience and Clinical Consensus

Case reports, case series, and clinical consensus, though not evidence-based, can aid suicide risk assessment. For example, in systematic review of the relevant literature, Hansen (2001) found that akathisia could not be definitively linked to suicidal behavior. In individual cases, however, clinical judgment may determine that akathisia adds to the patient's total illness burden, thus potentially increasing suicide risk. Evidence-based studies must be interpreted through the lens of the clinician's education, training, experience, and reasoned clinical judgment.

Lore, tradition, myths, caprice, anxiety, defensiveness, preconceptions, and other factors can lead to uncritical acceptance and perpetuation of substandard, pseudo-suicide assessments. Mental health professionals must do more than merely ask patients if they are suicidal and then record, "No SI, HI, or CFS (no suicidal ideation, homicidal ideation, and contracts for safety)." Suicide risk assessment necessitates identifying multiple risk and protective factors and ranking their relative importance. The so-called "suicide prevention contract" (SPC), also referred to as a "no-harm" contract, is a classic example of misconception. The SPC often masquerades as a protective factor but it can be an iatrogenic suicide risk factor. The SPC can falsely reassure the clinician, preempting adequate suicide risk assessments and increasing the patient's risk for suicide (Simon, 2004). No studies demonstrate that the SPC is effective in preventing suicide attempts or completions (Stanford, Goetz, & Bloom, 1994). Clinician anxiety is unavoidable in the treatment of suicidal patients. It is a reality of clinical practice. Evidence-based suicide risk assessments can help increase the clinician's comfort in treating and managing suicidal patients.

Managed care settings can become a potential suicide risk factor, if clinicians permit third-party payer dictated short length of stay, that results in the premature discharge of suicidal patients. Safety contracts are often relied upon with severely mentally ill suicidal patients, who are rapidly treated and discharged, compounding suicide risk.

Beyond evidence-based general suicide risk factors, suicidal patients have individual "signature" symptoms and behaviors that are associated with suicide risk. "Signature" risk factors recur during subsequent suicide crises. A patient's distinctive suicide risk factor patterns should receive high priority in the identification and assessment of suicide risk (Simon, 2008). For example, a guarded, schizophrenic patient with a severe stutter would speak clearly, when at high risk for suicide. Once his stutter returned, he was discharged from the hospital at low suicide risk. This individual-specific behavior was repeated a number of times. It was considered by the clinician to be a reliable behavioral indicator of suicide risk. The assessment of behavioral risk factors is important, especially with guarded or deceptive suicidal patients (Simon, 2006). Employing evidence-based risk factors in suicide assessment is essential, but knowing a patient's unique suicide risk profile is critical.

Conclusion

Suicide risk assessment is a core competency that psychiatrists are expected to possess. The purpose of suicide risk assessment is to identify treatable and modifiable risk and protective factors that inform the patient's treatment and safety management requirements. Unaided clinical experience can lead to impressionistic, substandard suicide risk assessments. The psychiatrist's diagnostic instrument is systematic suicide risk assessment, that is, informed by evidence-based psychiatry.

Clinician anxiety is unavoidable in the treatment of suicidal patients. Evidence-based suicide risk assessments can help increase clinicians' confidence in their assessments. Ultimately, evidence-based studies must be interpreted through the psychiatrist's reasoned clinical judgment.

References

Beautrais, L., Joyce, P. R., Mulder, R. T., Fergusson, D. M., Deavoll, B. J., & Nightingale, S. K. (1996). Prevalence and comorbidity of mental disorders in persons making serious suicide attempts: A case control study. *American Journal of Psychiatry, 153*, 1009–1014.

Brown, J., Cohen, P., Johnson, J. G., & Smailes, E. M. (1999). Childhood abuse and neglect: Specificity of effects on adolescent and young adult depression and suicidality. *Journal of the American Academy of Child and Adolescent Psychiatry, 38*, 1490–1496.

Conner, K. R., Cox, C., Duberstein, P. R., Tian, L., Nisbet, P. A., & Conwell, Y. (2001). Violence, alcohol, and completed suicide: A case control study. *American Journal of Psychiatry, 158*, 1701–1705.

Cooper, J., Kapur, N., Webb, R., Lawlor, M., Guthrie, E., Mackway-Jones, K., et al. (2005). Suicide after deliberate self-harm: A 4-year cohort study. *American Journal of Psychiatry, 162*, 297–303.

Dervic, K., Oquendo, M. A., Grunebaum, M. F., Ellis, S., Burke, A. K., & Mann, J. J. (2004). Religious affiliation and suicide attempt. *American Journal of Psychiatry, 161*, 2303–2308.

Dube, S. R., Anda, R. F., Whitfield, C. L., Brown, D. W., Felitti, V. J., Dong, M., et al. (2005). Long-term consequences of childhood sexual abuse by gender of victim. *American Journal of Preventive Medicine, 28*, 430–438.

Dumais, A., Lesage, A. D., Alda, M., Rouleau, G., Dumont, M., Chawky, N., et al. (2005). Risk factors for suicide completion in major depression: A case control study of impulsive and aggressive behaviors in men. *American Journal of Psychiatry, 162*, 2116–2124.

Fawcett, J. (2001). Treating impulsivity and anxiety in the suicidal patient. *Annals of the New York Academy of Sciences, 932*, 94–105.

Fawcett, J., Scheftner, W. A., Fogg, L., Clark, D. C., Young, M. A., Hedeker, D., et al. (1990). Time related predictors of suicide in major affective disorder: A controlled study. *American Journal of Psychiatry, 147*, 1189–1194.

Fergusson, D. M., Horwood, L. J., & Lynsky, M. T. (1996). Childhood sexual abuse and psychiatric disorder in young adulthood: Psychiatric outcomes of childhood sexual abuse. *Journal of the American Academy of Child and Adolescent Psychiatry, 35*, 1365–1374.

Gray, G. E. (2004). *Evidence-Based Psychiatry*. Washington, DC: American Psychiatric Publishing.

Grunebaum, M. F., Galfalvy, H. C., Oquendo, M. A., Burke, A. K., & Mann, J. J. (2004). Melancholia and the probability and lethality of suicide attempts. *British Journal of Psychiatry, 184*, 534–535.

Hansen, L. (2001). A critical review of akathisia and its possible association with suicidal behavior. *Human Psychopharmacology, 116*, 495–505.

Harris, C. E., & Barraclough, B. (1997). Suicide as an outcome for mental disorders. *British Journal of Psychiatry, 170*, 205–228.

Hawton, K., Houston, K., Haw, C., Townsend, E., & Harris, L. (2003). Comorbidity of axis I and axis II disorders in patients who attempted suicide. *American Journal of Psychiatry, 160*, 1494–1500.

Hawton, K., & Zahl, D. A. (2003). Suicide following deliberate self-harm: Long-term follow-up of patients who presented to a general hospital. *British Journal of Psychiatry, 182*, 537–542.

Kessler, R. C., Borges, G., & Walters, E. E. (1999). Prevalence of and risk factors for lifetime suicide attempts in the National comorbidity study. *Archives of General Psychiatry, 56*, 614–626.

Linehan, M. M., Goodstein, J. L., Nielsen, S. L., & Chiles, J. A. (1983). Reasons for staying alive when you are thinking of killing yourself: The reasons for living inventory. *Journal of Consulting and Clinical Psychology, 51*, 276–286.

Malone, K. M., Oquendo, M. A., Hass, G. L., Ellis, S. P., Li, S., & Mann, J. J. (2000). Protective factors against suicidal acts in major depression: Reasons for living. *American Journal of Psychiatry, 157*, 1084–1088.

Mann, J. J., Ellis, S. P., Waternaux, C. M., Liu, X., Oquendo, M. A., Malone, K. M., et al. (2008). Classification trees distinguish suicide attempters in major psychiatric disorders: A model of clinical decision making. *Journal of Clinical Psychiatry, 69*, 23–31.

Quan, H., Arboleda-Florez, J., Fick, G. H., Stuart, H. L., & Love, E. J. (2002). Association between physical illness and suicide among the elderly. *Social Psychiatry and Psychiatric Epidemiology, 37*, 190–197.

Sackett, D. L., Rosenberg, W. M. C., Gray, J. A. M., Haynes, R. B., & Richardson, W. S. (1996). Evidence-based medicine: What it is and what it isn't. *British Journal of Psychiatry, 312*, 71–71.

Scheiber, S. C., Kramer, T. S. M., & Adamowski, S. E. (2003). *Core competence for psychiatric practice: What clinicians need to know.* American Psychiatric Publishing: Washington, DC.

Simon, R. I. (2004). *Assessing and managing suicide risk: Guidelines for clinically based risk management.* Arlington, VA: American Psychiatric Publishing.

Simon, R. I. (2006). Suicide risk assessment: Assessing the unpredictable. In R. I. Simon & R. E. Hales (Eds.), *American Psychiatric Publishing textbook of suicide and assessment management.* Arlington, VA: American Psychiatric Publishing.

Simon, R. I. (2008). Behavioral risk assessment of the guarded suicidal patient. *Suicide Life Threatening Behavior, 38*, 517–522.

Stanford, E. J., Goetz, R. R., & Bloom, J. D. (1994). The no harm contract in the emergency assessment of suicide risk. *Journal of Clinical Psychiatry, 55*, 344–348.

Sullivan, G. R., & Bongar, B. (2006). Psychological testing in suicide risk management in avoiding malpractice litigation. In R. I. Simon & R. E. Hales (Eds.), *Textbook of suicide and assessment and management.* Arlington, VA: American Psychiatric Publishing.

About the Author

Robert I. Simon, MD, is Clinical Professor of Psychiatry, Director of the Program in Psychiatry and Law at the Georgetown University School of Medicine in Washington, DC, and Chairman of the Department of Psychiatry at the Suburban Hospital/Johns Hopkins Medicine in Bethesda, MD.

Robert I. Simon
8008 Horseshoe Lane
Potomac
MD 20854
USA
Tel.: +1 301 983 1270
E-mail: RISIMONMD@aol.com

The World Health Organization*

Approach to Evidence-Based Suicide Prevention

Diego De Leo

Australian Institute for Suicide Research and Prevention,
National Centre of Excellence in Suicide Prevention,
WHO Collaborating Centre for Research and Training in Suicide Prevention, and
Life Promotion Clinic, Griffith University, Mt. Gravatt Campus, Australia

In Western societies, structured suicide prevention efforts have been known for more than a century. Examples are represented by the *National Save-A-Life League* (New York, USA) and the constitution of a *Suicide Prevention Department*, by The Salvation Army, in London, UK, both originating in 1906. Competing priorities and lack of reliable information on epidemiological dimension of suicide worldwide have kept the World Health Organization for a long time away from major involvement in the suicide prevention activities (De Leo, Bertolote, & Lester, 2002). However, a United Nations document of 1996 entitled "Prevention of suicide: Guidelines for the formulation and implementation of national strategies" represents a convincing landmark in the commitment to the problem of suicide. Then, a WHO Technical Report (1999) entitled "Figures and facts about suicide" set the scene for epidemiology and trends of suicide around the world.

In 1999, WHO had also launched *SUPRE* (SUicide PREvention), the WHO worldwide initiative for the prevention of suicide, with the following objectives:

1. To bring about a lasting reduction in the frequency of suicidal behaviors, with emphasis on developing countries and countries in social and economic transitions.
2. To identify, assess, and eliminate in the early stages, as far as possible, factors that may result in young people taking their own lives.
3. To raise the general awareness about suicide and provide psychosocial support to people with suicidal thoughts or attempted suicide, and to their relatives and close

* This chapter represents an adaptation of the article WHO Research and Intervention Projects into Suicidal Behaviors: The WHO/SUPRE-MISS and the WHO/START Studies submitted for publication in the *Journal of Clinical Neuropsychiatry* (2009).

friends, as well as those of people who committed suicide (quoted in WHO, 2002).

Activities of the WHO dealt with surveillance of suicide mortality; production and dissemination of information; *Multisite Intervention Study on Suicide Behaviours – SUPRE-MISS*; and technical support to countries. After 1999, the data on suicide are being regularly updated on the WHO SUPRE website. A number of booklets were brought out on supporting the education and awareness of suicide prevention (*Preventing Suicide: A Resource for: 001 – General Physicians; 002 – Media Professionals; 003 – Teachers and Other School Staff; 004 – Primary Health care Workers; 005 – Prison Officers; 006 – How to Start a Survivors' Group, Counsellors, At work, Police, firefighters and other first line interveners*). A detailed description of the SUPRE-MISS study is presented below. Technical support to countries was offered through the WHO Headquarters, the six Regional Offices (with particular support from the WHO Regional Office in Copenhagen), and the WHO Collaborating Centres for Research and Training in Suicide Prevention, in Brisbane, Stockholm, and Beijing.

The WHO Department of Violence and Injury Prevention published the *World Report on Violence and Health* (Krug, Dahlberg, Mercy, Zwi, & Lozano, 2002) (prefaced by Nelson Mandela), subdividing the matter into interpersonal violence and self-directed violence. Thus, suicide phenomena could benefit from more international attention, even because the official launch took place in Brussels, at the Royal Palace, in the presence of King Albert II and a sizeable number of Nobel laureates, and was broadcasted live by the CNN. The writer of this paper, at that time the President of the International Association for Suicide Prevention and one of the panelists at the Brussels launch, was then in the best position for promoting the realization of the World Suicide Prevention Day, which was officially instituted for the first time on September 10, 2003, after several years of preparation. The World Suicide Prevention Day, since its first inception, has been a major booster of suicide prevention activities throughout the globe, with more than 70 countries organizing formal celebrations in 2007 (De Leo, 2008).

WHO Collaborative Studies on Suicidal Behavior

The World Health Organization, since its creation in 1948, has nurtured a substantial tradition of collaborative studies. Actually, the first cooperation in the area of suicide was promoted by the WHO Regional Office for Europe, Copenhagen, thanks to the long-sighted public health interests of Dr. John Henderson, who promoted and oversaw the founding of the study during a meeting in York (UK) in 1986. The *WHO/EURO Multicentre Study on Parasuicide* (renamed as WHO/EURO Multicentre Study on *Suicidal Behaviour* in Athens in 1999) started on the field in 1988 with 13 centers and ended formally in 2001 with 35 centers enrolled (Platt et al., 1992; Schmidtke, Bille-Brahe, De Leo, & Kerkhof, 2004; Schmidtke et al., 1996). The study was a by-product of the "Health for

All by the Year 2000" (a program with 32 targets voted by the World Health Assembly), whose Target 12 was specifically aimed at reversing the current trends of suicide and attempted suicide (Bille-Brahe, Schmidtke, Kerkhof, & De Leo, 2004). Needless to say, the study was enormously influential in fostering suicide research and education, not only in European countries (Schmidtke et al., 1998). The study originated more than 250 scientific publications, both at national and international levels, including three international books and three WHO Technical Reports. The study also stimulated the creation of the biannual European Symposia on Suicide and Suicidal Behavior, which rapidly became the natural stage for highest quality standard presentations in suicide research worldwide (the first meeting held in Munich in 1986 and the most recent one in Glasgow, 2008).

In 1995 in Berne, Switzerland, during a WHO/EURO meeting, the advantages and disadvantages of international cooperations in suicide research and prevention were the object of an intense debate (De Leo, 1995). Positive issues embedded with these types of studies present following features:

- Larger samples allow for bigger statistical power (extremely important for a low-base phenomenon such as suicide).
- Transcultural differences may instruct prevention.
- Large cooperative efforts could lead to better sensitization and awareness among the community members and health authorities.
- Creation of stable research units by highly specialized researchers.
- Implementation of suicide prevention programs at local, regional, and national levels.
- The opportunity for implementing suicidology courses in academic settings.
- Increased competency of researchers through international exchange.
- Stimulation of innovative research.

On the contrary, at the level of disadvantages, the following features were identified:

- Obtained data refer only to health facility referrals.
- Local data do not necessarily mirror national trends.
- Epidemiology is often perceived as detached from the clinical practice, even with the WHO "Tag."
- Comparability among the centers is often problematic.
- Diagnostic processes are influenced by cultural contexts and could lead to erroneous conclusions on pooled data sets.
- Study impact is often problematic to evaluate in terms of direct benefits.
- New treatment protocols are not necessarily an implicit outcome of any study.
- Cooperation among the team members could be problematic or even disruptive if personality factors or behavior attitudes are not properly controlled and managed.

The WHO/EURO Multicentre Study on Suicidal Behaviour formally ended in 2001, with its transformation into WHO/EURO Network for Suicide Prevention. The European Office of WHO was then the promoter of the European Assembly in Helsinki on

Mental Health, which promulgated a set of directions on suicide prevention, as reported below:

Suicide prevention strategies are concerned with

- identifying and reducing availability of and access to the means of suicide;
- improving health care services and promoting supportive and rehabilitation;
- functions for persons affected by suicidal behavior;
- improving diagnostic procedures and subsequent treatment;
- increasing the awareness of health care staff of their own attitudes and taboos towards suicide prevention and mental illness;
- increasing knowledge through public education about mental illness and its recognition at an early stage;
- supporting media reporting on suicide and attempted suicide;
- promoting research on suicide prevention and encouraging the collection of data on the causes of suicide by avoiding duplication of statistical records (WHO, 2005a, 2005b).

The ending of the WHO/EURO Multicentre Study on Suicidal Behaviour convinced WHO officers, and particularly Dr. José Bertolote (a very important player in many advancements of suicide prevention activities), to support the implementation of a new collaborative effort in the area of suicide (the advantages being far superior to the disadvantages), possibly focusing on a rather neglected – but extremely important – topic: The role of cultural factors in suicide phenomena (De Leo, 2002).

The WHO/SUPRE-MISS Study

Proposed by the author of this chapter, the idea of SUPRE-MISS study mainly originated by observing the marked disparities in suicide and attempted suicide rates in the countries that participated in the WHO/EURO Multicentre Study on Suicidal Behaviour. For example, the above-mentioned study demonstrated in men the rates of parasuicide to be sevenfold higher in Helsinki (Finland) compared to Guipúzcoa (Spain) (Schmidtke et al., 1996). On the other hand, the rates of suicide were notoriously very different among the European countries, with the rates in Finnish men being 40 times higher than in Albanian men (WHO, 1999). The idea of a study involving those countries in representation of the six WHO regions was launched on October 22, 1999, in Brisbane, Australia, during a WHO Regional Meeting on SUPRE, and this idea was accepted by all the participants. The background documents (De Leo & Broers, 2000; De Leo, Burless, & Broers, 2000) were prepared and discussed during the first meeting of the principal investigators of the WHO/SUPRE-MISS Project (April 5–7, 2000, WHO, Geneva). The study (the name of which meant Suicide Prevention: Multisite Intervention Study on Suicidal Behaviours) pertained to three different areas of investigation: (1) a transcultural description of the communities participating in the study; (2) a community survey of suicidal ideation and behavior on a representative sample of subjects from each community; and

(3) a randomized controlled trial of treatment as usual (TAU) of suicide attempters at health facilities versus TAU plus a brief form of contact and intervention (BIC) with attempters. The assumption on this specific part of the study was that a necessarily simple intervention (given the enormous variability of type and availability of care among countries) performed with some continuity (9 follow-ups in an 18-month trial) could elicit different results from routine forms of treatment. The feasibility of the community study and the structure of all questionnaires were first piloted in Queensland (De Leo, Cerin, Spathonis, & Burgis, 2005).

The study, globally, was meant:

- To contribute to increasing the awareness about the burden of suicidal behaviors.
- To identify reliable and valid indicators of risk for fatal and nonfatal suicidal behavior, with special emphasis on sociocultural factors.
- To describe the patterns of suicidal behavior.
- To identify variables that determine the presentation or not at health facilities following a suicide attempt.
- To improve the efficiency of general health care services through the identification of specific interventions effective for the reduction of suicide attempts.

Eight countries, in representation of the six regions of WHO, were selected to participate in the study: Estonia (EURO), South Africa (AFRO), Brazil (AMRO), Iran (EMRO), India and Sri Lanka (SEARO), and Vietnam and China (WPRO). For Iran, Vietnam, and South Africa, it was the first occasion of an international cooperation in the area of suicidal behaviors (Fleischmann et al., 2005). The main results from the community surveys are presented in Table 1.

The most relevant results of the SUPRE-MISS are those related to the randomized controlled trial involved in the pooling of all data of the TAU versus TAU + BIC on suicide attempters in all centers. Given the size of the two samples (945 subjects in TAU versus 922 in TAU + BIC, after randomization), the results obtained were particularly

Table 1. Results of the community surveys within the WHO/SUPRE-MISS Study (Bertolote et al., 2005)

Country	Ss	Suicide ideation* (%)	Suicide plans* (%)	Attempted suicide* (%)
Australia (Brisbane)	11,572	14.9	4.4	4.2
Estonia (Tallin)	498	12.4	5.4	3.6
Sri Lanka (Colombo)	670	7.3	1.5	2.1
Brazil (Campinas)	516	18.6	5.2	3.1
Iran (Karaj)	504	14.1	6.7	4.2
Vietnam (Hanoi)	2,266	8.9	1.1	0.4
South Africa (Durban)	500	25.4	15.6	3.4
India (Chennai)	500	2.6	2.0	1.6
China (Yuncheng)	503	18.5	7.4	2.4

*Lifetime.

convincing: In the group that received the series of planned follow-ups, mortality for cases of suicide was significantly reduced ($p < .0001$) compared to the TAU only subjects. Specifically, at 18-month follow-up, there were only two deaths due to suicide in the first group compared to 18 deaths in the group that received the routine care only. Furthermore, even the mortality for all other causes was higher in the group that received only TAU: 22 subjects versus 11 individuals in the TAU + BIC group ($p < .037$) (Fleischmann et al., 2008). Several articles were originated by the SUPRE-MISS study, the data of which are still being analyzed, both locally and centrally (pooled dataset).

The WHO/START Study

The WHO/START Study arose out of a perceived and identified need to address the problem of suicidal behaviors within the WHO Western Pacific Region (WPR). There is a paucity of information on suicide rates within the WPR, with only eight nations providing official national data to the WHO (De Leo & Evans, 2004). However, the 2004 edition of the World Health Report estimates that in 2002 there were 331,000 cases of suicide in this Region of the World Health Organization (WHO, 2004). This number represents more than one third (i.e., 38%) of all suicides occurring in the world every year for a corresponding population that is much less than one third of the global population [1,745,620 in 2005 (estimated)] (WHO, 2005a, 2005b). The suicide rate for this region in 2002 was 19/100,000, which is more than 30% higher than the average world rate for the same year (14/100,000). With 272,647 cases as the estimated number of deaths due to suicide in 2002, China contributes approximately 80% of the total number of deaths in the WPR (WHO, 2004). Suicide is among the top five causes of injury-related deaths, accounting for more than road accidents and falls combined, as well as more than all homicide deaths and war victims put together. Globally, suicide represents 1.4% of the global burden of diseases, but in the WPR the burden reaches 2.5% (WHO, 2004).

Most of the 37 Member States (28 countries, 9 territories) that belong to the WHO WPR are represented by low-income countries, with a small number of those countries currently witnessing booming expansions, like China and Malaysia. For many of the countries, the globalization process is imposing radical changes to the structure of societies and traditional values, and the loss of life due to suicide has increased.

In August 2005, 21 countries participated in a meeting in Manila WHO Offices, convened by the WHO Regional Adviser, Dr. Wang Xiangdong. The aim of the meeting was to ascertain the real extent of the problem of suicidal behaviors within the region and verify the feasibility of stimulating and implementing suicide prevention activities. The consensus among the participants of the meeting was that the development of a valid and reliable monitoring system was essential for health planning and resource allocation. It was accepted that the use of standardized nomenclature to effectively promote the implementation of surveillance systems and the launch of a regionally based study from coordinated efforts would provide substantial benefit. This would enable a starting point for the individual nation's public health systems with regard to monitoring suicide and other suicidal behaviors.

The study, called START (Suicide Trends in At-Risk Territories) also to emphasize the beginning of formal recording practices for many participating countries, was officially launched in Brisbane on March 3, 2006 by Dr. Shigeru Omi (Director of the WPRO) and Dr. José Bertolote (WHO-HQ, Coordinator, Department of Mental Health and Substance Abuse). Of the 37 WPR nations and territories, 22 of them agreed to take part in the study. The WHO/START study is the only officially endorsed study of the International Association for Suicide Prevention (IASP), with the Australian Institute for Suicide Research and Prevention (AISRAP) currently managing the project in all its components.

The tasks of the above-mentioned study are

1. Standardized collection of suicide mortality and morbidity (attempts/self-harm) from 22 nations in the Region (9 countries do not actually run any official data collection).
2. A randomized controlled trial of treatment and aftercare of suicide attempters (interventions study) following the example of SUPRE-MISS.
3. A psychological autopsy of suicide victims (transcultural comparison of risk factors for suicide).
4. A longitudinal evaluation of medically serious suicide attempters.

This large-scale study will provide significant insights into the cultural factors of suicidal behaviors and create a powerful network of researchers, clinicians, and public health administrators. The increased awareness and sensitivity toward suicide phenomena will be able to generate innovative research, develop education and training, and actively encourage regional and national suicide prevention strategies to develop and evaluate consequent impact. Clearly, the overall goal is to reduce suicide in the 22 World Health Organization Western Pacific nations and associate members, areas, and territories through the four phases of the study and its longer-term outcomes. In fact, the START Study is initially planned for a 3-year duration, but it is expected that a number of countries will commence at a later stage than the official starting on the field, which was January 2008. Twenty-two countries have so far agreed to participate in the START Study. They are Australia, Cambodia, China, Fiji, French Polynesia, Guam, Hong Kong (China), Japan, Lao People's Democratic Republic, Micronesia, Mongolia, New Caledonia, New Zealand, Northern Mariana Islands, Papua New Guinea, Republic of Korea, Samoa, Singapore, Solomon Islands, Tonga, Vanuatu, and Vietnam. This number is destined to increase, with more countries inside and outside the region seeking to participate, including India, Thailand, and Italy.

The project underpins the ability of WPR nations to develop local strategies to reduce suicide in their communities. The establishment of an efficient and standardized means of collection and record keeping is imperative to the later dissemination and interpretation of results. This data collection will be able to provide information on the social and economic impact of suicide with the database to reflect among a range of requirements – age, culture, income, language, mental health services available, literacy, and life expectancy. An atlas will finally be established, consisting of the profiles of the characteristics of each nation, associate member, area, and territory within the area and territory within the WPR.

Acknowledgment

The author is indebted to Dr. Alexandra Fleischman, WHO Department of Mental Health and Substance Abuse, Geneva, for her careful revision of this manuscript.

References

Bertolote, J. M., Fleischmann, A., De Leo, D., Bolhari, J., Botega, N., De Silv, D., et al. (2005). Suicide attempts, plans, and ideation in culturally diverse sites: The WHO SUPRE-MISS community survey. *Psychological Medicine, 35*, 1457–1465.

Bille-Brahe, U., Schmidtke, A., Kerkhof, A., & De Leo, D. (2004). The WHO/EURO multi-centre study on suicidal behavior: Its background, history, aims and design. In D. De Leo, B. Bille-Brahe, A. Kerkhof, & A. Schmidtke (Eds.), *Suicidal behavior: Theories and research findings* (pp. 5–13). Göttingen: Hogrefe & Huber.

De Leo, D. (1995). International collaborative studies: Advantages and disadvantages, Speech held at the meeting of the principal investigators of the WHO/EURO multicentre study on parasuicide, Berne, Switzerland (unpublished).

De Leo, D. (2002). Why are we not getting any closer to preventing suicide? (Editorial). *British Journal of Psychiatry, 181*, 372–374.

De Leo, D. (2008). Crisis: The road ahead (Editorial). *Crisis, 29*, 171–172.

De Leo, D., Bertolote, J. M., & Lester, D. (2002). Self-directed violence. In E. G. Krug, L. L. Dahlberg, J. A. Mercy, et al. (Eds.), *World report on violence and health* (pp. 185–212). Geneva: WHO.

De Leo, D., & Broers, M. (2000). *Intervention study.* Background document to the meeting of principal investigators of the WHO/SUPRE-MISS Project, 5–7 April 2000, Geneva, Switzerland. Geneva: WHO.

De Leo, D., Burless, C., & Broers, M. (2000). *Community survey.* Background document to the meeting of principal investigators of the WHO/SUPRE-MISS Project, 5–7 April 2000, Geneva, Switzerland. Geneva: WHO.

De Leo, D., Cerin, E., Spathonis, K., & Burgis, S. (2005). Lifetime risk of suicide ideation and attempts in an Australian community: Prevalence, suicidal process, and help-seeking behaviour. *Journal of Affective Disorders, 86*, 215–225.

De Leo, D., & Evans, R. (2004). *International suicide rates and prevention strategies*. Göttingen: Hogrefe & Huber.

Fleischmann, A., Bertolote, J. M., De Leo, D., Botega, N., Phillips, M., Sisak, M., et al. (2005). Characteristics of attempted suicides seen in emergency-care settings of general hospitals in eight low- and middle-income countries. *Psychological Medicine, 35*, 1467–1474.

Fleischmann, A., Bertolote, J. M., Wasserman, D., De Leo, D., Bolhari, J., Botega, N. J., et al. (2008). Effectiveness of brief intervention and contact for suicide attempters: A randomized controlled trial in five countries. *Bulletin of the World Health Organization, 86*, 703–709.

Krug, E. G., Dahlberg, L. L., Mercy, J. A., Zwi, A. B., & Lozano, R. (Eds.). (2002). *World report on violence and health*. Geneva: WHO.

Platt, S., Bille-Brahe, U., Kerkhof, A., Schmidtke, A., Bjerke, T., Crepet, P., et al. (1992). Parasuicide in Europe: The WHO/EURO multicentre study on parasuicide. Introduction and preliminary analysis for 1989. *Acta Psychiatrica Scandinavica, 85*, 97–104.

Schmidtke, A., Bille-Brahe, U., De Leo, D., & Kerkhof, A. (2004). The WHO/EURO multicentre study on suicidal behaviour. History and aims of the study. In A. Schmidtke, U. Bille-Brahe, et al. (Eds.), *Suicidal behaviour in Europe. Results from the WHO/EURO multicentre study on suicidal behaviour* (pp. 7–10). Göttingen: Hogrefe & Huber.

Schmidtke, A., Bille-Brahe, U., De Leo, D., Kerkhof, A. F. J. M., Bjerke, T., Crepet, P., et al. (1996). Attempted suicide in Europe: Rates, trends and sociodemographic characteristics of suicide attempters during the period 1989–1992. Results of the WHO/EURO multicentre study on parasuicide. *Acta Psychiatrica Scandinavica, 93*, 327–338.

Schmidtke, A., De Leo, D., Bille-Brahe, U., Crepet, P., Hjemeland, H., Kerkhof, A., et al. (1998). The fall downs of the WHO/EURO multicentre study on parasuicide. *European Psychiatry, 13*(Suppl. 4), 142s–143s(2).

United Nations. (1996). *Prevention of suicide: Guidelines for the formulation and implementation of national strategies*. New York: United Nations.

World Health Organization. (1999). *Figures and facts about suicide*. Geneva: WHO Technical Report.

World Health Organization. (2002). *Multi-site intervention study on suicide behaviour – SUPRE-MISS*. Geneva: WHO.

World Health Organization. (2004). *The world health report, 2004: Changing history*. Geneva: WHO.

World Health Organization. (2005). *Mental health: Facing the challenges, building solutions. Report from the WHO European Ministerial Conference*. Copenhagen: WHO, European Office.

World Health Organization. (2005). *The world health report, 2005: Make every mother and child count*. Geneva: WHO.

About the Author

Diego De Leo is Professor of Psychiatry and Director of the Australian Institute for Suicide Research and Prevention at Griffith University, Brisbane, which was designated as the National Centre of Excellence in Suicide Prevention in November 2008. At Griffith he also directs the World Health Organization (WHO) Collaborating Centre for Research and Training in Suicide Prevention. He is a graduate of the University of Padua (Italy) School of Medicine, where he then specialized in Psychiatry. He obtained his PhD degree in Social and Behavioral Sciences at the University of Leiden (The Netherlands). He was the founder of the first Psychogeriatric Service of Italy and also the first suicide research unit, both are at the University of Padua. Professor de Leo is Past President of the International Association for Suicide Prevention (IASP) and co-founder and Past President of the International Academy for Suicide Research (IASR) of which he also co-founded the journal *Archives of Suicide Research*. He has been the initiator of the World Suicide Prevention Day (2003). Member of the Editorial boards for several internationally renowned refereed journals, he is Editor-in-Chief of the journal *Crisis*. Professor de Leo has published extensively, with more than 220 refereed journal articles, 145 book chapters, and 30 volumes published in the past 25 years and over 200 conference presentations. Winner of six international awards, in 2007 he was given the title of Doctor of Science by Griffith University for his work on Suicide and Psychogeriatrics. Current research topics are diverse, and include definitional issues and data quality in suicide statistics, as well as suicide in the mentally well and suicidal behavior across different cultures.

Diego De Leo
Griffith University
Mt. Gravatt Campus
176 Messines Ridge Rd
QLD 4122
Australia
Tel.: +61 7 3735 3382
E-mail: D.DeLeo@griffith.edu.au

Evidence-Based Strategies for Suicide Prevention

Evidence-Based Suicide Prevention Strategies*

An Overview

J. John Mann and Dianne Currier

Division of Molecular Imaging and Neuropathology, Department of Psychiatry, Columbia University, NY, USA

Suicide Prevention Strategies

Suicide and attempted suicide are major public health issues, and prevention strategies to reduce the mortality and morbidity due to suicidal behavior are urgently required. Risk factors for suicidal behavior have been identified in multiple domains including biological, genetic, environmental, cognitive, personality, behavioral, and clinical (see Mann & Currier, 2008 for an overview). Given the variability and multidetermined nature of suicidal behavior, quantifying the attributable risk to various factors is a challenge and needs to be done in different populations such as different countries, urban versus rural populations, and different socioeconomic groups. Prevention strategies, interventions, and programs must rely on the existent knowledge base of potentially modifiable risk factors. A systematic review of suicide prevention strategies described five key areas on which prevention strategies were focused: education and awareness; screening for at-risk individuals; treatment of psychiatric disorders; restricting access to lethal means; and media reporting of suicide (Mann et al., 2005). Preventive interventions in these domains span the population (education and awareness, media reporting, and means access), institutional and professional (education and awareness, screening), and individual levels (treatment of psychiatric disorders) and may be multilevel. Evidence for many commonly accepted prevention strategies is sometimes sparse or absent, particularly for the key but less common outcome of suicide.

One of the reasons for the dearth of evidence are the methodological difficulties involved in evaluating prevention interventions using suicide as a primary outcome due to its low base rate. Nonfatal suicide attempt and suicidal ideation are more frequent

* This work was supported by MH048514.

and therefore more amenable to investigation, although there is considerable variability across interventions and studies in the definition and method of data collection for both these outcomes. Moreover, the relationship between ideation and even nonfatal suicide attempts with suicide is particularly remote for younger age groups where the ratio of fatal to nonfatal attempts is about 1:20 and declines to about 1:4 in older age groups. For these reasons, support for intervention efficacy often draws on suicidal ideation or nonfatal attempts or even secondary or intermediate outcomes, including help-seeking behavior, identification of at-risk individuals, entry into treatment, and antidepressant prescription rates. The findings from these more distant or secondary outcome-based studies need to be interpreted with caution.

This chapter outlines five key domains of prevention strategies listed above and presents a brief overview of current evidence supporting the effectiveness of interventions in those domains in terms of primary and intermediary outcomes. That evidence is derived from reports published in the biomedical literature in the English language where prevention programs are evaluated in terms of efficacy or effectiveness in prevention of suicide, suicide attempt or suicidal ideation, or intermediate outcomes as described above. Evidence presented is derived from a variety of study designs, as is necessary when investigating such a diversity of interventions, including those never subject to a randomized controlled trial (RCT). Thus, we include evidence from experimental and quasi-experimental studies as the most robust indicators, ecological studies examining changing rates of suicide and suicide attempts in populations, and systematic reviews and meta-analyses that consider the methodological quality of primary studies. This chapter is organized around level of prevention strategy: population level strategies, institutional and professional level strategies, and individual level interventions.

Population Level Strategies

Public Awareness and Education

Public education is a central plank of a public health approach to suicide prevention at the population level. Lack of knowledge about the causes and risk factors for suicidal behavior and treatment options, particularly with respect to mental illness, can prevent at-risk individuals seeking treatment or families appreciating the risk of suicide in a family member. Moreover, such knowledge gaps can support attitudes that create barriers to treatment seeking such as the stigmatization of those with mental illness or suicidal behavior that discourages seeking help. Other beliefs or attitudes that hinder prevention efforts include the acceptance of suicide as inevitable, as a national character trait or cultural practice, or accepting suicide as an appropriate solution to life problems, for example serious medical illness. Stigma is considered the most prevalent and problematic of these attitudes, as stigma associated with mental illness is a deterrent to seeking treatment and can also increase distress of the sufferer, both of which may increase suicide risk. Therefore, reducing the stigma associated with mental illness by education and thereby encouraging treatment seeking is frequently a part of suicide prevention efforts (Goldsmith, Pellmar, Kleinman, & Bunney, 2002). Most population level suicide prevention strategies contain education and awareness components aimed at creating a public awareness of mental illness as commonplace and treatable, and suicide as a preventable complication of mental illness. Some such plans focus public education and destigmatization programs on mental illness, particularly depression, rather than specifically on suicide prevention. This is in part due to concerns that overexposure to suicide may normalize or inadvertently encourage suicidal behavior. With respect to the effectiveness of public awareness and education campaigns in reducing suicidal behavior, there has been relatively little systematic evaluation.

Large-scale public education campaigns focused on depression in Germany (Hegerl, Althaus, & Stefanek, 2003), the UK (Paykel, Hart, & Priest, 1998), Australia (Hickie, 2004), and New Zealand (Akroyd & Wyllie, 2002) suggest modest effects of public education campaigns on attitudes regarding the causes and treatment of depression. In terms of effects of large-scale public education and awareness campaigns on the primary outcomes of decreasing suicide or suicide attempts, there has been only one study reporting a beneficial effect. Evaluation of the multifaceted Nuremberg Alliance against Depression program (Hegerl et al., 2003) reported declines in suicide attempts of 26.5% in the intervention region, which was significantly greater than the control region (Hegerl, Althaus, Schmidtke, & Niklewski, 2006), but did not have adequate statistical power to detect change in suicide rates. However, the beneficial change is not attributable to the improved public awareness or knowledge about depression because attitudes and knowledge in the intervention region did not improve compared to the control region (Hegerl et al., 2003). Likewise there is little evidence indicating a beneficial effect of such campaigns on intermediary outcomes such as increases in more treatment seeking or increased antidepressant use (Akroyd & Wyllie, 2002; Hickie, 2004; Paykel et al., 1998). An evaluation of changes in public attitudes over the course of the 1991–1996 UK Defeat Depression Campaign reported improvements in attitudes toward depression but less success regarding antidepressant treatment (Paykel et al., 1998). Goldney and Fisher (2008) conducted a large community survey in Australia of changes in mental health literacy and treatment seeking among depressed individuals with and without suicidal ideation from 1998 to 2004, a period in which there had been a number of public education campaigns on depression and suicide. They found that despite increasing awareness and understanding of treatment options for depression, there was little change in treatment seeking among the most at-risk group, depressed individuals with suicidal ideation (Goldney & Fisher, 2008).

Restriction of Lethal Means

Groups that attempt suicide using highly lethal means, for example men with firearms in the USA or women with pesticides in rural China, India, and Sri Lanka, have much higher rates of death per attempt, than those who use less lethal means. In other words, the suicide attempter's intent is revealed by the method chosen. The most determined individuals choose the most lethal method or use a less lethal method more determinedly such as taking an overdose of a larger number of pills. Alternatively, more impulsive individuals who use a very lethal method will show a higher rate of death than if they had chosen a less lethal method, for example, they will not go to the extra trouble of accumulating the additional pills to reach a fatal dose. It is this latter group that will have the most benefit from means restriction. The question is whether restricting access to more lethal methods results in method substitution, such that another equally lethal method is used resulting in no change in suicide rates, or if less lethal methods are used and survival is more likely or the attempt is abandoned altogether, both outcomes resulting in fewer suicides. There is a substantial body of evidence showing that restricting access to more lethal means leads to reduction in the number of suicides by that method. Norway, Canada, New Zealand, and certain regions in Australia and the United States have recorded a drop in firearm suicides following legislation restricting access to firearms (Bridges & Kunselman, 2004; Cantor & Slater, 1995; Lester & Leenaars, 1993; Loftin, McDowall, Wiersema, & Cottey, 1991; Ludwig & Cook, 2000; Snowdon & Harris, 1992). In all cases, the effect was stronger on male suicides who favor this method. The detoxification of domestic gas was followed by sharp decreases in suicide by that method in England, Australia, Switzerland, Japan, the Netherlands, Germany, and the US (Kreitman, 1976; Lester, 1990b, 1991; Whitlock, 1975; Wiedenmann & Weyerer, 1993). In Sri Lanka and Finland, restricting access to pesticides led to a decrease in pesticide suicides (Gunnell et al., 2007; Ohberg, Lonnqvist, Sarna, Vuori, & Penttila, 1995). Restrictions on the sale or changing prescription patterns of barbiturates in Australia, the UK, Denmark, Norway, Japan, and Sweden were accompanied by a sharp decline in barbiturate overdose suicides, although not in Finland (Carlsten, Allebeck, & Brandt, 1996; Crome, 1993; Nielsen & Nielsen, 1992; Oliver & Hetzel, 1972; Retterstol, 1989; Whitlock, 1975; Yamasawa, Nishimukai, Ohbora, & Inoue, 1980), and limits on analgesic package size and changing to blister packs reduced the number of overdoses in the UK (Hawton, 2002). The use of catalytic converters led to a reduction in suicides using vehicle emissions in the UK and the USA, but not in Australia (Kelly & Bunting, 1998; McClure, 2000; Motto et al., 2002; Shelef, 1994). Barriers at jumping sites such as bridges, tall buildings, train stations, and other "hot spots" have reduced suicides from those sites (Beautrais, Gibb, Fergusson, Horwood, & Larkin, 2009; Skegg & Herbison, 2009). Finally, the use of new lower toxicity antidepressants has led to a decrease in the number of suicides through antidepressant overdose (Gibbons, Hur, Bhaumik, & Mann, 2005; Kapur, Mieczkowski, & Mann, 1992).

Effects on overall suicide rates will depend on how widely the restricted method is used and whether method substitution involving a method of comparable lethality occurs. Correlational studies have shown that in certain cases the restriction of a particular method has been accompanied by a decline in overall suicide rates. This was the case for firearm restriction in Canada (Carrington, 1999) and Washington, DC (Loftin et al., 1991), barbiturate restriction in Australia (Oliver & Hetzel, 1972), detoxification of domestic gas in the UK (Kreitman, 1976) and Switzerland (Lester, 1990a), and regulation of vehicle emissions in England for the male suicide rate (Kelly & Bunting, 1998). While not a suicide method *per se*, restrictions on alcohol availability coincided with decreases in overall suicide rates in Iceland (Lester, 1999), in the USSR during the perestroika period (Wasserman & Varnik, 1998), and in Slovenia among males (Pridemore & Snowden, 2009). However, assessing the extent to which method control contributes to overall declines in suicide rates requires consideration of other factors that may influence long-term trends such as increased use of antidepressants. Where a decline is observed in suicides by the restricted method, but no overall decline in suicide rates observed, it may be that substitution of methods occurs, as was the case for domestic gas detoxification in the UK (Gunnell, Middleton, & Frankel, 2000), Germany (Wiedenmann & Weyerer, 1993), and among males in the US (Lester, 1990b), and banning the pesticide parathion in Finland (Ohberg et al., 1995). Despite unresolved questions about method substitution, the majority of these studies demonstrate the life-saving potential of restricting lethal means. Since people go through a suicide crisis when risk is high, making a more lethal method less available may result in nonfatal suicide attempts and then successful treatment.

Media Reporting of Suicide

Media contribute to misinformation about the causes and preventability of suicide through both the choice and presentation of suicide-related material. For example, particular types of suicide deaths are more likely to be reported including those by young people or where sensational methods are employed. Moreover, often a single event is presented as the precipitating factor, the role of stress overemphasized and that of mental illness often omitted, or suicide is presented as a realistic or inevitable option, romanticized, or idealized. Such misinformation is also problematic as many policymakers obtain their information on suicide from the media, and it can misdirect the focus of community-based prevention and lobbying activities. Beyond influencing opinion in the public arena, there are concerns that media coverage of suicide may precipitate suicidal behavior in vulnerable individuals. The theory of contagion suggests that exposure to suicide through the media glamorizing the act or promoting it as a solution to life's problems used by famous people such as pop stars, or just by more ordinary individuals with whom a person may identify, may induce vulnerable individuals to engage in suicidal behavior. The theory of imitation is concerned with suicidal individuals adopting methods or being attracted to suicide "hot spots" portrayed in the media. There is a body of evidence in support of both theories (see Pirkis & Blood, 2001; Gould, 2001 for reviews) which support interventions in media coverage as a preventative strategy, both to decrease detrimental coverage and to enlist media in educational campaigns.

Programs in journalist education or the production of media guidelines for reporting suicide have had mixed results. In Hong Kong, following the distribution of the WHO media guidelines "Preventing Suicide: A Resource for Media Professionals" and an awareness campaign, content analysis revealed changes in reporting of suicide in line with the recommendations (Fu & Yip, 2008). An evaluation of media content following the issuing of media guidelines for reporting suicide in Australia found improvement in the appropriateness of reporting (Pirkis et al., 2009). In Nuremberg after journalist education on suicide that there was some improvement in two of the three main newspapers, specifically there were fewer articles on suicides and less prominent placement of articles (Schafer, Althaus, Brosius, & Hegerl, 2006). In the USA, the Center for Disease Control endorsed recommendations for the responsible reporting of suicide; however, there has been no systematic evaluation of their impact (O'Carroll & Potter, 1994). These programs have not been evaluated in terms of potential effect of alterations in media reporting on rates of suicide or suicide attempts. However, evidence of an effect of restriction of media coverage is suggested by reports that media blackouts on reporting suicide, whether by negotiation or circumstance, have coincided with decreases in suicide rates. Motto documented a significant decrease in the suicides of females, most markedly in those under 35 years of age, during a 268-day complete newspaper blackout in Detroit in 1967 compared with the previous 3 years (Motto, 1970). Following a 1987 campaign to decrease media reporting of subway deaths in Austria, subway suicides and attempted suicides declined immediately by 80% and have remained at a low level since (Etzersdorfer, Sonneck, & Nagel-Kuess, 1992; Niederkrotenthaler & Sonneck, 2007). Media intervention programs have largely neglected the Internet, a source of increasing concern due to the deleterious effects of suicide chat rooms, the provision of instruction in methods for suicide, and the active solicitation of suicide pact partners.

Institutional/Professional Strategies

Gatekeeper Education and Interventions

There are many professional and community groups who have contact with at-risk populations or individuals and have the potential to refer at-risk individuals to mental health professionals for assessment and treatment as needed. These "gatekeepers" include clergy, first responders, pharmacists, nurses, geriatric caregivers, staff in personnel departments of large businesses, and staff in institutional settings such as the military, police, prisons, and schools. Education of psychiatric care staff in suicide prevention resulted in significant improvement in attitudes toward attempted suicide patients and suicide prevention in the intervention clinics compared with control clinics (Ramberg & Wasserman, 2004). However, in terms of effect on suicidal behavior outcomes, systematic evaluation of outcomes in suicide prevention strategies targeted at gatekeepers has largely been limited to programs conducted in institutional settings such as the military. Two military programs for which outcome data are available have shown some success. The United States Air Force instituted a comprehensive multimodal suicide prevention strategy in 1996 that included an extensive gatekeeper education component directed at supervisors and community agents including chaplains, family support centers, and so on. Suicide rates declined from 16.4/100,000 in 1994 to 5.6/100,000 in 1999, constituting a 33% decline in risk for suicide (Knox, Litts, Talcott, Feig, & Caine, 2003). In 1993, Norway conducted suicide prevention education in the military involving conscripts, officers, and commanders.

Due to the small number of suicides annually, rates are calculated for 8-year periods. Following the 1993 intervention, there was a decrease in suicide rates in conscripts from 15/100,000 in the 1985–1992 period to 9/100,000 in 1993–1999 (Melhem, L., unpublished data). In addition to gatekeeper training, these multimodal programs also promoted organization wide awareness of mental health and suicide, and facilitated access to mental health services.

Community gatekeeper education programs are frequent in suicide prevention programs that are aimed at youth including school- and community-based programs (Gould, Greenberg, Velting, & Shaffer, 2003). These programs are most often conducted in schools and are seldom systematically evaluated and consequently their effectiveness largely unknown. Moreover, some of these programs are a cause of concern for suicide prevention professionals as they are not evidence-based, do not reflect the current state of knowledge in suicide prevention, and do not include plans to evaluate their effectiveness and safety. Additionally, a sizeable population of at-risk youth is not captured by school-based programs, either because it is older or because absenteeism and/or drop-out rates are higher in at-risk youth. Given the identification of youth as a key target population in suicide prevention strategies and plans, and the prominence of including school-based education programs, the lack of provision for evaluation of outcomes is disturbing, particularly as reviews of existing programs are mixed at best. A review of published studies on school-based programs in Canada found that while knowledge on suicide improved, there were both beneficial and harmful effects, and overall insufficient evidence to support ongoing implementation of curriculum-based suicide prevention programs in schools (Ploeg et al., 1996). A more recent review of Canadian studies of school-based prevention programs also found improvements in knowledge and skills but did not demonstrate impact on suicidal ideation or attempts in any study (Guo & Harstall, 2002). Burns and Patton reviewing evidence from youth prevention programs found little evidence of efficacy for school-based suicide education programs (Burns & Patton, 2000). An analysis of US state-level youth suicide prevention initiatives from 1980 to 1996 found that the inclusion of a mandated or recommended school-based suicide prevention curriculum had no relationship to changes in youth suicide rates over that period (Metha, Weber, & Webb, 1998).

Results from individual studies of existing school-based youth education programs indicate that they increase knowledge and improve attitudes to mental illness and suicide (Aseltine & DeMartino, 2004; Breton et al., 2002; Metha et al., 1998; Shaffer, Garland, Vieland, Underwood, & Busner, 1991; Vieland, Whittle, Garland, Hicks, & Shaffer, 1991). In terms of suicidal behavior outcomes, only a few studies report benefits. Aseltine and DeMartino (2004) report lower suicide attempt rates, greater knowledge, and more adaptive attitudes about depression and suicide in the intervention group compared with controls in the three months after the intervention, but no significant effects on suicidal ideation or help-seeking. Zenere and Lazarus (1997) reported a decline in the rate of student suicides in Florida from 12.9% per year to 4.6% over the intervention period, 1990–1994, compared to the preceding 10 years, as well as a drop in suicide attempts from 87/100,000 in 1989/1990 to 31/100,000 in 1993/1994. That program was multifaceted with student, staff, and parent education and a mental health worker in schools. However, there was no control group and it remains to be seen if the effect is sustained or represents a chance fluctuation in the rate. Others found no difference between control and intervention group in suicide attempt rates in an 18-month follow-up (Vieland et al., 1991).

Primary Care Physician Education and Awareness

Improved treatment of mental illness is a prominent component of most national suicide prevention plans. Depression and other psychiatric disorders are under-recognized and undertreated in the general practice setting. Moreover, general practitioners or primary care physicians (PCPs) are commonly the most proximal and often only medical contact suicidal patients have. They are frequently the entry point into health care for those in distress and often are better positioned to offer continuity of care. In developing countries, they are often the only available health care provider. Studies have shown that there is an opportunity for suicide prevention in primary care settings because up to 83% of those who die by suicide have had contact with a PCP within a year of their death, and up to 66% within a month (Andersen, Andersen, Rosholm, & Gram, 2000; Luoma, Martin, & Pearson, 2002). Educating PCPs about the diagnosis and treatment of depression and risk factors for suicide must address a number of barriers to better health care. PCPs' lack of knowledge about and/or failure to screen patients for depression may underlie failure to diagnose and adequately treat depression (Goldman, Nielsen, & Champion, 1999; Hirschfeld et al., 1997) and the nonrecognition of those at risk for suicidal behavior. Additionally, lack of time for consultations may result in focus on other manifest major medical pathology, or a disdainful attitude toward mental illness and suicide reflecting the stigmatization of psychiatric illness may also contribute to undertreatment.

Results are mixed on the effectiveness of PCP education with respect to increasing the detection and treatment of depression. Education programs resulted in improved detection and increased treatment of depression in intervention compared to control groups in the UK (Hannaford, Thompson, & Simpson, 1996) and Australia (Naismith, Hickie, Scott, & Davenport, 2001). A Northern Ireland study found improvement in the short term but a fading of the effect after 12 months (Kelly, 1998). Other studies did not observe improvement in detection and treatment of depression following PCP education including in the US (Lin, Simon, Katzelnick, & Pearson, 2001), Brazil (Valentini et al., 2004), and the UK (Thompson et al., 2000).

Despite mixed reports with respect to depression outcomes, programs educating PCPs on the recognition and treatment of depression have shown promise for suicide prevention. The 1983/1984 Gotland study in Sweden is one of the earliest and best documented. In the 2 years after PCPs were provided education on recognizing and treating depression, there was a 50% increase in antidepressant prescription and a 60% decline in suicide rate (Rutz, 2001). When suicide rates began to increase subsequently, about 2 years after the educational program, perhaps because PCPs who did 2-year rotations on the island had now all left, booster and continuing education programs were conducted and once again suicide rates declined to the lowest levels since records were kept. Similarly in the Kiskunhalas region in Hungary, where the suicide rate was 50% higher than the national average (Hungary has averaged the highest national suicide rate worldwide over the last 100 years) comparing the 3 years before and after a PCP training program that started in 2000, there was a 58% increase in the prescription of antidepressants and a 22% decline in total suicide mortality (Rihmer, Belso, & Kalmar, 2001). Over that period nationally there was a 70% increase in antidepressant prescription rates and a 7% drop in suicide rates (Rihmer et al., 2001). In Japan, PCP education programs must contend with a strong stigma associated with mental illness and widespread reluctance to seek psychiatric treatment. PCP and community outreach campaigns in two towns resulted, after 10 years of implementation, in a 64–70% reduction in suicide risk for women compared to control regions, but no change for men (Oyama, Fujita, Goto, Shibuya, & Sakashita, 2006; Oyama, Goto, Fujita, Shibuya, & Sakashita, 2006).

PCP education is often just one component of broader organizational interventions which may also include introducing nurse case management, providing collaborative care, quality improvement initiatives, and improving the recognition and management of depression (Gilbody, Whitty, Grimshaw, & Thomas, 2003). In a US program for late-life depression in primary care, a controlled trial comparing treatment algorithm plus depression care management with treatment-as-usual found greater improvement in suicidal ideation as well as a more favorable course of illness in the intervention group compared with the treatment-as-usual group (Bruce et al., 2004). An Australian program that trained PCPs to recognize and respond to psychological distress and suicidal ideation in young people resulted in a 130% increase in the identification of suicidal patients; however, increased identification did not result in changes in treatment or management strategies (Pfaff, Acres, & McKelvey, 2001). A regional educational intervention for health care workers in suicide risk assessment and management in the UK was not associated with any decline in suicide rates in the post-intervention period compared to the pre-intervention period in the region (Morriss, Gask, Webb, Dixon, & Appleby, 2005).

Screening

Screening programs aim to identify at-risk individuals and direct them to treatment. Screening may focus directly on suicidal behavior or on risk factors such as aggressive behaviors, depression, or substance abuse. In youth populations, screens for depression, suicidal ideation or behaviors have been conducted in high school students (Shaffer et al., 2004), juvenile offenders (Cauffman, 2004), and youth in the community (Joiner, Pfaff, & Acres, 2002). These programs have demonstrated good reliability and validity in identifying individuals at increased risk for suicidal behavior and are reported to double the known number of at risk individuals (Scott, Shaffer, & Wilcox, 2004). In the US, 1,729 teens screened for depression identified 42% with suicidal ideation in the past 6 months and 37% who had made a suicide attempt that were unknown to school professionals (Scott et al., 2004). While screening may increase the case identification, it does not guarantee that identified individuals will move into treatment. A college Internet-based interactive screening program for depression and other psychiatric disorders identified 84.4% of respondents as at high or moderate risk for suicidal behaviors, of these 19% attended follow-up in-person counseling and 13.5% entered treatment (Haas et al., 2008). Screening youth for suicide does not induce suicidal thinking or behavior (Gould et al., 2005).

In adults, the use of depression screening instruments, often as an element of GP education plans, has shown some benefit in improving recognition of depression, though not necessarily treatment. The US Preventive Services Task Force (USPSTF) review of studies of depression screening in primary health care settings noted increases in rates of detection and diagnosis of depression of 10–47% with the use of screening tools (Pignone et al., 2002). The effects on treatment were found to be mixed, due to differences in study methodology. A recent meta-analysis suggested that screening resulted in small improvements in case detection but had no effect on treatment and management approach or on prescription of antidepressants (Gilbody, Sheldon, & House, 2008). Neither report commented on effects of screening on suicidal behavior. In terms of screening directly for suicide risk, the 2004 USPSTF review of evidence found some limited evidence for the accuracy of suicide screening in primary care and no published studies in English which directly addressed whether screening for suicide risk in primary care reduces morbidity or mortality (Gaynes et al., 2004). Screening by PCPs in localized geographic areas does appear to result in more treatment of depression and lower suicide rates (Oyama, Koida, Sakashita, & Kudo, 2004; Rutz, 2001; Szanto, Kalmar, Hendin, Rihmer, & Mann, 2007).

Individual Level Strategies

Psychiatric disorders are present in at least 90% of suicides, and over 80% of individuals who die by suicide are untreated at time of death (Henriksson, Boethius, & Isacsson, 2001; Lonnqvist et al., 1995). Depression is untreated or undertreated in general (Coyle et al., 2003; Hirschfeld et al., 1997), even after a suicide attempt (Oquendo, Malone, Ellis, Sackeim, & Mann, 1999). Not surprisingly, improving treatment of mood and other psychiatric disorders is an important suicide prevention strategy (Goldsmith et al., 2002).

Pharmacotherapy

There is ample evidence that antidepressant medications alleviate depression and other psychiatric disorders in adults (Agency for Health Care Policy Research, 1999). However, it has been difficult to demonstrate benefit for suicide or suicide attempts in studies of antidepressants in mood and other psychiatric disorders has been identified in meta-analyses and systematic reviews of RCTs (Fergusson et al., 2005; Gunnell, Saperia, & Ashby, 2005; Khan, Khan, Kolts, & Brown, 2003). The Food and Drug Administration analysis of about 100,000 adults in RCTs found an antisuicidal effect for older adults in terms of nonfatal attempts (Levinson, 2006). RCTs show benefit for lithium in terms of suicide and nonfatal suicide attempts in mood disorders (Cipriani, Pretty, Hawton, & Geddes, 2005; Guzzetta, Tondo, Centorrino, & Baldessarini, 2007; Tondo, Hennen, & Baldessarini, 2001) and for clozapine in terms of nonfatal attempts or suicide crises in schizophrenia (Glick et al., 2004; Meltzer et al., 2003).

Methodological issues limit the amount of available data such as the low base rate for suicidal behavior, particularly in short-term efficacy drug trials, as well as the fact that these studies routinely excluded suicidal individuals and are not designed to collect data on suicidal behavior and so do not systematically assess participants for suicidal outcomes. A reliance on suicide-related spontaneous adverse event reporting as outcome measures lowers the base rate partly because of an underestimation of rates of suicidal behavior (Malone, Szanto, Corbitt, & Mann, 1995).

Despite the lack of direct evidence from RCTs of an antisuicidal effect of antidepressants, there is evidence from population level studies that increased treatment of depression has an effect on suicide rates. There are reports of correlation between higher antidepressant prescription rates and declines in suicide rates, in adults or youth, from Hungary (Rihmer et al., 2001), Sweden (Carlsten, Waern, Ekedahl, & Ranstam, 2001; Isacsson, Holmgren, Osby, & Ahlner, 2009), a region of Italy (Castelpietra, Morsanutto, Pascolo-Fabrici, & Isacsson, 2008), Japan (Nakagawa et al., 2007), Australia (Hall et al., 2003), and the United States (Gibbons et al., 2005; Olfson, Shaffer, Marcus, & Greenberg, 2003). Studies in some other countries and regions do not find the same pattern (Barbui, Campomori, D'Avanzo, Negri, & Garattini, 1999; Helgason, Tomasson, & Zoega, 2004), and a systematic review of ecological studies of suicide rates and antidepressant rates finds the evidence inconclusive (Baldessarini et al., 2007). This is in part due to the difficulty in accounting for the influence of multiple other risk factors such as level of medication compliance, preexisting low suicide rates, and alcoholism. Recent large population studies report lower suicide attempt rates in both adult and adolescent populations diagnosed and then treated with antidepressant medication (Simon, Savarino, Operskalski, & Wang, 2006; Valuck, Libby, Sills, Giese, & Allen, 2004). The risk of ecological fallacy, that is inferring individual level causality from population level correlations, prevents attributing decreases in suicide rates solely to antidepressant use; nevertheless, there is a strong correlation and plausible mechanism linking antidepressant use to declining rates of untreated major depression and thus suicide.

Psychotherapy

While several trials of psychotherapies have produced promising results in terms of reducing repetition of suicidal behavior and/or improving depression treatment adherence, long-term reduction in suicide attempt and suicide rates following psychotherapy has yet to be demonstrated (Goldsmith et al., 2002). In individuals receiving therapeutic interventions following a suicide attempt or self-injury, problem-solving therapy (Hawton et al., 2000), intensive care plus outreach (Hawton et al., 2000), dialectical behavioral therapy

(DBT) (Linehan et al., 2006), cognitive behavioral therapy (Brown et al., 2005), and interpersonal psychotherapy (Guthrie et al., 2001; Tang, Jou, Ko, Huang, & Yen, 2009) have all shown benefits for reducing repetition of suicidal behavior and/or improving adherence compared to standard aftercare. Compared to standard aftercare, DBT (Hawton et al., 2000) and psychoanalytically oriented partial hospitalization (Bateman & Fonagy, 2001) improved treatment adherence and reduced suicidal behavior in individuals with borderline personality disorder. A systematic review of psychotherapies and suicidal behavior found improvement in intermediate outcomes such as hopelessness and depressive symptoms with problem-solving therapy, and that interpersonal psychotherapy, cognitive behavioral therapy, and DBT improved suicidal ideation (see Gaynes et al., 2004 for a review). There has been no evidence regarding reduction in completed suicide rates attributable to psychotherapy.

Follow-up Care for Suicide Attempters

Many depressed individuals who make a nonfatal suicide attempt will go on to make further attempts (Oquendo et al., 2004), with the period immediately following a psychiatric hospitalization being one of high risk (Angst, Stassen, Clayton, & Angst, 2002; Goldacre, Seagroatt, & Hawton, 1993). Moreover, many psychiatric disorders, including depression, are chronic and recurrent (Tasman & Leiberman, 2003) and given that compliance with maintenance medication is often poor, continuation and maintenance care of those with recurrent or chronic psychiatric disorders, particularly suicide attempters, is a target area for prevention interventions. Primary care-based treatment interventions for depression have been shown to be more effective in ensuring treatment compliance when a case manager is employed to follow up patients who miss appointments or need prescription renewals (Vergouwen, Bakker, Katon, Verheij, & Koerselman, 2003). In a Norwegian program, multidisciplinary chain-of-care networks provided follow-up care to suicide attempters after hospitalization. After a 1-year follow-up, there was a lower repetition rate and fewer overall suicide attempts in the intervention group compared to the control group (Hvid & Wang, 2009). Programs following up suicide attempters by mail (Motto & Bostrom, 2001) and issuing an emergency contact "green card" (Morgan, Jones, & Owen, 1993), both reported lower rates of reattempt, suggesting that even minimal follow-up can be beneficial. In an Australian project, where a suicide intervention counselor coordinated assessment and long-term treatment, there were three and a half times fewer hospital admissions for repeated suicide attempts compared to standard aftercare (Aoun, 1999). Other follow-up programs for suicide attempters, including intensive follow-up, telephone follow-up, intensive psychosocial follow-up, and video education plus family therapy, resulted in no difference between standard aftercare and intervention groups in rate of reattempt or reemergent suicidal ideation (Allard, Marshall, & Plante, 1992; Cedereke, Monti, & Ojehagen, 2002; Rotheram-Borus, Piacentini, Cantwell, Belin, & Song, 2000). One international multisite RCT of a brief intervention for suicide attempters comprising patient education and regular follow-up contact reported a significantly lower rate of suicide in the intervention group compared to the treatment-as-usual group over the 3-year trial period (Fleischmann et al., 2008).

Conclusions

While much progress has been made identifying risk factors for suicidal behavior and developing strategies to mitigate those risks, there remain substantial deficits in the evidence base with regard to the effectiveness of even some of the most widely accepted strategies. Moreover, it has generally not been possible to assess the relative impact of different strategies on suicide rates. To date, the strongest evidence is available for physician education, means restriction, and gatekeeper education intervention. This is not to say that other interventions are not effective, but that there has been insufficient evaluation of their effectiveness with respect to key outcomes of reducing suicide and suicide attempt rates. Moreover, given the multidetermined nature of suicidal behavior, many interventions tend to be multifaceted and it is not clear which components produce the desired outcome. Nevertheless, certain interventions show promise for reducing suicide and should be further developed, while more research is necessary to establish the evidence base for those interventions and strategies for which efficacy and effectiveness is unclear.

References

Agency for Health Care Policy Research. (1999). *Evidence report on treatment of depression – Newer pharmacotherapies*. Washington, DC: AHCPR, Evidence-Based Practice Centers.

Akroyd, S., & Wyllie, J. (2002). *Impacts of National Media Campaign to Counter Stigma and Discrimination Associated with Mental Illness: Survey 4*. Auckland: Phoenix Research.

Allard, R., Marshall, M., & Plante, M. C. (1992). Intensive follow-up does not decrease the risk of repeat suicide attempts. *Suicide & Life-Threatening Behavior, 22*, 303–314.

Andersen, U. A., Andersen, M., Rosholm, J. U., & Gram, L. F. (2000). Contacts to the health care system prior to suicide: A comprehensive analysis using registers for general and psychiatric hospital admissions, contacts to general practitioners and practising specialists and drug prescriptions. *Acta Psychiatrica Scandinavica, 102*, 126–134.

Angst, F., Stassen, H. H., Clayton, P. J., & Angst, J. (2002). Mortality of patients with mood disorders: Follow-up over 34–38 years. *Journal of Affective Disorders, 68*, 167–181.

Aoun, S. (1999). Deliberate self-harm in rural Western Australia: Results of an intervention study. *Australian and New Zealand Journal of Mental Health Nursing, 8*, 65–73.

Aseltine, R. H. Jr., & DeMartino, R. (2004). An outcome evaluation of the SOS suicide prevention program. *American Journal of Public Health, 94*, 446–451.

Baldessarini, R. J., Tondo, L., Strombom, I. M., Dominguez, S., Fawcett, J., Licinio, J., et al. (2007). Ecological studies of antidepressant treatment and suicidal risks. *Harvard Review of Psychiatry, 15*, 133–145.

Barbui, C., Campomori, A., D'Avanzo, B., Negri, E., & Garattini, S. (1999). Antidepressant drug use in Italy since the introduction of SSRIs: National trends, regional differences and impact on suicide rates. *Social Psychiatry and Psychiatric Epidemiology, 34*, 152–156.

Bateman, A., & Fonagy, P. (2001). Treatment of borderline personality disorder with psychoanalytically oriented partial hospitalization: An 18-month follow-up. *American Journal of Psychiatry, 158*, 36–42.

Beautrais, A. L., Gibb, S. J., Fergusson, D. M., Horwood, L. J., & Larkin, G. L. (2009). Removing bridge barriers stimulates suicides: An unfortunate natural experiment. *Australian and New Zealand Journal of Psychiatry, 43*, 495–497.

Breton, J. J., Boyer, R., Bilodeau, H., Raymond, S., Joubert, N., & Nantel, M. A. (2002). Is evaluative research on youth suicide programs theory-driven? The Canadian experience. *Suicide & Life-Threatening Behavior, 32*, 176–190.

Bridges, F. S., & Kunselman, J. C. (2004). Gun availability and use of guns for suicide, homicide, and murder in Canada. *Perceptual and Motor Skills, 98*, 594–598.

Brown, G. K., Ten Have, T., Henriques, G. R., Xie, S. X., Hollander, J. E., & Beck, A. T. (2005). Cognitive therapy for the prevention of suicide attempts: A randomized controlled trial. *Journal of the American Medical Association, 294*, 563–570.

Bruce, M. L., Ten Have, T. R., Reynolds, C. F., III, Katz, I. I., Schulberg, H. C., Mulsant, B. H., et al. (2004). Reducing suicidal ideation and depressive symptoms in depressed older primary care patients: A randomized controlled trial. *Journal of the American Medical Association, 291*, 1081–1091.

Burns, J. M., & Patton, G. C. (2000). Preventive interventions for youth suicide: A risk factor-based approach. *Australian and New Zealand Journal of Psychiatry, 34*, 388–407.

Cantor, C. H., & Slater, P. J. (1995). The impact of firearm control legislation on suicide in Queensland: Preliminary findings. *Medical Journal of Australia, 162*, 583–585.

Carlsten, A., Allebeck, P., & Brandt, L. (1996). Are suicide rates in Sweden associated with changes in the prescribing of medicines? *Acta Psychiatrica Scandinavica, 94*, 94–100.

Carlsten, A., Waern, M., Ekedahl, A., & Ranstam, J. (2001). Antidepressant medication and suicide in Sweden. *Pharmacoepidemiology and Drug Safety, 10*, 525–530.

Carrington, P. J. (1999). Gender, gun control, suicide and homicide in Canada. *Archives of Suicide Research, 5*, 71–75.

Castelpietra, G., Morsanutto, A., Pascolo-Fabrici, E., & Isacsson, G. (2008). Antidepressant use and suicide prevention: A prescription database study in the region Friuli Venezia Giulia, Italy. *Acta Psychiatrica Scandinavica, 118*, 382–388.

Cauffman, E. (2004). A statewide screening of mental health symptoms among juvenile offenders in detention. *Journal of American Academy of Child and Adolescent Psychiatry, 43*, 430–439.

Cedereke, M., Monti, K., & Ojehagen, A. (2002). Telephone contact with patients in the year after a suicide attempt: Does it affect treatment attendance and outcome? A randomised controlled study. *European Psychiatry, 17*, 82–91.

Cipriani, A., Pretty, H., Hawton, K., & Geddes, J. R. (2005). Lithium in the prevention of suicidal behavior and all-cause mortality in patients with mood disorders: A systematic review of randomized trials. *American Journal of Psychiatry, 162*, 1805–1819.

Coyle, J. T., Pine, D. S., Charney, D. S., Lewis, L., Nemeroff, C. B., Carlson, G. A., et al. (2003). Depression and bipolar support alliance consensus statement on the unmet needs in diagnosis and treatment of mood disorders in children and adolescents. *Journal of American Academy of Child and Adolescent Psychiatry, 42*, 1494–1503.

Crome, P. (1993). The toxicity of drugs used for suicide. *Acta Psychiatrica Scandinavica Supplementum, 371*, 33–37.

Etzersdorfer, E., Sonneck, G., & Nagel-Kuess, S. (1992). Newspaper reports and suicide. *New England Journal of Medicine, 327*, 502–503.

Fergusson, D., Doucette, S., Glass, K. C., Shapiro, S., Healy, D., Hebert, P., et al. (2005). Association between suicide attempts and selective serotonin reuptake inhibitors: Systematic review of randomised controlled trials. *British Medical Journal, 330*, 396.

Fleischmann, A., Bertolote, J. M., Wasserman, D., De, L. D., Bolhari, J., Botega, N. J., et al. (2008). Effectiveness of brief intervention and contact for suicide attempters: A randomized controlled trial in five countries. *Bulletin of the World Health Organization, 86*, 703–709.

Fu, K. W., & Yip, P. S. (2008). Changes in reporting of suicide news after the promotion of the WHO media recommendations. *Suicide & Life-Threatening Behavior, 38*, 631–636.

Gaynes, B. N., West, S. L., Ford, C. A., Frame, P., Klein, J., & Lohr, K. N. (2004). Screening for suicide risk in adults: A summary of the evidence for the U.S. Preventive Services Task Force. *Annals of Internal Medicine, 140*, 822–835.

Gibbons, R. D., Hur, K., Bhaumik, D. K., & Mann, J. J. (2005). The relationship between antidepressant medication use and rate of suicide. *Archives of General Psychiatry, 62*, 165–172.

Gilbody, S., Sheldon, T., & House, A. (2008). Screening and case-finding instruments for depression: A meta-analysis. *Canadian Medical Association Journal, 178*, 997–1003.

Gilbody, S., Whitty, P., Grimshaw, J., & Thomas, R. (2003). Educational and organizational interventions to improve the management of depression in primary care: A systematic review. *Journal of the American Medical Association, 289*, 3145–3151.

Glick, I. D., Zaninelli, R., Hsu, C., Young, F. K., Weiss, L., Gunay, I., et al. (2004). Patterns of concomitant psychotropic medication use during a 2-year study comparing clozapine and olanzapine for the prevention of suicidal behavior. *Journal of Clinical Psychiatry, 65*, 679–685.

Goldacre, M., Seagroatt, V., & Hawton, K. (1993). Suicide after discharge from psychiatric inpatient care. *Lancet, 342*, 283–286.

Goldman, L. S., Nielsen, N. H., & Champion, H. C. (1999). Awareness, diagnosis, and treatment of depression. *Journal of General Internal Medicine, 14*, 569–580.

Goldney, R. D., & Fisher, L. J. (2008). Have broad-based community and professional education programs influenced mental health literacy and treatment seeking of those with major depression and suicidal ideation? *Suicide & Life-Threatening Behavior, 38*, 129–142.

Goldsmith, S. K., Pellmar, T. C., Kleinman, A. M., & Bunney, W. E. (2002). *Reducing suicide. A National imperative*. Washington, DC: The National Academies Press.

Gould, M. S. (2001). Suicide and the media. *Annals of the New York Academy of Sciences, 932*, 200–221.

Gould, M. S., Greenberg, T., Velting, D. M., & Shaffer, D. (2003). Youth suicide risk and preventive interventions: A review of the past 10 years. *Journal of American Academy of Child and Adolescent Psychiatry, 42*, 386–405.

Gould, M. S., Marrocco, F. A., Kleinman, M., Thomas, J. G., Mostkoff, K., Cote, J., et al. (2005). Evaluating iatrogenic risk of youth suicide screening programs: A randomized controlled trial. *Journal of the American Medical Association, 293*, 1635–1643.

Gunnell, D., Fernando, R., Hewagama, M., Priyangika, W. D., Konradsen, F., & Eddleston, M. (2007). The impact of pesticide regulations on suicide in Sri Lanka. *International Journal of Epidemiology, 36*, 1235–1242.

Gunnell, D., Middleton, N., & Frankel, S. (2000). Method availability and the prevention of suicide – A re-analysis of secular trends in England and Wales 1950–1975. *Social Psychiatry and Psychiatric Epidemiology, 35*, 437–443.

Gunnell, D., Saperia, J., & Ashby, D. (2005). Selective serotonin reuptake inhibitors (SSRIs) and suicide in adults: Meta-analysis of drug company data from placebo controlled, randomised controlled trials submitted to the MHRA's safety review. *British Medical Journal, 330*, 385.

Guo, B., & Harstall, C. (2002). *Efficacy of suicide prevention programs for children and youth.* Edmonton: Alberta Heritage Foundation for Medical Research, Health Technology Assessment, Report No. HTA 26.

Guthrie, E., Kapur, N., Kway-Jones, K., Chew-Graham, C., Moorey, J., Mendel, E., et al. (2001). Randomised controlled trial of brief psychological intervention after deliberate self poisoning. *British Medical Journal, 323*, 135–138.

Guzzetta, F., Tondo, L., Centorrino, F., & Baldessarini, R. J. (2007). Lithium treatment reduces suicide risk in recurrent major depressive disorder. *Journal of Clinical Psychiatry, 68*, 380–383.

Haas, A., Koestner, B., Rosenberg, J., Moore, D., Garlow, S. J., Sedway, J., et al. (2008). An interactive web-based method of outreach to college students at risk for suicide. *Journal of American College Health, 57*, 15–22.

Hall, W. D., Mant, A., Mitchell, P. B., Rendle, V. A., Hickie, I. B., & McManus, P. (2003). Association between antidepressant prescribing and suicide in Australia, 1991–2000: Trend analysis. *British Medical Journal, 326*, 1008.

Hannaford, P. C., Thompson, C., & Simpson, M. (1996). Evaluation of an educational programme to improve the recognition of psychological illness by general practitioners. *British Journal of General Practice, 46*, 333–337.

Hawton, K. (2002). United Kingdom legislation on pack sizes of analgesics: Background, rationale, and effects on suicide and deliberate self-harm. *Suicide & Life-Threatening Behavior, 32*, 223–229.

Hawton, K., Townsend, E., Arensman, E., Gunnell, D., Hazell, P., House, A., et al. (2000). Psychosocial versus pharmacological treatments for deliberate self harm. *Cochrane Database of Systematic Reviews,* CD001764.

Hegerl, U., Althaus, D., Schmidtke, A., & Niklewski, G. (2006). The alliance against depression: Two-year evaluation of a community-based intervention to reduce suicidality. *Psychological Medicine, 36*, 1225–1233.

Hegerl, U., Althaus, D., & Stefanek, J. (2003). Public attitudes towards treatment of depression: Effects of an information campaign. *Pharmacopsychiatry, 36*, 288–291.

Helgason, T., Tomasson, H., & Zoega, T. (2004). Antidepressants and public health in Iceland. Time series analysis of national data. *British Journal of Psychiatry, 184*, 157–162.

Henriksson, S., Boethius, G., & Isacsson, G. (2001). Suicides are seldom prescribed antidepressants: Findings from a prospective prescription database in Jamtland county, Sweden, 1985–95. *Acta Psychiatrica Scandinavica, 103*, 301–306.

Hickie, I. (2004). Can we reduce the burden of depression? The Australian experience with beyondblue: The national depression initiative. *Australasian Psychiatry, 12*(Suppl.), S38–S46.

Hirschfeld, R. M. A., Keller, M., Panico, S., Arons, B. S., Barlow, D., Davidoff, F., et al. (1997). The national depressive and manic-depressive association consensus statement on the undertreatment of depression. *Journal of the American Medical Association, 277*, 333–340.

Hvid, M., & Wang, A. G. (2009). Preventing repetition of attempted suicide – I. Feasibility (acceptability, adherence, and effectiveness) of a Baerum-model like aftercare. *Nordic Journal of Psychiatry, 63*, 148–153.

Isacsson, G., Holmgren, A., Osby, U., & Ahlner, J. (2009). Decrease in suicide among the individuals treated with antidepressants: A controlled study of antidepressants in suicide Sweden 1995–2005. *Acta Psychiatrica Scandinavica, 40*, 471–480.

Joiner, T. E., Jr., Pfaff, J. J., & Acres, J. G. (2002). A brief screening tool for suicidal symptoms in adolescents and young adults in general health settings: Reliability and validity data from the Australian National General Practice Youth Suicide Prevention Project. *Behaviour Research and Therapy, 40*, 471–481.

Kapur, S., Mieczkowski, T., & Mann, J. J. (1992). Antidepressant medications and the relative risk of suicide attempt and suicide. *Journal of the American Medical Association, 268*, 3441–3445.

Kelly, C. (1998). The effects of depression awareness seminars on general practitioners knowledge of depressive illness. *Ulster Medical Journal, 67*, 33–35.

Kelly, S., & Bunting, J. (1998). Trends in suicide in England and Wales 1982–96. *Population Trends, 92*, 29–41.

Khan, A., Khan, S., Kolts, R., & Brown, W. A. (2003). Suicide rates in clinical trials of SSRIs, other antidepressants, and placebo: Analysis of FDA reports. *American Journal of Psychiatry, 160*, 790–792.

Knox, K. L., Litts, D. A., Talcott, G. W., Feig, J. C., & Caine, E. D. (2003). Risk of suicide and related adverse outcomes after exposure to a suicide prevention programme in the US Air Force: Cohort study. *British Medical Journal, 327*, 1376.

Kreitman, N. (1976). The coal gas story. United Kingdom suicide rates, 1960–71. *British Journal of Preventive & Social Medicine, 30*, 86–93.

Lester, D. (1990a). The effects of detoxification of domestic gas on suicide in the United States. *American Journal of Public Health, 80*, 80–81.

Lester, D. (1990b). The effect of the detoxification of domestic gas in Switzerland on the suicide rate. *Acta Psychiatrica Scandinavica, 82*, 383–384.

Lester, D. (1991). Effects of detoxification of domestic gas on suicide in The Netherlands. *Psychological Reports, 68*, 202.

Lester, D. (1999). Effect of changing alcohol laws in Iceland on suicide rates. *Psychological Reports, 84*, 1158.

Lester, D., & Leenaars, A. (1993). Suicide rates in Canada before and after tightening firearm control laws. *Psychological Reports, 72*, 787–790.

Levinson. (2006). Antidepressants and suicidality in adults: Statistical evaluation. http://www.fda.gov/ohrms/dockets/ac/06/slides/2006-4272s1-04-FDA_files/frame.htm [On-line]. Available: http://www.fda.gov/ohrms/dockets/ac/06/slides/2006-4272s1-04-FDA_files/frame.htm.

Lin, E. H., Simon, G. E., Katzelnick, D. J., & Pearson, S. D. (2001). Does physician education on depression management improve treatment in primary care? *Journal of General Internal Medicine, 16*, 614–619.

Linehan, M. M., Comtois, K. A., Murray, A. M., Brown, M. Z., Gallop, R. J., Heard, H. L., et al. (2006). Two-year randomized controlled trial and follow-up of dialectical behavior therapy vs therapy by experts for suicidal behaviors and borderline personality disorder. *Archives of General Psychiatry, 63*, 757–766.

Loftin, C., McDowall, D., Wiersema, B., & Cottey, T. J. (1991). Effects of restrictive licensing of handguns on homicide and suicide in the District of Columbia. *New England Journal of Medicine, 325*, 1615–1620.

Lonnqvist, J. K., Henriksson, M. M., Isometsa, E. T., Marttunen, M. J., Heikkinen, M. E., Aro, H. M., et al. (1995). Mental disorders and suicide prevention. *Psychiatry and Clinical Neurosciences, 49*(Suppl. 1), S111–S116.

Ludwig, J., & Cook, P. J. (2000). Homicide and suicide rates associated with implementation of the Brady Handgun Violence Prevention Act. *Journal of the American Medical Association, 284*, 585–591.

Luoma, J. B., Martin, C. E., & Pearson, J. L. (2002). Contact with mental health and primary care providers before suicide: A review of the evidence. *American Journal of Psychiatry, 159*, 909–916.

Malone, K. M., Szanto, K., Corbitt, E. M., & Mann, J. J. (1995). Clinical assessment versus research methods in the assessment of suicidal behavior. *American Journal of Psychiatry, 152*, 1601–1607.

Mann, J. J., Apter, A., Bertolote, J., Beautrais, A., Currier, D., Haas, A., et al. (2005). Suicide prevention strategies: A systematic review. *Journal of the American Medical Association, 294*, 2064–2074.

Mann, J. J., & Currier, D. (2008). Suicide and attempted suicide. In S. H. Fatemi & P. J. Clayton (Eds.), *The medical basis of psychiatry* (3rd ed., pp. 561–576). Philadelphia, PA: Humana Press.

McClure, G. M. (2000). Changes in suicide in England and Wales, 1960–1997. *British Journal of Psychiatry, 176*, 64–67.

Meltzer, H. Y., Alphs, L., Green, A. I., Altamura, A. C., Anand, R., Bertoldi, A., et al. (2003). Clozapine treatment for suicidality in schizophrenia: International suicide prevention trial (InterSePT). *Archives of General Psychiatry, 60*, 82–91.

Metha, A., Weber, B., & Webb, L. D. (1998). Youth suicide prevention: A survey and analysis of policies and efforts in the 50 states. *Suicide & Life-Threatening Behavior, 28*, 150–164.

Morgan, H. G., Jones, E. M., & Owen, J. H. (1993). Secondary prevention of non-fatal deliberate self-harm. The green card study. *British Journal of Psychiatry, 163*, 111–112.

Morriss, R., Gask, L., Webb, R., Dixon, C., & Appleby, L. (2005). The effects on suicide rates of an educational intervention for front-line health professionals with suicidal patients (the STORM Project). *Psychological Medicine, 35*, 957–960.

Motto, J. A. (1970). Newspaper influence on suicide. A controlled study. *Archives of General Psychiatry, 23*, 143–148.

Motto, J. A., & Bostrom, A. G. (2001). A randomized controlled trial of postcrisis suicide prevention. *Psychiatric Services, 52*, 828–833.

Motto, J. A., Wolfe, M. I., Alverson, C. J., Macdonald, S. C., Bailey, C. R., Ball, L. B., et al. (2002). National vehicle emissions policies and practices and declining US carbon monoxide-related mortality. *Journal of the American Medical Association, 288*, 988–995.

Naismith, S. L., Hickie, I. B., Scott, E. M., & Davenport, T. A. (2001). Effects of mental health training and clinical audit on general practitioners' management of common mental disorders. *Medical Journal of Australia, 175*(Suppl.), S42–S47.

Nakagawa, A., Grunebaum, M. F., Ellis, S. P., Oquendo, M. A., Kashima, H., Gibbons, R. D., et al. (2007). Association of suicide and antidepressant prescription rates in Japan, 1999–2003. *Journal of Clinical Psychiatry, 68*, 908–916.

Niederkrotenthaler, T., & Sonneck, G. (2007). Assessing the impact of media guidelines for reporting on suicides in Austria: Interrupted time series analysis. *Australian and New Zealand Journal of Psychiatry, 41*, 419–428.

Nielsen, A. S., & Nielsen, B. (1992). Pattern of choice in preparation of attempted suicide by poisoning – with particular reference to changes in the pattern of prescriptions. *Ugeskrift For Laeger, 154*, 1972–1976.

O'Carroll, P. W., & Potter, L. B. (1994). Suicide contagion and the reporting of suicide: Recommendations from a national workshop. United States Department of Health and Human Services. *Morbidity and Mortality Weekly Report. Recommendations and Reports, 43*, 9–17.

Ohberg, A., Lonnqvist, J., Sarna, S., Vuori, E., & Penttila, A. (1995). Trends and availability of suicide methods in Finland. Proposals for restrictive measures. *British Journal of Psychiatry, 166*, 35–43.

Olfson, M., Shaffer, D., Marcus, S. C., & Greenberg, T. (2003). Relationship between antidepressant medication treatment and suicide in adolescents. *Archives of General Psychiatry, 60*, 978–982.

Oliver, R. G., & Hetzel, B. S. (1972). Rise and fall of suicide rates in Australia: Relation to sedative availability. *Medical Journal of Australia, 2*, 919–923.

Oquendo, M. A., Galfalvy, H., Russo, S., Ellis, S. P., Grunebaum, M. F., Burke, A., et al. (2004). Prospective study of clinical predictors of suicidal acts after a major depressive episode in patients with major depressive disorder or bipolar disorder. *The American Journal of Psychiatry, 161*, 1433–1441.

Oquendo, M. A., Malone, K. M., Ellis, S. P., Sackeim, H. A., & Mann, J. J. (1999). Inadequacy of antidepressant treatment for patients with major depression who are at risk for suicidal behavior. *The American Journal of Psychiatry, 156*, 190–194.

Oyama, H., Fujita, M., Goto, M., Shibuya, H., & Sakashita, T. (2006). Outcomes of community-based screening for depression and suicide prevention among Japanese elders. *The Gerontologist, 46*, 821–826.

Oyama, H., Goto, M., Fujita, M., Shibuya, H., & Sakashita, T. (2006). Preventing elderly suicide through primary care by community-based screening for depression in rural Japan. *Crisis, 27*, 58–65.

Oyama, H., Koida, J., Sakashita, T., & Kudo, K. (2004). Community-based prevention for suicide in elderly by depression screening and follow-up. *Community Mental Health Journal, 40*, 249–263.

Paykel, E. S., Hart, D., & Priest, R. G. (1998). Changes in public attitudes to depression during the Defeat Depression Campaign. *British Journal of Psychiatry, 173*, 519–522.

Pfaff, J. J., Acres, J. G., & McKelvey, R. S. (2001). Training general practitioners to recognise and respond to psychological distress and suicidal ideation in young people. *Medical Journal of Australia, 174*, 222–226.

Pignone, M. P., Gaynes, B. N., Rushton, J. L., Burchell, C. M., Orleans, C. T., Mulrow, C. D., et al. (2002). Screening for depression in adults: A summary of the evidence for the U.S. Preventive Services Task Force. *Annals of Internal Medicine, 136*, 765–776.

Pirkis, J., & Blood, R. W. (2001). Suicide and the media. Part I: Reportage in nonfictional media. *Crisis, 22*, 146–154.

Pirkis, J., Dare, A., Blood, R. W., Rankin, B., Williamson, M., Burgess, P., et al. (2009). Changes in media reporting of suicide in Australia between 2000/01 and 2006/07. *Crisis, 30*, 25–33.

Ploeg, J., Ciliska, D., Dobbins, M., Hayward, S., Thomas, H., & Underwood, J. (1996). A systematic overview of adolescent suicide prevention programs. *Canadian Journal of Public Health, 87*, 319–324.

Pridemore, W. A., & Snowden, A. J. (2009). Reduction in suicide mortality following a new national alcohol policy in Slovenia: An interrupted time-series analysis. *American Journal of Public Health, 99*, 915–920.

Ramberg, I. L., & Wasserman, D. (2004). Suicide-preventive activities in psychiatric care: Evaluation of an educational programme in suicide prevention. *Nordic Journal of Psychiatry, 58*, 389–394.

Retterstol, N. (1989). Norwegian data on death due to overdose of antidepressants. *Acta Psychiatrica Scandinavica, 80*, 61–68.

Rihmer, Z., Belso, N., & Kalmar, S. (2001). Antidepressants and suicide prevention in Hungary. *Acta Psychiatrica Scandinavica, 103*, 238–239.

Rotheram-Borus, M. J., Piacentini, J., Cantwell, C., Belin, T. R., & Song, J. (2000). The 18-month impact of an emergency room intervention for adolescent female suicide attempters. *Journal of Consulting and Clinical Psychology, 68*, 1081–1093.

Rutz, W. (2001). Preventing suicide and premature death by education and treatment. *Journal of Affective Disorders, 62*, 123–129.

Schafer, R., Althaus, D., Brosius, H. B., & Hegerl, U. (2006). Media coverage on suicide in Nuremberg's daily papers – Frequency and form of the reporting before and during media-intervention with guidelines. *Psychiatrische Praxis, 33*, 132–137.

Scott, M., Shaffer, D., & Wilcox. H. (2004). *The Columbia suicide screen: Does screening identify new teens at risk?* Washington, DC: American Academy of Child and Adolescent Psychiatry.

Shaffer, D., Garland, A., Vieland, V., Underwood, M., & Busner, C. (1991). The impact of curriculum-based suicide prevention programs for teenagers. *Journal of American Academy of Child and Adolescent Psychiatry, 30*, 588–596.

Shaffer, D., Scott, M., Wilcox, H., Maslow, C., Hicks, R., Lucas, C. P., et al. (2004). The Columbia suicide screen: Validity and reliability of a screen for youth suicide and depression. *Journal of American Academy of Child and Adolescent Psychiatry, 43*, 71–79.

Shelef, M. (1994). Unanticipated benefits of automotive emission control: Reduction in fatalities by motor vehicle exhaust gas. *Science of the Total Environment, 146–147*, 93–101.

Simon, G. E., Savarino, J., Operskalski, B., & Wang, P. S. (2006). Suicide risk during antidepressant treatment. *American Journal of Psychiatry, 163*, 41–47.

Skegg, K., & Herbison, P. (2009). Effect of restricting access to a suicide jumping site. *Australian and New Zealand Journal of Psychiatry, 43*, 498–502.

Snowdon, J., & Harris, L. (1992). Firearms suicides in Australia. *Medical Journal of Australia, 156*, 79–83.

Szanto, K., Kalmar, S., Hendin, H., Rihmer, Z., & Mann, J. J. (2007). A suicide prevention program in a region with a very high suicide rate. *Archives of General Psychiatry, 64*, 914–920.

Tang, T. C., Jou, S. H., Ko, C. H., Huang, S. Y., & Yen, C. F. (2009). Randomized study of school-based intensive interpersonal psychotherapy for depressed adolescents with suicidal risk and parasuicide behaviors. *Psychiatry and Clinical Neurosciences, 2*, 25–33.

Tasman, A. & Leiberman, J. A. (Eds.). (2003). *Psychiatry*. Chichester, UK: Wiley.

Thompson, C., Kinmonth, A. L., Stevens, L., Peveler, R. C., Stevens, A., Ostler, K. J., et al. (2000). Effects of a clinical-practice guideline and practice-based education on detection and outcome of depression in primary care: Hampshire depression project randomised controlled trial. *Lancet, 355*, 185–191.

Tondo, L., Hennen, J., & Baldessarini, R. J. (2001). Lower suicide risk with long-term lithium treatment in major affective illness: A meta-analysis. *Acta Psychiatrica Scandinavica, 104*, 163–172.

Valentini, W., Levav, I., Kohn, R., Miranda, C. T., Mello, A. A., Mello, M. F., et al. (2004). An educational training program for physicians for diagnosis and treatment of depression. *Revista de saude publica, 38*, 522–528.

Valuck, R. J., Libby, A. M., Sills, M. R., Giese, A. A., & Allen, R. R. (2004). Antidepressant treatment and risk of suicide attempt by adolescents with major depressive disorder: A propensity-adjusted retrospective cohort study. *CNS Drugs, 18*, 1119–1132.

Vergouwen, A. C., Bakker, A., Katon, W. J., Verheij, T. J., & Koerselman, F. (2003). Improving adherence to antidepressants: A systematic review of interventions. *Journal of Clinical Psychiatry, 64*, 1415–1420.

Vieland, V., Whittle, B., Garland, A., Hicks, R., & Shaffer, D. (1991). The impact of curriculum-based suicide prevention programs for teenagers: An 18-month follow-up. *Journal of American Academy of Child and Adolescent Psychiatry, 30*, 811–815.

Wasserman, D., & Varnik, A. (1998). Suicide-preventive effects of perestroika in the former USSR: The role of alcohol restriction. *Acta psychiatrica Scandinavica Supplementum, 394*, 1–4.

Whitlock, F. A. (1975). Suicide in Brisbane, 1956 to 1973: The drug-death epidemic. *Medical Journal of Australia, 1*, 737–743.

Wiedenmann, A., & Weyerer, S. (1993). The impact of availability, attraction and lethality of suicide methods on suicide rates in Germany. *Acta Psychiatrica Scandinavica, 88*, 364–368.

Yamasawa, K., Nishimukai, H., Ohbora, Y., & Inoue, K. (1980). A statistical study of suicides through intoxication. *Acta Medicinae Legalis et Socialis, 30*, 187–192.

Zenere, F. J., III, & Lazarus, P. J. (1997). The decline of youth suicidal behavior in an urban, multicultural public school system following the introduction of a suicide prevention and intervention program. *Suicide & Life-Threatening Behavior, 27*, 387–402.

About the Authors

Dr. John Mann is the Paul Janssen Professor of Translational Neuroscience (in Psychiatry and Radiology) at Columbia State University, NY, and Director of the Division of Molecular Imaging and Neuropathology. He has recently been President of the Society of Biological Psychiatry in the US and is Past President of the International Academy for Suicide Research.

Dianne Currier obtained her PhD at Monash University, Australia. She is currently a senior staff associate in the Division of Molecular Imaging and Neuropathology, Department of Psychiatry, at Columbia University, NY.

Dianne Currier
Division of Molecular Imaging and Neuropathology
Columbia University
Unit #42
1051 Riverside Drive
New York, NY
USA
Tel.: +1 212 543 6846
E-mail: dmc2111@columbia.edu

Evidence-Based Psychotherapy With Suicidal People

A Systematic Review

Antoon A. Leenaars

Private Practice in Windsor, Canada

Psychotherapy has a long history (Freedheim, 1992). One could find expressions of it throughout the ages and places. Yet, to define the "it" that I am writing about is complex, if not daunting. Psychotherapy is a human exchange. The relationship is what Martin Buber (1970) called an "I-Thou," not "I-it" relationship. To define psychotherapy, it has to be broadly defined (Lambert, 2004). One of many possible ways to do so is Frank and Frank's (1991) definition:

> Attempts to relieve suffering and disability are usually labelled treatment, and every society trains some of its members to apply this form of influence. Treatment typically involves a personal relationship between healer and sufferer. Certain types of therapy rely primarily on the healer's ability to mobilize healing forces in the sufferer by psychological means. These forms of treatment may be generically termed psychotherapy (p. 1).

Yet, even this definition may not be sufficiently broad (Orlinsky, Rønnestad, & Willutzki, 2004); yet, it is the one found in Lambert's fifth edition of Bergin and Garfield's classic reference text on evidence-based psychotherapy (Lambert, 2004). It is both historical and culturally inclusive. Psychotherapy is a form of treatment. Psychotherapy is concerned with what kind of person the individual is, not simply focused on a disease or a mental disorder. However, as Orlinsky, Rønnestad, and Willutzki point out:

> . . .therapy also is, or can be (1) a form of remedial or higher education in the social-emotional sphere of functioning (what in the nineteenth century might have been termed "moral education"), (2) a nonviolent form of social control for deviant behavior (a substitute or adjunct form of "correctional" influence for those who offend against others or themselves), and (3) a facilitator of meaningful personal orientation and philosophy of life (or "spiritual" development, for those whom Maimonides might have found "perplexed" or Durkheim "anomic"). Many who seek psychotherapy in fact do not qualify for a diagnosable form

> of suffering or disability. Some are constrained to do so as a result of having transgressed against a basic social norm (e.g., marital infidelity, to avoid divorce) or against a legal norm (e.g., youthful delinquency, to avoid prison or as a condition of parole). Many more do so because they are unhappy with their lives, their relationships, and their selves. Thus, "functioning as persons" ought to include terms such as deviance and deficient well-being in addition to suffering and disability (p. 311).

This will be our view when we talk about psychotherapy. Psychotherapy with suicidal people is no different. The intent of the therapy is to reduce the sufferer's psychological pain. To quote Edwin Shneidman, a lead figure in the 20th century in suicidology:

> If the villain is psychological pain then we need something that fights that pain. There is a word for that: *anodyne*. An anodyne is a substance that (or an agent or person who) assuages pain. Psychotherapy in general ought to be anodynic. But with a highly suicidal patient – with *perturbation* and, even more seriously, high *lethality* – the anodynic function of the therapist is vital (Shneidman, 2001, p. 182).

Our method with our suicidal patient is to serve as an anodynic agent "to relieve the pain so that the patient's *raison d'être* for suicide is mollified and the need to end the inner suffering is no longer pressing" (p. 182) (Shneidman, 1981, 1984; see Leenaars, 1999). The purpose of this review paper is to outline the research basis for an evidence-based approach to psychotherapy with suicidal people (Leenaars, 2004, 2006; Leenaars, Maltsberger, & Neimeyer, 1994).

The question that is posed in this review is, "Is psychotherapy effective?" or more specifically, "Is psychotherapy effective with suicidal people?" Today, in fact, as for millennia, this has been *the* question about an anodyne for "a mind disease" or "deficient well-being." The question is: What is the "best" evidence-based psychotherapy with suicidal people? However, before we could address that question, we have to ask the more general one: What is the "best" evidence-based psychotherapy? The specific question should flow from the more general one. Yet, we must first begin with an even more *a priori* question here: What is suicide? After all, we ought to know what we are treating.

We Ought to Know What We Are Treating

We need to clarify what we are talking about. What is suicide? Briefly defined, suicide is the human act of self-inflicted, self-intentional cessation (Shneidman, 1973). Suicide is complex (World Health Organization [WHO], 2002); yet, it would be accurate to state that "intent" is central. Suicide is intentional cessation. Intent is defined as to have suicide or deliberate self-killing as one's purpose. Suicide is not self-injurious behavior or self-harm behavior with no intentional cessation. These are behaviors that involve deliberate self-inflicted physical harm with no intent of cessation. There is no intent to die as a consequence of this behavior (We thus, exclude discussion of this topic. See below). This is very different from suicide; the suicidal person intends at some level, to kill him- or herself

(Leenaars et al., 1997; O'Carroll et al., 1996; Silverman, Berman, Sanddal, O'Carroll, & Joiner, 2007). Suicide has a fatal outcome. A suicide attempt is like a suicide, but there is no fatal outcome. There is no cessation. Yet, there is intent. The person intended to kill him- or herself. The person intended to die, again very different than self-harm behavior. This is also quite different from the intent of people with Borderline Personality Disorder (BPD); in such people, one often sees recurrent suicidal behavior, gestures or threats, or self-mutilating behavior. Thus, to avoid confusion, I also exclude discussion here of people with BPD (see more below). I focus on suicide, something that is complex enough.

Some years ago, I had the opportunity to chair a task force of the International Academy for Suicide Research (IASR) on the very topic (although the complete report extends beyond the topic of definition – the focus is on future direction for study in suicide). I hereby quote what was stated about definitions (the complete text was published in *Archives of Suicide Research,* 1997, *3*, 139–151). I cannot write it any better than on that occasion:

> A. Definitions. Suicide today is defined differently depending on the purpose of the definition – medical, legal, administrative, etc. In most countries reporting to the World Health Organisation (WHO), suicide is defined as one of four possible modes of death. An acronym for the four modes of death is NASH: natural, accidental, suicidal, and homicidal. This fourfold classification of all deaths has its problems. Its major deficiency is that it treats the human being in a Cartesian fashion. It obscures the individual motivations, intentions and much more, never mind the degree of these characteristics.
>
> Yet, it is essential that matters relating to suicide be operationally defined to facilitate comparisons and to measure the efficacy of interventions both intranationally and internationally. Even if we simply divided suicide into (a) suicide and (b) nonfatal suicidal behavior (or simply, suicidal behavior), obscurity would occur. Nonfatal suicidal behavior would encompass suicidal ideas and suicidal acts; yet here, the issues of nomenclature are rife.
>
> Clustering of suicidal ideation among suicidal behavior has and may continue to increase confusions. Ideas are separate from actions, which is equivalent to saying that ideation *per se* does not imply any consequent behavior. Obviously, defining in a simple, clinically sounding way nonfatal suicidal behavior (or just suicidal behavior) is a much more complicated issue.
>
> Suicidal ideas, for example, may themselves be divided into those signifying that life is not worth living and those signifying that death is preferable. The hierarchy of ideas is further extended by active consideration of methods including the where, the when, the how, and the consequences. There is a further step in the hierarchy if the methods and attendant circumstances are both practical and accessible. This hierarchical model of suicidal ideas should not presuppose that the individual moves up or down the hierarchy in a linear manner, but the clear definition of where his/her ideas rest on such a continuum would clarify comparisons. To begin this clarification, a major international project is needed to clearly define terms, concepts, etc.
>
> Efforts to begin to address these issues have promised hope; yet, to date, there is no accepted nomenclature (Leenaars et al., 1997, pp. 141–142).

Let it suffice to state once more Shneidman's definition: Suicide is a human act of self-inflicted, self-intentioned cessation. That is what we will be talking about here: Suicide and suicidal behaviour.

What Is Evidence-Based?

What is evidence-based practice? This is equally a complex question, not a simple one as many espouse. Fortunately with the foresight of the editors of this volume, we have some direction. I quote verbatim:

> Evidence-based medicine (EBM) involves the conscientious, explicit, and judicious use of current best evidence in making decisions about the care of individual patients. The practice of evidence-based medicine means integrating individual clinical expertise with the best available external clinical evidence from systematic research. By individual clinical expertise we mean the proficiency and judgment that individual clinicians acquire through clinical experience and clinical practice (Pompili & Tatatrelli, personal communication, December 24, 2008).

They suggest the following appropriate methods for our topic:

1. Systematic reviews and meta-analyses.
2. Randomized controlled trials with definitive results (i.e., confidence intervals that do not overlap the threshold clinically significant effect).
3. Randomized controlled trials with nondefinitive results (i.e., a point estimate that suggests a clinically significant effect but with confidence intervals overlapping the threshold for this effect).

My intent is to present the evidence from those methods. This is in keeping with the aim of evidence-based practice (Evidence-Based Medicine Working Group, 1992). We begin with the question in general with people and then the specific one with suicidal people.

What Is the "Best" Psychotherapy?

I hold to the tenet that evidence-based psychotherapy is *the* key to effective treatment. If we are empirically based, we can better treat our patient effectively. The purpose of this section is to outline some of the major research-based issues in the field of psychotherapy in general. The core question is, "Is psychotherapy effective?" and "What is empirically-based or evidence-based practice?"

Psychotherapy research is well established today (Strupp & Howard, 1992). As soon as Freud developed his analytic therapy (1916/1974), he advanced the claim that his psychological treatment was uniquely "*superior.*" He was immediately asked, where the empirical evidence was. "Does the treatment work?" was then and is now the question. The most current empirical answer to this question can be found in Michael Lambert's fifth edition (2004) of Bergin and Garfield's classic in the field of research, *Handbook of Psychotherapy and Behavior Change* (see also Garfield & Bergin, 1978). Not only Freud, but also others, have claimed that their treatment is uniquely effective. Polarization, defensiveness, closed-mindedness, and so on (somewhat akin to the suicidal constricted mind) in claims have occurred. This is singularly responsible for a slowness of progress in this science (Lambert, 2004). To allow the reader to get a better understanding, I highlight the work of Saul Rosenzweig, Hans Eysenck, Michael Lambert, and some others.

Rosenzweig (1936) is most famous in the field for quoting *Alice in Wonderland's* Dodo bird, "*Everybody* has won, and *all* must have prizes." Rosenzweig made the now obvious point that if you claim that your psychotherapy is unique or superior, you suggest, "all others false." He noted that rather than arguing for superiority, we should look for commonalities. He writes,

> ...it is justifiable to wonder (1) whether the factors *alleged to be* operating in a given therapy are identical with the factors *that actually are* operating and (2) whether the factors that actually are operating in several different therapies may not have much more in common than have the factors alleged to be operating (p. 412).

He presented data that all psychotherapies were equally effective. Rosenzweig reframed the field (Kuhn, 1962) and asked the obvious question, "What do these therapies actually have in common that makes them equally successful?" He suggested that the therapist should be person-centered, what the individual needed. Even if Rosenzweig's 1936 original statement about the Dodo bird did not have sufficient empirical data then, it does now. Thus, Rosenzweig's quote, "At last the Dodo said, '*Everybody* has won, and *all* must have prizes.' " remains.

Without question, the best-known researcher in the modern era who studied effectiveness in psychotherapy was Hans Eysenck. His paper entitled, "The effectiveness of psychotherapy: An evaluation," published in 1952, was a classic and remains widely quoted. Yet, the paper is wrong; Eysenck's findings have been "ultimately refuted" (Bergin & Lambert, 1978; Lambert, 2004; Lambert & Bergin, 1992; Strupp & Howard, 1992). Eysenck examined 24 studies on psychotherapy's effectiveness. Based on that review, he concluded:

> In general, certain conclusions are possible from these data. They fail to prove that psychotherapy, Freudian or otherwise, facilitate the recovery of neurotic patients. They show that roughly two-thirds of a group of neurotic patients will recover or improve to a marked extent within about two years of the onset of their illness, whether they are treated by means of psychotherapy or not (p. 322).

Eysenck concluded that, "These results and conclusions will no doubt contradict the strong feeling of usefulness and therapeutic success which many psychiatrists and clinical psychologists hold" (p. 323). He stated that there is no "definite proof"; indeed, many quoted him then and now that, "Psychotherapy causes negative effects."

The problem is that Eysenck is wrong! Indeed, it is worse – his work on psychotherapy has been discredited for decades (Bergin & Lambert, 1978; Freedheim, 1992). Strupp and Howard (1992) have stated:

> The modern era of outcome research is generally dated to Eysenck's (1952) broadside attack on all forms of psychotherapy. Ironically, his results supported the efficacy of psychotherapy, but his conclusion – to abandon the training of psychotherapists – was very damning. The field responded with a variety of attacks on the database, methodology, and motives of this

> piece and finally with an explosion of research activity. Bergin and Lambert (1978) reanalyzed Eysenck's data and showed that ... 67% of those who do seek psychotherapy are improved in about 2 *months* (Howard, Kopta, Krause, & Orlinsky, 1986; McNeilly & Howard, 1991). This was a clear demonstration of the efficacy of psychotherapy (p. 312).

The main valid conclusion, in fact, from Eysenck's study is Psychotherapy works!

There are many studies and systematic reviews to date (Lambert, 2004), but probably one of the best early studies was by Luborsky, Singer, and Luborsky (1975). They analyzed the studies comparing psychotherapies and suggested a verdict similar to the Dodo bird: "Everyone has won." Lambert (2004) also gives the same verdict.

Yet, the question remains, "Is one treatment preferable to another?" Today, the discussion is most polarized between researchers, albeit a reductionist group, and the rest, including practitioners, some of whom find little value in research, including scientific journals (Cohen, Sargent, & Sechrest, 1986; Morrow-Bradley & Elliott, 1986).

"Several dynamics" have resulted in a renewed interest in outcome research (Lambert, Bergin, & Garfield, 2004). These forces included the increasing specification of the *Diagnostic and Statistical Manual of Mental Disorders* (DSM) of the American Psychiatric Association (1994); managed care organizations, associated solely with cost-effectiveness; the application of psychopharmacological models, for example, placebo designs, on other health factors; and the introduction of highly specialized therapies and manuals (cookbooks). "The most notorious effects," stated the best-known editors in the field of research on psychotherapy, Lambert et al. (2004), "in the area were those developed by Division 12 of the American Psychological Association (the Division of Clinical Psychology)" (p. 8). The agenda of Division 12's original Task Force was to impact education, disseminate information, and the like, but the group quickly turned to developing a list of *the best* treatments. The push was to establish *the* list of effective psychotherapies. This resulted in a highly controversial list of what they called, empirically supported therapies (EST) (Chambless, 1996; Chambless & Ollendick, 2001), not to be confused with our intent to look at the broader application of evidence-based research (such as randomized controlled trials). Lists of EST manuals were drawn up and widely distributed, including in the media (Woody & Sanderson, 1998).

To quote Lambert et al. (2004):

> The controversies generated from the initial report came mainly from practitioners who saw the report as rigid, if not dogmatic, and as having an agenda that was biased in favor of therapies promoted by Task Force members (e.g., criteria were set up that would give an advantage to highly structured short-term behavioral and cognitive behavioral treatments advocated by many Task Force members). But strong criticism came from psychotherapy researchers as well (Garfield, 1996; Nathan, 1998; Strupp, 1997) (p. 8).

The initial response of the Task Force to their list was quite "defensive." "Members seemed to lack the humility of recognizing the limitations of their own work" (Lambert et al., 2004, p. 8). Their work has been appropriately called "methodolatry" (something not rare in science). This is *not* evidence-based psychotherapy. It is, moreover, too narrow vis-à-vis the broad definition of psychotherapy that we plan to adhere to. Greater distances were created not only between scientists and practitioners, but also even more so among scientists (something true for Copernicus too). Fortunately, a current committee of APA is reexamining the facts and hopefully the damage done can be repaired. As an aside, much of this has to do with the very frame or paradigm of the scientist (Kuhn, 1962; Lambert, 2004; Leenaars, 2004). The main paradigm of a few EST researchers was modeled after the US Food and Drug Administration criteria for certifying drugs. The original APA Task Force espoused a simple linear model that favored treatments that were psychological analogs to drugs and fit within a narrow medical framework. The psychopharmacological paradigm may not be, however, the best! Holmes (2002) has strongly criticized the use of research being modeled after criteria of certifying drugs. Psychotherapy cannot be reduced to a pill (Leenaars, 2004), probably some in the CBT movement have. Holmes states:

> ...cognitive behaviour therapy is usually compared with waiting list controls, no therapy at all, or some sort of bland pseudotherapy rather than with another form of psychotherapy. As in drug trials, comparing good treatments with those that may be better is a much greater research challenge than demonstrating that a treatment is better than nothing (p. 289).

He further argues:

> The drug treatment paradigm has enormous power in medicine. Research in psychological therapies, especially cognitive behaviour therapy, has been shaped by the "drug metaphor." This implies specific treatments for specific conditions – and that anything that lies outside the paradigm lies beyond the bounds of science (p. 290).

He argues:

> However, the drug metaphor has also had a distorting and potentially damaging effect in psychological medicine. Psychotherapy is essentially concerned with people, not conditions, or disorders, and its methods arise out of an intimate relationship between two people that cannot easily be reduced to a set of prescribed techniques. One of the most robust findings in psychotherapy research is that a good therapeutic alliance is the best predictor of outcome in psychotherapy (p. 290).

I agree.

The whole issue is much more complex (and, of course, space is limited). Chambless and Ollendick (2001) argue that their empirically supported treatments (ESTs) are based on a broader paradigm that arose in the United Kingdom, known as evidence-based medicine (The Evidence-Based Medicine Working Group, 1992; Saskett, Richardson, Rosenberg, & Haynes, 1997). However, they argue for limited evidence-based research, not consistent with our definition earlier, nor that of The Evidence-Based Medicine Working Group (1992), or as defined in this edited volume, for that matter. It was extreme Occam's Razor reductionism. Chambless and Ollendick (2001) dismiss qualitative research, clinical process research, and/or case studies. They write,

> ...it is clear that there is much to be learned about the application of EST's and the benefits in clinical practice. Whatever the reluctance of some to embrace EST's, we expect that the

> economic and societal pressures on practitioners for accountability, will encourage continued attention to these treatments (pp. 711–712).

Will economics, thus, dictate "best" practice? Of course, however, the research of empirically based psychotherapy is more complex – ESTs (also called empirically validated treatments or EVTs) are only one part of the research. I am not suggesting that they may not be of value, only that they are not all of evidence-based research (Henry, 1998; Koocher, 2003).

I am, of course, not opposed to empirically supported treatment research; I oppose, however, Chambless' Razor. I, in fact, review the evidence-based research on the "best" psychotherapy with suicidal people. However, in its narrow-minded form, it is "a mess" (Wm. James). It is not what psychotherapy is (see definition). There are others, including researchers associated with evidence-based psychotherapy that state the same, such as Aaron T. Beck (Beck, 1976; Beck & Freeman, 1990). Psychotherapy research must be more complex than what is still called ESTs; we need a paradigm switch to answer our question. The main task according to Henry (1998) is the following: "We must not lose sight of the *people* in this people oriented endeavor" (p. 138).

Before I turn to the studies on randomized controlled trials, I need to make explicit one more point; the claim of "superiority." The whole issue remains at the head of polemics. Bergin and Lambert (1978) write:

> Competing approaches to psychotherapy have traditionally been pitted against one another. Presumably, the one shown to be most effective will prove that position to be correct and will serve as a demonstration that the "losers" should be persuaded to give up their views. Under the broad question of "which treatment is more efficacious?" are more meaningful and productive questions. Which specific procedure obtains which results, with which patients, in what amount of time, and are these differential results equally enduring? These more specific questions do not set up a *win-lose* situation and, therefore, serve the more mature interests of inquiry (p. 162).

Many researchers have presented on the issue of no superiority; for example, a collaborative effort of the American National Institute of Mental Health (Elkin et al., 1989) strongly supports the view that there is *no* superiority of one therapy, cognitive or psychoanalytic or interpersonal or otherwise. Many have come to the realization of the fact of equivalence and the empirically supported view of common factors; that is, *commonalities* (Lambert & Bergin, 1992; Leenaars, 2004).

Common Versus Unique (Specific) Factors in the Best Evidence-Based Psychotherapy

Freud (1916/1974) was at pains to differentiate his psychotherapy from others; the *modus operandi* of psychoanalytic psychotherapy was to be unique (Strupp & Howard, 1992). The claim to "superiority" has been, however, as false and narrow-minded as the claims of the original APA Division 12 Task Force. Other systems of psychotherapy also claimed to be unique and superior – Beck, Ellis, Rogers, Shneidman, Wolpe, to name a few. Yet, to quote Strupp and Howard (1992), "The seeming uniqueness of each system might simply be semantic or stylistic or reflect previous fashions" (p. 313). The view is "that common factors may be of overriding importance in all forms of psychotherapy" (Strupp & Howard, 1992, p. 313). There is evidence for many forms of psychotherapy.

The issue "Is psychotherapy effective?" is like asking, "Is surgery effective?" A better question would be Bruce Wampold's (1997): "Which treatments are most efficacious for which patients under which conditions?" (p. 21). What is the "best" psychotherapy? (A good surgeon asks the same about procedures, of course). Wampold offers a shift in paradigms; he writes:

> The case could be made that a discussion of the causal factors related to efficacy is irrelevant to the empirical validation of a treatment. That is, if treatment A is proven to be efficacious, then it is unimportant to identify exactly what characteristics of the treatment led to this conclusion. As appealing as this argument sounds, relatively few would adhere to it. First, treatment developers develop treatment operations to be consistent with theory and research and believe that the actions prescribed by the treatment lead to therapeutic change. Second, when that treatment is shown to be efficacious, the proponents believe that these specific operations were responsible for the positive outcomes and typically will argue to that end. Third, the very essence of looking for a set of empirically validated treatments supposes a belief that some treatments are not efficacious and consequently operations common to therapies cannot be responsible for treatment effects. Finally, knowledge of factors related to outcome leads to refining treatments and increased potency (Wampold, 1997, pp. 24–25).

Many will have difficulty accepting that there is no evidence for treatment specificity. There is no "the best" psychotherapy. Indeed, Wampold's and others' meta-analytic work clearly supports common factors, not unique. There is evidence for the conclusion: there are commonalities in psychotherapy that make psychotherapies effective. Wampold (1997) offers the following definition of commonalities: "The features that are shared by all these therapies . . . are designated as common features" (p. 25). The wedding of being evidence-based and psychotherapy will allow many of us to be more effective with suicidal people. This is what makes psychotherapy effective (Leenaars, 2004).

Wampold (1997) has proposed if the common factor thesis were true, then we need to shift the paradigm from a simplistic drug metaphor model of psychotherapy to a contextual or process model (Saunders, 2003; Orlinsky et al., 2004). "Process" research is more associated to this contextual view than to the linear deterministic "drug metaphor" model. We need to add process research to our list of evidence-based studies. This research, some 50 years thereof, has clearly demonstrated that "effectiveness is clearly more than a set of technical procedures," and, once more, the more important common factors are noted (Orlinsky et al., 2004). Yet again, it is not simple, but complex. A warm, supportive therapeutic relationship, for example, by itself is not sufficient, even if it is a key ingredient. This is the common factor paradigm, something espoused by Rosenzweig, Luborsky, and many others. Luborsky et al. (1975), for example, suggest a verdict similar to Wampold's.

Lambert et al. (2004) in the most recent update of the research study supports the common factors. They write:

> ...process research aimed at examining the in-session behavior of therapists across different theoretical orientations indicates that the distinctiveness of approaches is less pronounced in practice than it is at the abstract level of theory (Ablan & Jones, 1999; Norcross & Goldfried, 1992). Thus, theories of change are somewhat independent of therapists' actual activities which show a large degree of overlap across treatments – sometimes referred to as common factors (p. 7).

The commonality movement reflects an attempt to being truly evidence-based. There is no the "best" psychotherapy. Yet, this begets a core question here: What is "the best" psychotherapy with suicidal people? I will next turn to an answer.

Method: Data Sources on Evidence-Based Psychotherapy With Suicidal People

Electronic literature searches of all articles available until January 2009 were conducted of all literature archived at the Centre for Suicide Prevention, Calgary, Alberta, Canada (Myra Morant, personal communication, February 12, 2009; April 14, 2009). It houses 38,997 documents on the topic of suicide, the SIEC database. We identified reports: evaluation.randomised controlled trials.psychotherapy.suicide (people, patients, and clients). We used a broad term for psychotherapy, such as cognitive-behavioral, psychodynamic, family, interpersonal, and problem solving, a vast array. We also searched out subject terms psychodrama, marital therapy, hypnosis, and existential therapies in combination with evaluation but none of these returned any results. In addition, we searched for articles targeting meta-analysis and systematic reviews. Six hundred eighty-two articles were identified. Yet, further searches were undertaken. Nine articles not yet entered on the SIEC database were identified, largely 2008 studies (searched January 12, 2009). We searched PUBMED/Medline and PsychInfo (we last searched these on September 11, 2009). After a general search, we located "Search efficacy suicide, plus inserted psychotherapy, counseling, psychological therapy, brief therapy, behavior therapy, family therapy, interpersonal therapy, and therapy." Three hundred seventy-five articles were identified.

In addition, the systematic review articles on "suicide" only (not excluded groups) (there were no meta-analyses found) were examined for further articles, and handsearched every article deemed relevant in all journals. These articles listed 23 studies (Rudd, 2000), 28 studies (Tarrier, Taylor, & Gooding, 2008), 25 articles (Hepp, Wittmann, Schnyder, & Michel, 2004), 2 studies (Hirsch, Walsh, & Draper, 1982), a total of 78 articles, with considerable agreement about the studies, however. Crawford, Thomas, Khan, and Aya (2007) also presented a systematic review, but they included studies of "patients who had harmed themselves," so it is unclear what we are discussing. Nevertheless, we searched their article; it had 38 references, all previously cited in other reviews. We did not *a priori* specify "relevant" journals or not; we did not exclude any journal (as opposed to some reviewers;

some even excluded journals such as *Crisis* and *Archives of Suicide Research*). We wanted to be as broad as possible. We, thus, initially identified 1,182 articles. Abstracts were reviewed and full text articles that met inclusive criteria were retrieved. Sixty-eight articles were retrieved and all reports were reviewed in detail, summarized, highlighted, and cataloged, the basis for the findings.

Inclusion criteria were the following: Any kind of suicide or suicide behavior as the identified subject (patient, person) and not self-harm only, as defined earlier; all systematic reviews and all meta-analyses were included; studies if they were published in a journal or as a chapter in a book and if they included randomized controls, a treatment group that consisted of a form of psychotherapy, as broadly defined before, a control group such as treatment as usual (TAU), no treatment, or other treatment.

Exclusion criteria were the following: Studies were excluded if they focused on BPD (we discuss more below, a complete separate review is needed on this topic) and self-harm studies (with no evaluation of intention or impossible to discern intention, but believed to be so, but offered limited information; otherwise we included them). We excluded studies that primarily studied the effect of psychopharmacology and other tests, including TAU or psychotherapy. Further, for the review here, we also excluded process research, clinical descriptions, and case studies. We attempted to search as far back as possible, but generally to the 1970s and excluded, if they were not published in English.

Results: The Search Findings

Studies were included if they reported on the primary outcome of interest, namely suicides, attempted suicides, and suicidal ideation, or, when applicable, intermediate outcomes, including help-seeking behavior, problem-solving skills, interpersonal relationships, hopelessness, and so on (see definition above, Leenaars et al., 1997; Mann et al., 2005; Tarrier et al., 2008; the latter two provide easily replicable methods for systematic review on the topic, such as those used here).

From the initial search, 1,182 articles were identified. Of these, 10 reviews were identified, but only 4 were systematic within our criteria (Hepp et al., 2004; Hirsch et al., 1982; Rudd, 2000; Tarrier et al., 2008; see Table 1 for list), and 16 randomized controlled trials literature on evidence-based psychotherapy with suicidal people were identified (see Table 2), with six cognitive-behavioral therapy (CBT), one on dialectical behavior therapy (DBT) (with BPD excluded here), and although consistent with the broad definition of psychotherapy, called here problem-solving training (PST), nine articles. The total of 16 is meager, given the claims made by some proponents of the old EST movement. We need to know what we really know.

The reviews and studies are listed in Tables 1 and 2; we owe these researchers much in developing evidence-based understanding of psychotherapy. Of course, the limited number of studies (never mind the conclusions to be made) suggest that we have to look even more broadly for an evidence-based approach. The limits make it so.

Table 1. Review of the literature on evidence-based psychotherapy with suicidal people

Comtois, K., & Linehan, M. (2006). Psychosocial treatments of suicidal behaviors: A practice-friendly review. *Journal of Clinical Psychology: In Session, 62,* 161–170.

Crawford, M., Thomas, O., Khan, N., & Aya, E. (2007). Psychosocial interventions following self-harm. *British Journal of Psychiatry, 190,* 11–17.

Hepp, U., Wittmann, L., Schnyder, U., & Michel, K. (2004). Psychological and psychosocial interventions after attempted suicide: An overview of treatment studies. *Crisis, 25,* 108–117.

Hirsch, S., Walsh, C., & Draper, R. (1982). Parasuicide: A review of treatment interventions. *Journal of Affective Disorders, 4,* 299–311.

Kerkhof, A., & Diekstra, R. (1995). The prevention of suicidal behaviour: A review of effectiveness. In R. Diekstra, W. Gulbinat, I. Kienhorst, & D. De Leo (Eds.). *Preventive strategies on suicide* (pp. 207–229). Leiden: E.J. Brill.

Links, P., Bergmans, Y., & Cook, M. (2003). Psychotherapeutic interventions to prevent repeated suicidal behavior. *Brief Treatment and Crisis Intervention, 3,* 445–464.

Mann, J., Apter, A., Bertolote, J., et al. (2005). Suicide prevention strategies: A systematic review. *Journal of the American Medical Association, 294,* 2064–2074.

Möller, H. (1992). Attempted suicide: Efficacy of different aftercare strategies. *International Clinical Psychopharmacology, 6S,* 58–69.

Rudd, M. (2000). Integrating science into the practice of clinical suicidology: A review of the psychotherapy literature and a research agenda for the future. In R. Maris, S. Canetto, J. McIntosh, & M. Silverman (Eds.). *Review of suicidology 2000* (pp. 47–83). New York: Guilford.

Tarrier, N., Taylor, K., & Gooding, P. (2008). Cognitive-behavioral interventions to reduce suicide behavior: A systematic review and meta-analysis. *Behavior Modification, 32,* 77–108.

Aside from the first obvious conclusion of limited studies, it should be noted that there were considerable variations in what was included as psychotherapy and how psychotherapy was delivered. There were further limits; one study only studied five people. There are Everest problems!

Discussion: Evidence-Based Psychotherapy for Suicidal People

Despite the Dodo bird's description, there is an astonishing lack of evidence. From a review of the research back in the early 1990s, Kerkhof and Diekstra (1995) had affirmed the dictum: "It can be concluded that there is no empirical evidence whatsoever." There were no documented substantial effects not only of psychotherapy, but also of any prevention effort. Despite these skeptics then, there is evidence-based literature today, and also in the early 1990s, for that matter. Mann et al. (2005) presented a more recent prototypical study on the evidence for effectiveness of specific suicide-prevention intervention. Not only was there solid evidence for such efforts as environmental (gun) control, they also concluded that there were primary results in reducing suicidal behavior from psychotherapy,

Table 2. Randomized controlled trials literature on evidence-based psychotherapy with suicidal people

Cognitive-behavioral therapy

Brown, G., Have, T., Henriques, G., et al. (2005). Cognitive therapy for the prevention of suicide attempts: A randomized controlled trial. *Journal of the American Medical Association, 294*, 563–570.

Donaldson, D., Spirito, A., & Esposito-Smythers, C. (2005). Treatment of adolescents following a suicide attempt: Results of a pilot trial. *Journal of the American Academy of Child & Adolescent Psychiatry, 44*, 113–120.

Liberman, R., & Eckman, T. (1981). Behavior therapy vs. insight-oriented therapy for repeated suicide attempters. *Archives of General Psychiatry, 38*, 1126–1130.

Power, P., Bell, R., Mills, R., et al. (2003). Suicide prevention in first episode psychosis: The development of a randomised controlled trial of cognitive therapy for acutely suicidal patients with early psychosis. *Australian and New Zealand Journal of Psychiatry, 37*, 414–420.

Rudd, M., Rajab, M., Orman, D., et al. (1996). Effectiveness of an outpatient intervention targeting suicidal young adults: Preliminary results. *Journal of Consulting and Clinical Psychology, 64*, 179–190.

Salkovskis, P., Atha, C., & Storer, D. (1990). Cognitive-behavioural problem-solving in treatment of patients who repeatedly attempt suicide: A controlled trial. *Journal of Psychiatry, 157*, 871–876.

Dialectical behavior therapy

Katz, L., Cox, B., Gunasekara, S., & Miller, A. (2004). Feasibility of dialectical behavior therapy for suicidal adolescent inpatients. *Journal of the American Academy of Child and Adolescent Psychiatry, 43*, 276–282.

Problem-solving training

Allard, R., Marshall, M., & Plante, M. (1992). Intensive follow-up does not decrease the risk of repeat suicide attempts. *Suicide and Life-Threatening Behavior, 22*, 303–314.

Chowdhury, N., Hicks, R., & Kreitman, N. (1973). Evaluation of an after-care service for parasuicide (attempted suicide) patients. *Social Psychiatry, 8*, 67–81.

Clum, G., Yang, B., Curtin, L., et al. (1992). Problem-solving treatment of severe ideators. In D. Lester (Ed.), *Suicide '92: Proceedings. Silver Anniversary Conference* (pp. 173–174). Chicago: American Association of Suicidology.

Eskin, M., Ertekin, K., & Demir, H. (2008). Efficacy of a problem-solving therapy for depression and suicide potential in adolescents and young adults. *Cognitive Therapy Research, 32*, 227–245.

Gibbons, J., Butler, J., Urwin, P., & Gibbons, J. (1978). Evaluation of social work service for self-poisoning patients. *British Journal of Psychiatry, 133*, 111–118.

Hawton, K., McKeown, S., Day, A., et al. (1987). Evaluation of outpatient counselling compared with general practitioner care following overdoses. *Psychological Medicine, 17*, 751–761.

Lerner, M., & Clum, G. (1990). Treatment of suicide ideators: A problem-solving approach. *Behavior Therapy, 21*, 403–411.

(continued on next page)

Table 2. Continued

McLeavey, B., Daly, R., Ludgate, J., & Murray, C. (1994). Interpersonal problem-solving skills training in the treatment of self-poisoning patients. *Suicide and Life-Threatening Behavior, 24,* 382–394.

Möller, H. (1989). Efficacy of different strategies of aftercare for patients who have attempted suicide. *Journal of the Royal Society of Medicine, 82,* 643–647.

Patsiokas, A., & Clum, G. (1985). Effects of psychotherapeutic strategies in the treatment of suicide attempters. *Psychotherapy, 22,* 281–290.

compared with standard care. Surprisingly, despite that being so, there is a lack of study and it is fraught with controversy (Rudd, 2000). The main one being, which is the *superior* psychotherapy with suicidal sufferers? Like me, Holmes (2002) has concluded that the argument for superiority is more apparent than real. Yet, the claim persists, with no evidence for. Liberman and Eckman (1981) have, in fact, concluded that the best method of psychotherapy has not yet emerged, but there is evidence that psychotherapy with suicidal people helps.

To answer the question posed, we did a systematic review of the literature. Table 1 presents the systematic review of the literature on evidence-based psychotherapy with suicidal people. Probably, one of the best is by David Rudd (2000). Rudd asked the obvious question: What do we really know about treating suicidal behavior? He also asked many more questions, a few examples of which are: What treatment has demonstrated effectiveness? Within identified treatments, are there common factors associated with positive outcomes? Negative harmful outcomes (see Barlow, 2010; Dimidijan & Hollon, 2010)? Do particular people require specific treatment approaches? Does short-term treatment work? Long-term? There are others; yet, it is obvious that these are the same ones that Lambert (2004) lists as the common ones in psychotherapy in general.

What Do We Know: Randomized Controlled Trials Literature on Evidence-Based Psychotherapy With Suicidal People

Next, I present the studies found, some 16 only. Table 2 lists the studies; I have subdivided the studies into three groups: CBT, DBT, and PST. CBT has six studies, DBT 1, and PST 9.

Cognitive-Behavioral Therapy

It would be a truism to state that the studies by Gregory Brown and his team, and by David Rudd and his team are some of the best randomized controlled trials literature. I thus present a summary, but also add one other study toward the end of this section.

Gregory Brown, Thomas Have, Gregg Henriques, and their colleagues (2005), in their article, Cognitive Therapy for the Prevention of Suicide Attempts: A Randomized Controlled Trial, present the following somewhat modified abstract:

> The empirical evidence for treatments that effectively prevent repetition of suicide attempts is limited. The objective of this study was to determine the effectiveness of a 10-session cognitive behavioral therapy (CBT) intervention designed to prevent repeated suicide attempts in adults. Randomized controlled trial of adults ($N = 120$) who attempted suicide was undertaken. Participants were followed up for 18 months. Intervention was cognitive therapy or enhanced usual care with tracking and referral services. From baseline to the 18-month assessment, 13 participants (24.1%) in the cognitive therapy group and 23 participants (41.6%) in the usual care group made at least one subsequent suicide attempt. Participants in the cognitive therapy group had a significantly lower reattempt rate and were 50% less likely to reattempt suicide than those in the usual care group. The severity of self-reported depression, hopelessness, and suicidal ideation was significantly lower. It was concluded that cognitive therapy was effective in preventing suicide attempts for adults who recently attempted suicide (p. 563).

This study is important because it was designed with adequate power to determine whether a brief psychosocial intervention could reduce the rate of repetition for suicide attempts over an 18-month interval, a longer period than previously reported in most randomized controlled trials. Cognitive therapy was selected as the psychosocial intervention for this study because it builds on clinical investigations with regard to the psychopathological characteristics of suicidal behaviors, and it has been shown to be successful in a wide variety of psychiatric disorders. In the method, Brown and his team studied 120 individuals who attempted suicide, with spelled-out inclusion criteria of what a suicide attempt is, consistent with our definition. The 120 people were randomly assigned to cognitive therapy or usual care (TAU). Participants in the cognitive therapy intervention were scheduled to receive 10 specifically developed sessions for preventing suicide attempts: the identification of proximal thoughts, images, and core beliefs. Cognitive and behavioral strategies were applied. Participants in both study groups received usual care from clinicians in the community. The primary outcome measure was the occurrence of a suicide attempt during the follow-up period. The sample size ($N = 120$) provided at least 80% power to detect a hazard ratio (.05). The impact on measures of depression, hopelessness, and suicidal ideation was also examined from 1 to 18 months following the baseline. There was significantly less suicidal ideation, depression, and hopelessness in the cognitive therapy group than in the control group. This is evidence.

Brown et al. concluded:

> The results of this randomized controlled trial indicated that a relatively brief cognitive therapy intervention was effective in preventing suicide attempts for adults who recently attempted suicide. Specifically, participants in the cognitive therapy group were approximately 50% less likely to attempt suicide during the follow-up period than participants in the usual care group (p. 567).

They further argue for the superiority of CBT; they state:

> The short-term feature of cognitive therapy would make it particularly applicable for the treatment of suicide attempters at community mental health centers, which typically provide relatively short-term therapy (p. 570).

The next study to be presented in detail is by David Rudd, Hasan Rajab, David Orman, and their team, in a 1996 paper, Effectiveness of an Outpatient Intervention Targeting Suicidal Young Adults: Preliminary Results. The verbatim abstract reads:

> This study evaluated the effectiveness of a time-limited, outpatient intervention targeting suicidal young adults. Participants (*N* = 264) were randomly assigned to either the experimental treatment or the control condition (i.e., treatment as usual). In addition to intake assessments, participants completed follow-ups at 1, 6, 12, 18, and 24 months. Both treatment and control participants evidenced significant improvement across all outcome measures throughout the follow-up period. Reductions were reported in suicidal ideation and behavior, associated symptomatology, and experienced stress, along with marked improvement in self-appraised problem-solving ability. Results also indicated that the experimental treatment was more effective than treatment as usual at retaining the highest risk participants. Available data demonstrate the efficacy of a time-limited, outpatient intervention for suicidal young adults. Implications of current findings for intervention with and treatment of this population are discussed (p. 179).

Rudd noted that, "The data that are available have led investigators to raise questions about ... our demonstrated ability to translate the limited knowledge available into coherent, theory-driven prevention and early intervention models and treatment programs" (p. 179).

More cautious than Brown, they noted a lack of empirical data. The findings to date, they concluded, were disappointing at best. Rudd concluded that, "Overall, research to date has failed to answer some of the most fundamental questions about early intervention and treatment of those exhibiting suicidal behavior" (p. 180). He wrote, "Can such interventions prove effective?" To answer the question, Rudd and his team evaluated the efficacy of time-limited, outpatient intervention targeting deficient problem solving and overall adaptive coping in suicidal adolescents and young adults. In the method, a design with randomization to treatment or control conditions (i.e., TAU) was used. They randomly assigned to groups. The measures were multiple: Suicidal ideation; life stress; negative expectations; depression; problem-solving behavior and attitudes; personality traits, character features, and acute symptomatology; intellectual functioning; and psychosocial history. Participants included 302 individuals (248 males and 54 females), with a total of 38 who withdrew (*N* = 264), 143 in the treatment group, and 121 in the control group. The results revealed a lack of identified between-group differences and indications. Treatment and control participants improved significantly across all measures. Perhaps, there are no differences in effective treatment. Yet, Rudd did state:

> Results also provide evidence that those presenting complex diagnostic pictures, with considerable comorbidity, can be treated effectively with approaches... Somewhat surprising given the brief and outpatient nature of the experimental treatment, observed gains were, for the

> most part, comprehensive and enduring, with initial gains maintained over the 12-month follow-up period (p. 188).

They argued that, "brief, albeit intensive, interventions can be effective over the long term for a percentage of those experiencing severe and potentially extreme pathology such as suicidal behavior" (p. 188). Yet, both groups evidenced quick remission of reported symptoms and significant improvement across all areas or domains assessed, including suicidal ideation and behavior, symptomatology, and general problem solving, raising the question whether there is a best therapy.

Liberman and Eckman (1981), in their paper, Behavior Therapy versus Insight-Oriented Therapy for Repeated Suicide Attempters, made the same conclusion:

> A behavior therapy package was compared with insight-oriented therapy in a clinical trial for repeated suicide attempters. Self-report measures of depression, anxiety, and assertiveness were obtained before and after ten days of inpatient treatment and at follow-up intervals for nine months. Interviews with patients during a two-year follow-up period elicited frequency of suicidal attempts and ideation. Results indicated the superiority of the behavior therapy package, with the structured, brief hospitalization and assertive follow-up likely contributing to the main effects (p. 1126).

Yet, Liberman concluded that the best method of treatment has not yet emerged, and I would add, Liberman only added an observation to the question, not a conclusion. In the clinical trial, *only* 8 men and 16 women were treated; too few to have any significant power. Actually, his conclusion can only be like Rudd's, no difference. In fact, he states:

> While both treatment groups showed marked and statistically significant improvements on each of the psychological tests at the end of the inpatient period, the magnitude of gains for the patients in the behavior therapy group were greater for each test (p. 1128).

How was that conclusion arrived at? 12 people? This study is very limited, so are the rest of CBT trials, but generally so.

Salkovskis, Atha, and Storer (1990), in a controlled trial of 20 patients at high risk of repeated suicide attempts, randomly allocated them to either cognitive-behavioral problem solving or a "treatment-as-usual" (TAU) control condition. The group practicing problem solving improved significantly more than controls on ratings of depression, hopelessness, suicidal ideation, and target problems at the end of treatment and at follow-up of up to 1 year. They concluded that the cognitive-behavioral approach to problem solving should be a useful short-term treatment. That may be true, but we can conclude little else.

Power, Bell, and Mills (2003) in a study, Suicide Prevention in First episode Psychosis, noted that young people with early psychosis are at particularly high risk of suicide. However, there is little evidence to suggest that early intervention could reduce this risk. In the method, 56 suicidal patients with first episode psychosis were randomly assigned to standard clinical care (TAU) or standard care plus a CBT. Clinical ratings and measures of suicidality and risk were assessed before, immediately after the intervention, and 6 months later. Benefits were noted in the treatment group on indirect measures of suicidality, for example, hopelessness. The treatment group showed a greater average improvement (though not significant) on a measure of suicidal ideation. They concluded that early intervention in psychosis for young people might well reduce the risk of suicide. That may be true, but we do not know what psychotherapy. It may not be relevant whether the person is diagnosed with this or that disease, say depression or a personality disorder, but what is relevant is that the person received quality care, and that means being person-centered, not diagnosis-centered (Leenaars, 2004).

I had suggested that the articles by Brown and Rudd were the best to date; yet, I would like to add a third, Deidre Donaldson, Anthony Spirito, and Christianne Esposito-Smythers, Treatment of Adolescents following a Suicide Attempt: Results of a Pilot Trial (2005). Despite some limitations such as low power (N = 39), it still presents a unique finding. Here is the abstract:

> **Objective:** To compare the efficacy of a skills-based treatment protocol to a supportive relationship therapy for adolescents after a suicide attempt. **Method:** Thirty-nine adolescents (12–17 years old) and parents who presented to a general paediatric emergency department or inpatient unit of a child psychiatric hospital after a suicide attempt were randomized to either a skills-based or a supportive relationship treatment condition. Follow-up assessments were conducted at intake and 3 and 6 months post-attempt. **Results:** In contrast to the low rates of treatment received by adolescent suicide attempters in the community, approximately 60% of this sample completed the entire treatment protocol. Significant decreases in suicidal ideation and depressed mood at 3- and 6-month follow-ups were obtained, but there were no differences between treatment groups. There were six reattempts in the follow-up period. **Conclusions:** When adolescents who attempt suicide are maintained in treatment, significant improvements in functioning can be realized for the majority of patients (p. 113).

The study actually compared *two* individual-based treatments with adolescent attempters. They provided a clear definition of suicide attempt, consistent with mine (O'Carroll et al., 1996). There were exclusions, such as psychosis, primary language other than English. All participants received standard medical care. Participants were 39 adolescents (12–17 years old); they were randomly assigned to one of the two groups (they stated that no treatment would be unethical). One group of people received a cognitive-behavioral mode of individual therapy (a specific-task-oriented treatment), and the other group received a nondirective mode (supportive relationship treatment), with details spelled out to allow replication. Both interventions included an active phase, six sessions, and one adjunct family session, if warranted due to family issues, during 3 months, followed by a 3-month maintenance follow-up. Evaluations were undertaken at 3 months and 6 months. Outcome measures included such measures as diagnostics, suicidal ideation, depression, anger expression, and problem solving (again, all clearly spelled out). Eighty percent completed the trials (N = 31). This is high retention. No significant differences were noted in demographics, suicide attempts, etc., between the groups. No differences were noted on outcome measures. No differences were found, even if prescribed medication, at 3 months, for depressed mood, suicidal ideation, and problem solving. No differences were observed at 6 months. There were no differences in suicide attempts. Thus, contrary to prediction, both treatments helped. I will go further. This research supports the claim that the relationship (attachment) that the therapist develops is central in effective psychotherapy with suicidal patients. What the researchers learned is that it did not matter what treatment the patients received. Patients in both groups showed positive response. Thus, this study replicated Luborsky, Singer, and Luborsky's (1975) finding, now with suicidal patients. It was hypothesized that the relationship was critical. Suicidal people were telling their narratives and someone was listening (after all, these patients were important; they were part of a research study). Keep in mind in this study, the same seven therapists did both treatments; maybe they were just good therapists. Psychotherapy is the attachment, not simply this, or that technique. What works is mollifying that sufferer's pain. What works is quality care.

Donaldson and his team made a few more observations, worthwhile repeating verbatim:

> . . .the therapists in this project had small case loads and were invested in maintaining subject participation in the study. These circumstances may be unlike those of community service agencies in which fewer supports exist to follow patients once a crisis is stabilized. Many of the patients in this study, regardless of treatment condition, reported their therapy experience to be positive and asked to continue treatment beyond the protocol schedule. Fostering these conditions in community treatment settings may enhance care for this population (p. 119).

> Improvements associated with both treatments also could be related to the fact that the same therapists conducted both treatments. Nonspecific therapist factors, e.g., therapist warmth and genuineness, may have led to improvement in both conditions. The therapists in the study may have been particularly skilled and especially effective in working with difficult populations (p. 119).

I agree; Donaldson, Spirito, and Overholser (2003), for the first time in a randomized controlled trial, have shown that what matters is psychotherapy, not this or that cookbook detail. All psychotherapies are "best."

Dialectical Behavior Therapy

There is one study on DBT and suicide. This is the 2004 study by Laurence Katz, Brian Cox, Shiny Gunasekara, and Alec Miller (2004), Feasibility of Dialectical Behavior Therapy for Suicidal Adolescent Inpatients. The abstract reads:

> OBJECTIVE: To evaluate the feasibility of dialectical behavior therapy (DBT) implementation in a general child and adolescent psychiatric inpatient unit and to provide preliminary effectiveness data on DBT versus treatment as usual (TAU). METHOD: Sixty-two adolescents with suicide attempts or suicidal ideation were admitted to one of two psychiatric inpatient units. One unit used a DBT protocol and the other unit relied on TAU. Assessments of depressive symptoms, suicidal ideation, hopelessness, parasuicidal behavior, hospitalizations, emergency room visits, and adherence to follow-up recommendations were conducted before and after treatment and at 1-year follow-up for both groups. In addition, behavioral incidents

> on the units were evaluated. RESULTS: DBT significantly reduced behavioral incidents during admission when compared with TAU. Both groups demonstrated highly significant reductions in parasuicidal behavior, depressive symptoms, and suicidal ideation at 1 year. CONCLUSIONS: DBT can be effectively implemented in acute-care child and adolescent psychiatric inpatient units. The promising results from this pilot study suggest that further evaluation of DBT for adolescent inpatients appears warranted (p. 276).

Problem-Solving Training

The largest set of studies is not on CBT, but on problem-solving therapy or training (PST). Nilima Chowdhury, R. Hicks, and Norman Kreitman, in the 1973 paper, Evaluation of an After-Care Service for Parasuicide (Attempted Suicide) Patients, present a classic study on PST. Here are some observations from the study: An experimental after-care program was provided for patients who had repeatedly attempted suicide. One hundred ninety-seven patients were identified as repeaters. Forty-two of these were rated as at high risk of further repetition and were excluded. Of the non-high-risk patients, 71 remained in the treatment group and 84 in the TAU control group. The treatment group, in addition to TAU, received treatment in problem solving, especially about social difficulties, although it is unclear how; domiciliary visits and a 24-h emergency service in addition to outpatient clinics were provided. At 6 months, no significant difference was found between the treatment and control groups in the proportion of patients with further acts of parasuicide during the follow-up: 24% and 23%, respectively. No significant differences were found in the follow-up assessments of psychiatric and behavioral states. The social circumstances of the treated group, especially the females, were significantly improved when compared with the controls. They concluded that the aftercare provided might have been of too short duration to permit full evaluation.

Yet, whom were we studying? Were self-harm patients included? Who was excluded? Forty-two high-risk patients were excluded from the evaluation of the program. There were 23 males and 19 females. There is a great deal of ambiguity. They state that:

"Some repeaters were considered to be at such high risk of further parasuicide that allocation to the control group could not be justified on ethical grounds."

They noted that this group had serious problems in the use of alcohol and dependency on sedative or stimulant drugs. That may be true, but it is true for many truly suicidal people. Are they not typical of suicidal people presented for psychotherapy?

There were further problems; a follow-up period of six months was probably unrealistically short. What is an adequate time line? How were measures, such as "psychiatric and behavioural states," assessed? Most of the studies, especially the early ones, on effective PST have such limitations and more.

Gibbons, Butler, Urwin, and Gibbons (1978) studied 400 patients, after deliberately poisoning themselves; they were randomly assigned between an experimental service (PST) and a control (routine) follow-up service (TAU). One hundred thirty-nine patients were excluded from the trial, most of whom were at high risk of suicide. After 1 year, there was no difference. Yet, are these patients really suicidal? Alternatively, were they self-harm patients, and thus, should be excluded? This is a major problem in the group of studies. Who are the subjects? Patients were excluded if they had a psychiatric illness, required psychiatric care (such as hospitalization), immediate risk for suicide, and not otherwise suitable? Are these not the very suicidal patients who present to our psychotherapy room? We need to ask, what is the best treatment for truly suicidal people?

Patsiokas and Clum (1985) studied 15 hospitalized suicide attempters. The patients were randomly assigned to cognitive therapy, PST, or nondirective control treatment, consisting of 10 one-hour individual therapy sessions. Results indicated that the three treatment conditions were comparable with regard to the nonspecific effects associated with expectancy of improvement, treatment demand characteristics, and therapist effects. At the completion of treatment, subjects in the problem-solving condition evidenced better problem-solving abilities than either the cognitive or nondirective control group on a measure of interpersonal problem solving. However, this may be no surprise, if I train patients in problem-solving skills, others not, and then I evaluate everyone on problem-solving skills, would I not expect the trained people to do better?

Patsiokas and Clum at least studied different therapies. They showed changes in hopelessness and suicidal intention in the three treatment conditions. There was no drop in suicidal ideation. (Why would there be?) At the completion of treatment, only the problem-solving and nondirective treatment groups were significantly different on hopelessness. Apparently the problem-solving approach provides individuals with a tool for dealing with future problems that resulted in a more optimistic appraisal of the future. That may be true, but are they less suicidal? In fact, no significant differences were found even between the treatment conditions on the interpersonal problem-solving measure. Is suicide not often interpersonal?

Allard, Marshall, and Plante (1992) carried out a randomized controlled trial to determine whether an intensive intervention after a suicide attempt could decrease by half the risk of a repeat attempt in the following 2 years. After initial assessment and randomization, experimental subjects attended 18 therapy appointments over 1 year, including one home visit, and measures to improve attendance (Are 18 sessions sufficient? 12? 3?). Control subjects received the usual care. Of 63 experimental subjects, 35% made a repeat attempt, and so did 30% of 63 control subjects. The study had a 99% power to detect the desired decrease of risk (30–15%). Clearly, the intervention did not achieve its objective.

Hawton et al. (1987) in a randomized prospective treatment study studied 80 overdose patients (with low risk) who either received brief outpatient problem-solving counseling or were returned to the care as usual (TAU) of their general practitioners. There was little difference in the outcome between the two groups. However, two subgroups of patients benefited more from outpatient counseling than from general practitioner care; they were as follows: (a) women and (b) patients with interpersonal problems. Counseling following overdoses should be focused on groups of patients such as these who are most likely to benefit from this counseling. Further work is needed to identify those treatment approaches that would help other groups who take overdoses, especially men. Therefore, counseling of this kind helps to solve some problems.

The randomized controlled trials studies by Clum et al. (1992), Eskin, Ertekin, and Demir (2008), Lerner and Clum (1990), McLeavey, Daly, Ludgate, and Murray (1994) generally made the same conclusion. PST could help, but it is not sufficient in the treatment of truly suicidal people. The studies have common problems; Lerner and Clum had 18 subjects, and McLeavey had 39. It is often unclear who the *subjects* are. What were the suicide risks? We especially question if some are more self-harm patients, than suicidal? McLeavey's is apparently so. Could PST be effective for suicidal people displaying tendencies with high lethality? Clum, Yang, Curtin, and their team performed such a study, but they are limited to 39 subjects. The question to be asked, as you read the following: What are we treating? Clum (1992) stated:

> Subjects were randomly assigned to treatment groups. Subjects received either (1) 10 sessions of a problem solving intervention, (2) 10 sessions of social support training, and (3) 5 sessions of a treatment designed to provide subjects with insight regarding the circumstances, situations.

They further stated:

> Subjects in the present study improved on measures of suicide ideation, depression and hopelessness regardless of the treatment employed. However, results were consistent with the constructs targeted by the respective treatments. Subjects in problem solving improved on both perceived social support and their perceptions of their ability to solve problems. Subjects in social support improved only on their perceived levels of social support. Subjects in the functional analysis group did not improve on any process measure. The possibility exists that the skills developed in the problem solving approach will continue.

The issue may be if we train in cognitive skills, the cognitive skills should improve. The real question is: Does it help in reducing suicide risk? Suicide attempts? Crawford et al. (2007), albeit in a very problematic systematic review, concluded, "no." There may be no primary evidence of reducing suicide. I am more optimistic; it all depends on the quality care, not this or that technique (see also Mann et al., 2005).

The Exclusions: What Does the Evidence-Based Research Say?

We excluded two major groups: the deliberate self-harm (DSH) group (see definition earlier, but mainly people with no suicidal intent) and the BPD group. The latter is excluded for a number of primarily specified reasons; mainly, they call for their own systematic review. They are different, but can be seen as a subsample of suicides sometimes. We let the leaders, Marsha Linehan and Anthony Bateman, speak about their studies.

Marsha Linehan, without a doubt, has advanced the study by randomized controlled trials the most, all with sound methodology. Linehan's therapy, as we have already learned, is called DBT. It is a cognitive-behavioral psychotherapy for suicidal patients with a diagnosis of BPD. Shearin and Linehan (1994) present a systematic review. The DBT treatment was shown to be effective; randomizing controlled trials show "superiority" (that word again) in reducing suicidal behavior, medical risk, hospitalization, dropout rates, and ability to adjust to/with anger. It is more effective than TAU, doing nothing and pure chance.

Linehan et al. (2006) show the effectiveness of DBT with a 1-year randomized controlled trial (yes, 1 year, not unexpected, if we are going to show effectiveness of psychotherapy with suicidal people. Ten sessions are not enough with suicidal patients with BPD too) plus 1-year post treatment follow-up! They studied 101 people (a significant number) with DSM criteria and recurrent suicidal behavior, all defined carefully. One year of DBT or 1 year of TAU with expert therapists was undertaken; 1-year follow-up assessment was undertaken for both the groups. DBT was associated with better outcomes during the 2 years of treatment and follow-up. Linehan concluded: "dialectical behaviour therapy appears to be unequivocally effective in reducing suicide attempts." There is no doubt that DBT can be effective; yet, is it the best psychotherapy for treating suicidal people with BPD? Is it "superior" or "unequivocally effective"?

Bateman and Fonagy (2001) reported that psychoanalytic (or psychodynamic) psychotherapy could be equally effective for treating suicidal patients with BPD. They studied, albeit a smaller sample, 44 patients, diagnosed so, over a period of 18 months. Patients were randomly assigned to psychoanalytic-oriented therapy with partial hospitalization group or to a TAU group, "standard psychiatric care." Over the 18 months, in an ongoing manner, they evaluated outcome variables: frequency of suicide attempts, number and duration of inpatient hospitalizations, service utilization, and self-reported measures of depression, anxiety, general symptom distress, interpersonal functioning, and social adjustment. The psychoanalytic group showed substantial gain compared to the control group on all measures. They concluded that they were the best, again the word *superiority* appears in the text, "The superiority of psychoanalytically oriented hospitalisation over standard psychiatric treatment found in previous randomized, controlled trials was maintained over an 18-month follow-up period." Not only Freud, thus, but also Linehan and Bateman claim their therapy to be the best. But so do Apsche, Bass, and Siv (2006) with a different treatment for suicidal people with BPD. Maybe all evidence-based psychotherapies, provided they render long-term care, are effective for treating suicidal patients with BPD (Leenaars, 2004). More research is obviously needed to answer the question, what type of psychotherapy is superior for treating suicidal people with BPD?

There is one more significant group excluded, the DSH group. Self-injurious behaviors or self-harm behaviors with no intentional cessation are not suicidal behaviors. These are behaviors that involve deliberate self-inflicted physical harm with no intent to die (see earlier discussion). Townsend et al. (2001) present a good systematic review of the topic. They undertook an extensive literature review of randomized controlled trials for DSH patients. They identified six studies, with variations in sample size, characteristics, and treatments; yet, all looked at whether PST (a brief 10-session PST) was effective with DSH people. Studies excluded people at risk for suicide; other exclusions occurred (e.g., hospitalization). They concluded, from the review, that training in a problem-solving approach was more effective than TAU. This was not only, however, true for occurrences of self-harm, but also for self-ratings on intermediate variables such as depression, hopelessness, and presence of problems. Testing for self-harm was not done, however. Yet, Townsend did caution, calling for the conclusion to be "confirmed by large trials, which will also allow adequate testing of the impact of this treatment on repetition of DSH." Tyrer et al. (2003) have shown "limited efficacy" of brief cognitive therapy versus TAU in reducing DSH. Guthrie et al. (2001) showed the same promise with group therapy versus TAU. Maybe all evidence-based therapies for people with self-harm behavior, like for people with suicidal behavior, are effective. Maybe there are commonalities that make them so (Leenaars, 2004; Lambert, 2004). To date, we would support the experts in this field.

On the method of study of DSH, Wood et al. (2001) concluded:

> Our preliminary study shows that it is feasible to conduct a randomised trial with this challenging group of patients, to the extent that the majority of cases agreed to enter the study and most agreed to have some treatment. However, our results also show that very large studies will be needed to detect reliably an effect of treatment on some indicators of repetition of self-harm. For example, we estimate that to detect a 33% reduction in the total number of episodes of repeated deliberate self-harm (which from a public health perspective is arguably the most important outcome), a sample size of approximately 150 cases in each arm would be required (p. 1252).

And, what needs to be done next to establish an evidence-based approach, Guthrie et al. (2001) concluded:

> These results are promising, but larger studies of interpersonal psychotherapies in different settings are needed to establish the potential costs and benefits of such treatments for patients who poison themselves. Studies comparing psychodynamic interpersonal therapy with placebo treatments and other psychological interventions may help to identify the active components of the therapy. Such research would inform our future approaches to a problem which is both difficult to manage and widespread (p. 4).

These are the same conclusions as for randomized controlled trials for suicide and suicidal behavior. It is true for studies of people with BPD too. The unanimous conclusion, whether included and/or excluded, in this systematic review is: *more study is needed.*

Effectiveness: Some Closing Arguments

"Is psychotherapy effective?" The topic has been central throughout this chapter. Psychotherapy is effective in helping people achieve their goal, such as being a better problem-solver, and overcome their psychopathology, even suicide risk (Lambert & Bergin, 1992). This is faster than TAU healing, leaving the sufferer alone, and the like (The critique of the Eysenck study shows that fact!). Of course, every psychotherapy has not been studied with every patient. Be that as it may, the average psychotherapy patient is better off than 80% of untreated people (Lambert & Bergin, 1992; Smith, Glass, & Miller, 1980).

The question of how much therapy is enough is important, both for practical and for theoretical reasons. Some espouse 10–12 sessions, but research shows that most patients would be underserved (Lambert & Ogles, 2004). This may not be psychotherapy, in fact (Freedheim, 1992; Leenaars, 2004; Lambert, 2004). For example, it may be PST, but is it psychotherapy? The answer is maybe; it fits our broader definition. Yet, this begets the question, "how much psychotherapy is needed?"

Lambert and Ogles, in fact, write:

> Research suggests that a sizable portion of patients reliably improve after 10 sessions and that 75% of patients will meet more rigorous criteria for success after about 50 sessions of treatment. Limiting treatment sessions to less than 20 will mean that about 50% of patients will not achieve a substantial benefit from therapy (p. 156–157).

Thus, even if we offer 10 sessions of PST, it is probably not enough. This fact is critical with *lethal* suicidal patients; indeed, I would suggest that accepting a highly lethal suicidal patient for brief intervention is suicidogenic (Leenaars, 2004). Indeed, most PST studies reviewed did not include really suicidal people. They did not allow such patients to be referred to the experimental group for 10 sessions of problem solving. Why? Simple: it is suicidogenic. These researchers knew that. Suicidal people often need long-term psychotherapy and more, not 10 sessions (Leenaars, 2004).

Are all patients helped by psychotherapy? Or are some patients not helped? Are there negative consequences? The literature is scant, and nothing on suicidal people in psychotherapy that do not benefit (Lambert & Bergin, 1992; Lambert & Ogles, 2004). Two variables that have been associated to negative outcomes in patients in psychotherapy are more severe problems at intake and significant interpersonal difficulties (both common in subjects excluded from almost all studies to date). The percentage of negative consequences may be as high as 5%, in fact (Lambert & Ogles, 2004), but then this is true with medication, hospitalization, or any treatment. Much greater research is needed; this, in fact, may well help in identifying those patients who benefit and those who do not.

What is ineffective? Are there common problems in psychotherapy with suicidal patients? This may well be one of the most important questions, namely because they can result – and have – resulted in deaths by suicide. There is only one, and most unique study on the question, the work of Hendin, Haas, Maltsberger, Koestner, and Szanto (2006). They examined the cases of patients who died by suicide while receiving psychotherapy (and most also medication and some hospitalization too). Therapists of 36 patients were studied by multiple methods. Hendin and his group isolated six recurrent problems: poor communication between therapists, permitting patients and their relatives to control the therapy, avoidance of issues related to sexuality, ineffective or coercive actions resulting from the therapist's anxiety, not recognizing the meanings of patients' communications, and untreated or undertreated symptoms. It would be important that all therapists, regardless of orientation, pay very careful attention to these *common* problems, not only in psychotherapy with suicidal people. Of course, much more process research is needed.

On one final point on effectiveness, change is multidimensional. Luborsky's work, for example, supports this fact (Strupp & Hadley, 1977); they emphasize the multiple effects of psychotherapy. It is not simply problem solving, although this may well be critical in some. Bergin and Lambert (1978) state:

> . . .divergent processes are occurring in therapeutic change; that people themselves embody divergent dimensions or phenomena; and that divergent methods of criterion measurement must be used to match the divergence in human beings and in the change processes that occur within them. This confirms the notion that any assumptions of uniformity in client characteristics or in changes thereof are simply mythical. (Kiesler, 1966, 1968) (pp. 171–172).

Once more, we are in the realm of complexity; thus, effectiveness too must be measured in complex and individual ways. Effectiveness means being person-centered.

How Much Do We Need To Know?

A key question that remains is how much do we need to know to be effective? The surgeon has the same question. This question is like, what aspects of therapy with suicidal people are common and effective? (Leenaars, 2004, 2006; Rudd, 2000). This is the need of process research; there are few studies on this topic. Surely we need to understand which factors are effective. The general research will guide us (Lambert, 2004).

Can we ever reduce effective psychotherapy to minute detail in a cookbook or manual? Or is knowledge of the general commonalities sufficient? Do we need absolute evidence? Or, at a given point of our randomized controlled trials studies, is more information better? My belief is that at a tipping point, we know enough about psychotherapy, as in surgery, to be effective (Gladwell, 2005), but then this is a general principle of learning (Saltz, 1971). The evidence-based therapist has enough knowledge and skills. He/she knows how to relieve suffering. He/she is a healer. He/she has the healer's ability to mobilize healing forces in the patient by psychological means (Frank & Frank, 1991). All you need is enough evidence-based medicine to be effective, and once you do, it comes knowingly. I will go further, past a point, the therapist might be more ineffective because there is too much information. The therapist is too dependent on the details of some manual or cookbook. Are we really going to need Occam's reductionistic psychotherapy? No. The reason is the common factors. I do not know how many, but we do know some core common factors and we know therapy, psychotherapy follows consequentially (Leenaars, 2006), and the therapist relationship (attachment) is central.

There is no question that some things in psychotherapy just happen. Like in any human exchange, the therapist relationship flows naturally. Of course, we should gather more information; we need to be evidence-based; yet, when a person's life is in imbalance, when a patient is truly suicidal, we have to do it knowingly. Too much detail may be suicidogenic; the reverse is true too. We have to be sure not to get muddled.

Evidence-based medicine can put some theory into our practice. It will sort out the mess. The *law* in effective psychotherapy with suicidal people is that truly effective healing relies on a balance between knowledge, such as randomized controlled trials and evidence-based psychotherapy, and natural healing. Those old enough among us will recognize this as the Boulder model (Freedheim, 1992). One has to be both a clinician and a scientist. A good clinician is a good clinician because he/she is evidence-based. He/she knows an I-Thou relationship. He/she can effectively engage in a human exchange. Second, to do so, he/she has to know the commonalities (Leenaars, 2006; Lambert, 2004). This is why no research has shown that one psychotherapy is best. Many are, not simply because of science, but also because of intuition's natural healing. One fact is clear: some people are good healers (Donaldson, Spirito, & Esposito-Smythers, 2005; Lambert, 2004).

Under what makes people good healers, there could be an endless list of factors. The research, in fact, has long shown that there is considerable consensus in studies that ask the patient what was most helpful; they will state the therapist (Lambert & Bergin, 1992). Some therapists are more effective than others (Lambert & Ogles, 2004); the influential early study of Luborsky, McLellan, Woody, O'Brien, & Auerbach (1985) has clearly demonstrated this fact. Lambert and Bergin (1992) agree; they cite some of the core conditions as empathy, worth, and positive regard. The list may seem like ones from Carl Rogers (1951), but Freud (1916/1974) and behavior therapists (Lazarus, 1971) too have embraced concepts such as warm, sensitive, and the like, and so have cognitive-behavioral therapists (Beck & Freeman, 1990). Lambert and Bergin (1992) stress these ingredients as essential means to establish rapport. Luborsky et al. (1985) state the same; they use such descriptions as "supportive," "liked very much by the patients," and "very persistent in trying to help." These are common factors in good healers.

We do not need to know everything about the best psychotherapy; we just need to know enough. We do need to learn more. What are the common factors that make psychotherapy with suicidal people effective? What stops suicide? What is an anodyne? What reduces pain and suicide attempts?

Concluding Thoughts

Of greatest importance, we must understand that the search for *a* singular universal response is a foolish and unrealistic fancy. There is no one evidence-based technique. There is no the "best" psychotherapy with suicidal people. The "best" does not exist, nor the "superior." The research (even the randomized controlled trials studies) strongly supports this opinion (Comtois & Linehan, 2006; Donaldson et al., 2005; Holmes, 2002; Lambert, 2004; Liberman & Eckman, 1981; Links, Bergmans, & Cook, 2003). How do we then effectively stop the lethal suicidal "pain"? How do we treat our suicidal patient? The answer from the research: there are many best evidence-based psychotherapies with suicidal people.

One can use an array of evidence-based psychotherapies with moderate to highly lethal individuals; many approaches are, in fact, effective (Donaldson et al., 2005; Lambert, 2004; Leenaars, 2006; Rudd, 2000; Rudd et al., 1996; Sudak, Ford, & Rushforth, 1984). Psychotherapy can be effective with suicidal people. This *FACT* is empirically supported/validated because there are common factors that make psychotherapy effective. The seeming uniqueness of a technique is simply semantic and stylistic. The common factors may be of overriding importance in effective psychotherapy (Leenaars, 2004). There are *commonalities*. This implies the need for process research (which has clinical implications). With the treatment of suicidal patients, this implies that our treatment should also be multimodal or multicomponent (Lambert et al., 2004; Leenaars et al., 1994; Shneidman & Farberow, 1957; Stengel, 1964; WHO, 2006). These measures may include support, cognitive-behavioral techniques, psychodynamic interpretation, medication, hospitalization, environmental control (I strongly believe this), a postcard (Carter et al., 2007), and especially the involvement of others in the community, not only others to whom the patient was (or is) close to but also "social" agencies – teachers, priests, elders, doctors, social workers, etc. – all of whom serve, directly or indirectly, to alleviate the pain (American Psychiatric Association, 2003; Lambert, 2004; Leenaars, 2004; Shneidman, 1985). There may well be many evidence-based adjuncts to psychotherapy that will result in greater effectiveness. One may well want to include 10 sessions of training in problem solving, but much more is needed with the truly suicidal sufferer. Treatment should often be multimodal, but what this *all* entails needs greater study.

A closer working alliance between therapists and researchers is needed (Strupp & Howard, 1992). This is not only true in psychotherapy with suicidal patients, but in the field in general. It is an essential ingredient. We need more collaborative efforts in evidence-based treatment with suicidal people. We need more research. However, as we learned, this does *not* mean that we should accept only randomized controlled trials studies, although they are essential, if we are going to be evidence-based. We need process research. This was a recommendation of the American Psychological Association's Task Force on Empirically Supported Therapy Relationships (2001). We need the Buddhist middle way. We need systematic reviews and meta-analyses, randomized controlled trials (with definitive and nondefinitive results), process research, and case reports (I strongly believe in this one). We need cultural sensitivity. We need all research, if we are going to be evidence-based in psychotherapy with suicidal people (Leenaars, 2004). Quantitative and qualitative studies are needed (Benjafield, 2002). We need to cultivate an approach in suicidology that attempts to reconcile and merge these modes. It is my belief, in fact, that by amalgamating the quantitative and qualitative approaches, the field of psychotherapy with suicidal people will become a more scientific enterprise. It will then become truly evidence-based. We need openness to knowledge and methods. I believe that the newer studies, reviewed above, have attempted to do so.

The current research supports the "openness" view (Holmes, 2002; Leenaars, 2004, 2006; Lambert, 2004; Rudd, 2000). This view is also supported by the recommendations of a task force of the IASR (Leenaars et al., 1997). Empirically supported psychotherapy does *not*, for example, mean randomized controlled trials *only*, as argued for by some quantitative researchers who only espouse such, but it does include them. Goldney (1998) in his review of effective strategies in suicide prevention concluded that research has, indeed, demonstrated that there are effective prevention strategies, but we have to be "creative" to show this. The same is true in psychotherapy, and thus, psychotherapy with suicidal people. Historically, in fact, the openness to methods of studying psychotherapy has been the most valuable paradigm (Lambert, 2004), not *methodolatry*. The use of simple linear drug treatment paradigm designs had limited value in psychotherapy research (Lambert, 2004; Lambert & Bergin, 1992). There is no *the* EST! Never was. A specific list of "proven" based treatments offer only "a false guarantee of effectiveness. Although many practitioners and the public may be comforted by the notion that they are offering or receiving an empirically supported psychotherapy, the fact is that the success of treatment appears to be largely dependent on the patient and the therapist, not on the use of "proven" empirically based treatments" (Lambert, 2004, p. 9). Beck, Lambert, Leenaars, Luborsky, Rudd, Shneidman, and Tarrier, as we learned, argue for being evidence-based. Evidence-based effectiveness in psychotherapy with suicidal people depends on individually tailored evidence-based therapy to the unique characteristics/qualities of each patient (*whom* we are treating). This is what the Evidence-Based Medicine Working Group (1992) stated too. This is the *best* psychotherapy with suicidal people.

Furthermore, The Task Force on Empirically Supported Therapy Relationships (2001) recommended – and Lambert (2004) and Leenaars (2004) agree – the concurrent use of evidence-based therapy within the context of research-based understanding of the person (*what and whom* we are treating) to generate the best clinical outcome. This is effective psychotherapy at its best. There is the *best* anodyne for *suicidal people*. This is "superior."

What works is quality care! This is as true in the therapy room as the operating room. There are *many* best psychotherapies with suicidal people. And, one final thought: To quote once more the Dodo bird, the wise one in *Alice in Wonderland*: "*Everybody* has won, and *all* must have prizes."

References

Ablan, J., & Jones, E. (1999). Psychotherapy process in the National Institute of Mental Health Treatment of Depression Collaborative Research Program. *Journal of Consulting and Clinical Psychology, 67*, 64–74.

Allard, R., Marshall, M., & Plante, M. (1992). Intensive follow-up does not decrease the risk of repeat suicide attempts. *Suicide & Life-Threatening Behavior, 22*, 303–314.

American Psychiatric Association. (1994). *Diagnostic and statistical manual of mental disorders* (4th ed., DSM-IV). Washington, DC: Author.

American Psychiatric Association. (2003, November). Practice guidelines for the assessment and treatment of patients with suicidal behavior. *Supplement to the American Journal of Psychiatry, 160*(11), 1–183.

Apsche, J., Bass, C., & Siv, A. (2006). A treatment study of suicidal adolescents with personality disorder or traits: Mood deactivation therapy as compared to treatment as usual. *International Journal of Behavioral Consultation and Therapy, 2*, 215–223.

Barlow, D. (2010). Negative effects from psychological treatments. *American Psychologist, 65*, 13–20.

Bateman, A., & Fonagy, P. (2001). Treatment of borderline personality disorder with psychoanalytically oriented partial hospitalization. An 18 month follow-up. *American Journal of Psychiatry, 158*, 36–42.

Beck, A. (1976). *Cognitive therapy and emotional disorders*. New York: International University Press.

Beck, A. & Freeman, A. (Eds.). (1990). *Cognitive therapy of personality disorders*. New York: Guilford Press.

Benjafield, J. (2002). Research methods: A history of some important strands. *Archives of Suicide Research, 6*, 5–14.

Bergin, A., & Lambert, M. (1978). The evaluation of therapeutic outcome. In S. Garfield & A. Bergin (Eds.), *Handbook of psychotherapy and behavior change: An empirical analysis* (2nd ed., pp. 139–189). Chichester, UK: Wiley.

Brown, G., Have, T., Henriques, G., Xie, S., Hollander, J., & Beck, A. (2005). Cognitive therapy for the prevention of suicide attempts: A randomised controlled trial. *Journal of the American Medical Association, 294*, 563–570.

Buber, M. (1970). I & thou (W. Kaufman, Trans.). New York: Charles Scribner's Sons.

Carter, G. L., Clover, K., Whyte, I. M., Dawson, A. H., & D'Este, C. (2007). Postcards from EDge: 24 month outcomes of a randomised controlled trial for hospital-treated self-poisoning. *British Journal of Psychiatry, 191*, 548–553.

Chambless, D. (1996). In defense of dissemination of empirically supported psychological interventions. *Clinical Psychology: Science and Practice, 3*, 230–235.

Chambless, D., & Ollendick, T. (2001). Empirically supported psychological interventions: Controversies and evidence. *Annual Review of Psychology, 52*, 685–716.

Chowdhury, N., Hicks, R., & Kreitman, N. (1973). Evaluation of an after-care service for parasuicide (attempted suicide) patients. *Social Psychiatry, 8*, 67–81.

Clum, G., Yang, B., Curtin, L., Pickett, C., Priester, T., Weaver, T., & Weiss, K. (1992). Problem-solving treatment of severe ideators. In D. Lester (Ed.), *Suicide '92: Proceedings. Silver Anniversary Conference* (pp. 173–174). Chicago: American Association of Suicidology.

Cohen, L., Sargent, M., & Sechrest, L. (1986). Use of psychotherapy research by professional psychologists. *American Psychologist, 41*, 198–206.

Comtois, K., & Linehan, M. (2006). Psychosocial treatments of suicidal behaviors: A practice-friendly review. *Journal of Clinical Psychology: In Session, 62*, 161–170.

Crawford, M., Thomas, O., Khan, N., & Aya, E. (2007). Psychosocial interventions following self-harm. *British Journal of Psychiatry, 190*, 11–17.

Dimidijan, S., & Hollon, S. (2010). How would we know psychotherapy were harmful? *American Psychologist, 65*, 21–33.

Donaldson, D., Spirito, A., & Esposito-Smythers, C. (2005). Treatment of adolescents following a suicide attempt: Results of a pilot trial. *Journal of the American Academy of Child & Adolescent Psychiatry, 44*, 113–120.

Donaldson, D., Spirito, A., & Overholser, J. (2003). Treatment of adolescent suicide attempters. In A. Spirito & J. Overholser (Eds.), *Evaluating and treating adolescent suicide attempters: From research to practice* (pp. 295–321). New York: Academic Press.

Elkin, I., Shea, M., Watkins, J., Imber, S., Stosky, S., Collins, J., et al. (1989). National Institute of Mental Health treatment of Depression Collaborative Research Program: General effectiveness of treatments. *Archives of General Psychiatry, 46*, 971–982.

Eskin, M., Ertekin, K., & Demir, H. (2008). Efficacy of a problem-solving therapy for depression and suicide potential in adolescents and young adults. *Cognitive Therapy Research, 32*, 227–245.

Evidence-Based Medicine Working Group. (1992, November 4). Evidence-based medicine. A new approach to teaching the practice of medicine. *Journal of the American Medical Association, 268*(17), 2420–2425.

Eysenck, H. (1952). The effects of psychotherapy: An evaluation. *Journal of Consulting Psychology, 16*, 319–324.

Frank, J., & Frank, J. (1991). *Persuasion and healing: A comparative study of psychotherapy* (3rd ed.). Baltimore, MD: John Hopkins University Press.

Freedheim, D. (Ed.). (1992). *History of psychotherapy.* Washington, DC: American Psychological Association.

Freud, S. (1974). Analytic therapy. In J. Strachey (Ed. & Trans.), *The standard edition of the complete psychological works of Sigmund Freud* (Vol. XVI, pp. 448–463). London: Hogarth Press (Original work published 1916).

Garfield, S. (1996). Some problems associated with "validated" forms of psychotherapy. *Clinical Psychology: Science and Practice, 3*, 218–229.

Garfield, S. & Bergin, A. (Eds.). (1978). *Handbook of psychotherapy and behavior change: An empirical analysis* (2nd ed.). Chichester, UK: Wiley.

Gibbons, J., Butler, J., Urwin, P., & Gibbons, J. (1978). Evaluation of social work service for self-poisoning patients. *British Journal of Psychiatry, 133*, 111–118.

Gladwell, M. (2005). *Blink*. New York: Back Bay Books.

Goldney, R. (1998). Suicide prevention is possible: A review of recent studies. *Archives of Suicide Research, 4*, 329–339.

Guthrie, E., Kapur, N., Machway-Jones, K., Chew-Graham, C., Moorey, J., Mendel, E., et al. (2001). Randomised controlled trial of brief psychological intervention after deliberate self-poisoning. *British Medical Journal, 323*, 135–138.

Hawton, K., McKeown, S., Day, A., Martin, P., O'Connor, M., & Yule, J. (1987). Evaluation of outpatient counselling compared with general practitioner care following overdoses. *Psychological Medicine, 17*, 751–761.

Hendin, H., Haas, A., Maltsberger, J., Koestner, B., & Szanto, K. (2006). Problems in psychotherapy with suicidal patients. *American Journal of Psychiatry, 163*, 67–72.

Henry, W. (1998). Science, politics, and the politics of science: The use and misuse of empirically validated treatment research. *Psychotherapy Research, 8*(2), 126–140.

Hepp, U., Wiltmann, L., Schnyder, U., & Michel, K. (2004). Psychological and psychosocial interventions after attempted suicide: An overview of treatment. *Crisis, 25*, 108–117.

Hirsch, S., Walsh, C., & Draper, R. (1982). Parasuicide: A review of treatment interventions. *Journal of Affective Disorders, 4*, 299–311.

Holmes, J. (2002). All you need is cognitive behaviour therapy? *British Medical Journal, 324*, 288–290.

Howard, K., Kopta, S., Krause, M., & Orlinsky, D. (1986). The dose effect relationship in psychotherapy. *American Psychologist, 41*, 159–164.

Katz, L., Cox, B., Gunasekara, S., & Miller, A. (2004). Feasibility of dialectical behavior therapy for suicidal adolescent inpatients. *Journal of the American Academy of Child and Adolescent Psychiatry, 43*, 276–282.

Kerkhof, A., & Diekstra, R. (1995). The prevention of suicidal behaviour: A review of effectiveness. In R. Diekstra, W. Gulbinat, I. Kienhorst, & D. De Leo (Eds.), *Preventive strategies on suicide* (pp. 207–229). Leiden: E.J. Brill.

Kiesler, D. (1966). Some myths of psychotherapy research and the search for a paradigm. *Psychological Bulletin, 65*, 110–136.

Kiesler, D. (1968). A grid model for theory and research in the psychotherapies. In L. Eron (Ed.), *The relationship of theory and technique in psychotherapy* (pp. 36–74). Chicago: Aldine.

Koocher, G. (2003). Three myths about empirically validated therapies. *Ontario Psychologist, 35*(3), 13.

Kuhn, T. (1962). *The structure of scientific revolutions*. Chicago: The University of Chicago Press.

Lambert, M. (Ed.). (2004). *Bergin and Garfield's handbook of psychotherapy and behavior change* (5th ed.). New York: Wiley.

Lambert, M., & Bergin, A. (1992). Achievements and limitations of psychotherapy research. In D. Freedheim (Ed.), *History of psychotherapy* (pp. 360–390). Washington, DC: American Psychological Association.

Lambert, M., Bergin, A., & Garfield, S. (2004). Introduction and historical overview. In M. Lambert (Ed.), *Bergin and Garfield's handbook of psychotherapy and behavior change* (5th ed., pp. 3–15). New York: Wiley.

Lambert, M., & Ogles, B. (2004). The efficacy and effectiveness of psychotherapy. In M. Lambert (Ed.), *Bergin and Garfield's handbook of psychotherapy and behavior change* (5th ed., pp. 139–193). New York: Wiley.

Lazarus, A. (1971). *Behavior therapy & beyond*. New York: McGraw-Hill.

Leenaars, A. (Ed.). (1999). *Lives and deaths: Selections from the works of Edwin S. Shneidman*. Philadelphia, PA: Brunner/Mazel.

Leenaars, A. (2004). *Psychotherapy with suicidal people: A person-centred approach*. Chichester, UK: Wiley.

Leenaars, A. (2006). Psychotherapy with suicidal people: The commonalties. *Archives of Suicide Research, 10*, 305–322.

Leenaars, A. (2009). *What is the "best" evidence-based psychotherapy with suicidal patients?* Manuscript submitted for publication.

Leenaars, A., De Leo, D., Diekstra, R., Goldney, R., Kelleher, M., Lester, D., et al. (1997). Consultations for research in suicidology. *Archives of Suicide Research, 3*, 139–151.

Leenaars, A., Maltsberger, J. & Neimeyer, R. (Eds.). (1994). *Treatment of suicidal people*. London: Taylor & Francis.

Lerner, M., & Clum, G. (1990). Treatment of suicide ideators: A problem-solving approach. *Behavior Therapy, 21*, 403–411.

Liberman, R., & Eckman, T. (1981). Behavior therapy vs. insight-oriented therapy for repeated suicide attempters. *Archives of General Psychiatry, 38*, 1126–1130.

Linehan, M., Comtois, K., Murray, A., Brown, M., Gallop, R., Heard, H., et al. (2006). Two year randomised controlled trial and follow up of dialectical behavior therapy vs. therapy by experts for suicidal behavior and borderline personality disorder. *Archives of General Psychiatry, 63*, 757–767.

Links, P., Bergmans, Y., & Cook, M. (2003). Psychotherapeutic interventions to preventing repeated suicidal behavior. *Brief Treatment and Crisis Intervention, 3*, 445–464.

Luborsky, L., McLellan, A., Woody, G., O'Brien, C., & Auerbach, A. (1985). Therapist success and its determinants. *Archives of General Psychiatry, 42*, 602–611.

Luborsky, L., Singer, B., & Luborsky, L. (1975). Comparative studies of psychotherapies. *Archives of General Psychiatry, 32*, 995–1008.

Mann, J., Apter, A., Bertolote, J., Beautrais, A., Carrier, D., Haas, A., et al. (2005). Suicide prevention strategies: A systematic review. *Journal of the American Medical Association, 294*, 2064–2074.

McLeavey, B., Daly, R., Ludgate, J., & Murray, C. (1994). Interpersonal problem-solving skills training in the treatment of self-poisoning patients. *Suicide & Life-Threatening Behavior, 24*, 382–394.

McNeilly, C., & Howard, K. (1991). The effects of psychotherapy: A reevaluation based on dosage. *Psychotherapy Research, 1*, 74–78.

Möller, H. (1989). Efficacy of different strategies of aftercare for patients who have attempted suicide. *Journal of the Royal Society of Medicine, 82*, 643–647.

Möller, H. (1992). Attempted suicide: Efficacy of different aftercare strategies. *International Clinical Psychopharmacology, 6S*, 58–69.

Morrow-Bradley, C., & Elliott, R. (1986). Utilization of psychotherapy research by practicing psychotherapists. *American Psychologist, 41*, 188–197.

Nathan, P. (1998). Practice guidelines: Not yet ideal. *American Psychologist, 53*, 290–299.

Norcross, J. & Goldfried, M. (Eds.). (1992). *Handbook of psychotherapy integration*. New York: Basic Books.

O'Carroll, P., Berman, A., Maris, R., Moscicki, E., Tanney, B., Silverman, M., et al. (1996). Beyond the tower of Babel: A nomenclature for suicidology. *Suicide & Life-Threatening Behavior, 26*, 237–252.

Orlinsky, D., Rønnestad, M. & Willutzki, U. (2004). Fifty years of psychotherapy process-outcome research: Continuity and change. In M. Lambert (Ed.), *Bergin and Garfield's handbook of psychotherapy and behavior change* (5th ed., pp. 307–389). New York: Wiley.

Patsiokas, A., & Clum, G. (1985). Effects of psychotherapeutic strategies in the treatment of suicide attempters. *Psychotherapy, 22*, 281–290.

Power, P., Bell, R., Mills, R., Herrman-Doig, T., Dovern, M., Henry, L., et al. (2003). Suicide prevention in first episode psychosis: The development of a randomised controlled trial of cognitive therapy for acutely suicidal patients with early psychosis. *Australian and New Zealand Journal of Psychiatry, 37*, 414–420.

Rogers, C. (1951). *Client-centered therapy.* Boston: Houghton Mifflin.

Rosenzweig, S. (1936). Some implicit common factors in diverse methods of psychotherapy. *American Journal of Orthpsychiatry, 6*, 412–415.

Rudd, M. (2000). Integrating science into the practice of clinical suicidology: A review of the psychotherapy literature and a research agenda for the future. In R. Maris, S. Canetto, J. McIntosh, & M. Silverman (Eds.), *Review of suicidology 2000* (pp. 47–83). New York: Guilford.

Rudd, M., Rajab, M., Orman, D., Stulman, D., Joiner, T., & Dixon, W. (1996). Effectiveness of an outpatient intervention targeting suicidal young adults: Preliminary results. *Journal of Consulting and Clinical Psychology, 64*, 179–190.

Salkovskis, P., Atha, C., & Storer, D. (1990). Cognitive-behavioural problem-solving in treatment of patients who repeatedly attempt suicide: A controlled trial. *Journal of Psychiatry, 157*, 871–876.

Saltz, E. (1971). *The cognitive bases of human learning*. Homewood, IL: The Dorsey Press.

Saskett, D., Richardson, W., Rosenberg, W., & Haynes, R. (1997). *Evidence-based medicine*. New York: Churchill Livingstone.

Saunders, S. (2003). Clients' assessment of affective environment of the psychotherapy sessions: relationship to session quality and treatment effectiveness. *Journal of Clinical Psychology, 54*, 597–605.

Shearin, E., & Linehan, M. (1994). Dialectical behavior therapy for borderline personality disorder: Theoretical and empirical foundation. *Acta Psychiatrica Scandivanica, 89*(Suppl. 379), 62–68.

Shneidman, E. (1973). Suicide. In *Encyclopedia Britannica* (Vol. 21, pp. 383–385). Chicago: Williams Benton.

Shneidman, E. (1981). Psychotherapy with suicidal patients. *Suicide & Life-Threatening Behavior, 11*, 341–348.

Shneidman, E. (1984). Aphorisms of suicide and some implications for psychotherapy. *American Journal of Psychotherapy, 38*, 319–328.

Shneidman, E. (1985). *Definition of suicide*. New York: Wiley.

Shneidman, E. (2001). Anodyne therapy: Relieving the suicidal patient's psychache. In H. Rosenthal (Ed.), *Favorite counselling and therapy homework assignments* (pp. 180–183). Philadelphia: Taylor & Francis.

Shneidman, E., & Farberow, N. (Eds.). (1957). *Clues to suicide*. New York: Harper & Row.

Silverman, M., Berman, A., Sanddal, N., O'Carroll, P., & Joiner, T. (2007). Rebuilding the tower of Babel: A revised nomenclature for the study of suicide and suicidal behaviors. Part 2: Suicide-related ideations, communications, and behaviors. *Suicide & Life-Threatening Behavior, 37*, 264–277.

Smith, M., Glass, G., & Miller, T. (1980). *The benefits of psychotherapy.* Baltimore: Johns Hopkins University Press.

Stengel, E. (1964). *Suicide and attempted suicide*. Baltimore, MD: Penguin.

Strupp, H. (1997). On the limitations of therapy manuals. *Clinical Psychological Science and Practice, 4*, 76–82.

Strupp, H., & Hadley, S. (1977). A tripartite model of mental health and therapeutic outcomes: With special reference to negative effects in psychotherapy. *American Psychologist, 32*, 187–196.

Strupp, H., & Howard, K. (1992). A brief history of psychotherapy research. In D. Freedheim (Ed.), *History of psychotherapy* (pp. 309–334). Washington, DC: American Psychological Association.

Sudak, H., Ford, A., & Rushforth, N. (1984). Therapies and intervention: A review. In H. Sudak (Ed.), *Suicide in the young*. Littleton, NY: John Wright.

Tarrier, N., Taylor, K., & Gooding, P. (2008). Cognitive-behavioral interventions to reduce suicide behavior: A systematic review and meta-analysis. *Behavior Modification, 32*, 77–108.

Task Force on Empirically Supported Therapy Relationships. (2001). Empirically supported therapy relationships: Conclusions and recommendations of Division 29 task force. http://academic.uofs.edu/faculty/NORCROSS/empir.htm.

Townsend, E., Hawton, K., Altman, D., Arensmon, E., Gunnell, D., Hazell, P., et al. (2001). The efficacy of problem solving treatments after deliberate self-harm: Meta-analysis of randomised controlled trials with respect to depression, hopelessness and improvement in problems. *Psychological Medicine, 31*, 979–988.

Tyrer, P., Thompson, S., Schmidt, U., Jones, V., Knapp, M., Davidson, K., et al. (2003). Randomised controlled trial of brief cognitive behaviour therapy versus treatment as usual in recurrent deliberate self-harm: The POMPACT study. *Psychological Medicine, 33*, 969–976.

Wampold, B. (1997). Methodological problems in identifying efficacious psychotherapies. *Psychotherapy Research, 7*, 21–43.

Wood, A., Trainor, G., Rothenwell, J., et al. (2001). Randomized trial of group therapy for repeated deliberate self-harm in adolescents. *Journal of the American Academy of Child and Adolescent Psychiatry, 40*, 1246–1253.

Woody, S., & Sanderson, W. (1998). Manuals for empirically supported treatments: 1998 updates. *Clinical Psychology Review, 51*, 17–21.

World Health Organization. (2002). *World report on violence and health*. Geneva: Author.

World Health Organization. (2006). *Preventing disease through healthy environments*. Geneva: Author.

About the Author

Dr. Antoon A. Leenaars, a psychologist, is in private practice in mental health, public health, and forensic sciences in Windsor, Canada, and is a Senior Advisor with the Norwegian Institute of Public Health, Norway. He is the first Past President of the Canadian Association for Suicide Prevention and a Past President of the American Association of Suicidology. He has collaborated with colleagues in over 35 nations and has published over 150 professional articles/chapters on violence, suicide, suicide notes, homicide, psychotherapy, gun control, ethical/legal issues, and related topics. He has published 12 books, including forthcoming *Suicide and Homicide-Suicide among Police*, and was the founding/first Editor-in-Chief of *Archives of Suicide Research*, the official journal of the International Academy for Suicide Research. He has served as an expert investigator/witness on cases of wrongful death, suicide, homicide, and homicide-suicide for police services, coroners, and lawyers, and lectures regularly worldwide on topics related to suicidology.

Antoon A. Leenaars
880 Ouellette Ave.
Suite 7806
Windsor, ON
Canada
N9A 1C7
Tel.: +1 519 253-9377
E-mail: draalee@sympatico.ca

Evidence-Based Psychosocial Interventions for Suicidal Behavior

What Is the Evidence?

James R. Rogers, Teri L. Madura, and Jennifer L. Hardy

Department of Counseling, The University of Akron, OH, USA

Suicide is clearly a major public health problem across the globe with over 1 million suicides occurring annually (DeLao, Bertolote, & Lester, 2002) and expectations that this figure will increase to 1.53 million deaths by 2020 (World Health Organization [WHO], 2009). Indeed, worldwide trends suggest a linear increase in suicide both as a function of historical time and as individuals age with highest rates for suicide generally evidenced among older adults. Although some of this apparent increase as reported by the WHO is likely a function of increased numbers of countries reporting suicide statistics and improvements in classification, the identification of suicide as a major, global public health problem is undeniable. Beyond deaths by suicide, the likely incidence and prevalence of nonfatal suicidal behaviors further highlight the critical need to address this worldwide phenomenon. Although accurate data on these behaviors are lacking, applying estimates of the ratio between deaths by suicide and nonfatal suicide attempts in the United States offered by the American Association of Suicidology (25:1; April 2009), a reasonable estimate of the global occurrence of nonfatal suicidal behavior for 2000 is 25 million.

In recognition of the vital need to address the problem of suicide, numerous approaches to prevention, intervention, and postvention have emerged. The purpose of this chapter is to provide perspective with regard to psychosocial interventions for suicide. Specifically, we focus our discussion on "evidence-based" "psychosocial" interventions identified in reviews of the literature and provide a context for considering further the status of research in this area.

Defining Psychosocial Interventions for Suicide

What initially appeared to be a relatively straightforward purpose, that is, identifying evidence-based psychosocial interventions for suicidal behavior, was complicated by the ambiguous definition of "psychosocial" in the literature. Specific to the literature related to suicidal behavior, the term psychosocial has lacked specificity and seems to encompass intervention strategies at the individual, group, and community levels. For example, Hawton et al. (1999) differentiated between "psychosocial" interventions and pharmacological approaches to treating suicidal individuals. Their review of psychosocial interventions included Problem Solving Therapy, Dialectical Behavior Therapy, inpatient behavior therapy, and the use of emergency cards as psychosocial interventions. Similarly, Crawford, Thomas, Khan, and Kulinskaya (2007), in addition to the interventions identified by Hawton et al., included such interventions as the use of self-help manuals in the context of brief cognitive behavioral therapy, psychodynamic interpersonal therapy, group psychotherapy, telephone interventions, and case management all under the rubric of psychosocial interventions.

Taking a somewhat different but equally inclusive approach to looking at psychosocial interventions for addressing the issue of suicide, Pompili, Angeletti, De Pisa, and Tatarelli (2006) distinguished between psychosocial "strategies" and psychosocial "treatments" in their discussion of interventions with individuals diagnosed with schizophrenia. These authors grounded their presentation of psychosocial strategies in a rehabilitation model and included cognitive therapy, psychoeducation, supported employment, social skills training, dual diagnosis treatment, and assertive community treatment as interventions under this model. In terms of psychosocial "treatments," Pompili et al. included family therapy, individual psychotherapy, self-help groups, group therapy, and community treatments and rehabilitation in this framework. Similar to the work of Hawton et al. (1999) and Crawford et al. (2007), Pompili and his colleagues have cast a wide net with regard to approaches that could be included under the general heading of "psychosocial" interventions for suicidal behavior.

Thus, it seems that the term "psychosocial" is employed in a very broad way that allows for many different treatment approaches and modalities to be considered. Because of its inclusive use in the literature, our initial undertaking was to search various databases to get a sense of the extent of the literature in this area. Despite the lack of definitional specificity with regard to the term "psychosocial," we employed that term in our search strategy. Thus, our own approach to identifying the literature related to psychosocial interventions for suicidal behavior included searches of the past 10 years using Medline, Academic Search Complete, and PsychNet. Table 1 provides a listing of the various searches we conducted across the three databases with the number of "hits" from each search. Across the search engines, we used the following four queries:

1. Psychosocial intervention and suicide.
2. Psychosocial intervention and suicide attempt.
3. Psychosocial intervention and suicidal behavior.
4. Psychosocial intervention and deliberate self-harm.

In the initial step of our search in Medline, PsychNet, and Academic Search Complete, we entered without any methodological specifications. Following this initial step, we identified studies in Medline that utilized specific methodologies (e.g., randomized controlled

Table 1. Psychosocial intervention searches within last 10 years (as of 4/16/2009)

Medline:

1. Psychosocial intervention and suicide = 1,187 total hits
   a. Clinical trial = 0 total hits
   b. Controlled clinical trial = 0 hits
   c. Meta-analysis = 0 hits
   d. RCT = 0 hits
   e. Review = 4 hits
2. Psychosocial intervention and suicide attempt = 204,196 total hits
   a. Clinical trial = 0 hits
   b. Controlled clinical trial = 0 hits
   c. Meta-analysis = 0 hits
   d. RCT = 0 hits
   e. Review = 0 hits
3. Psychosocial intervention and suicidal behavior = 403,248 total hits
   a. Clinical trial = 0 hits
   b. Controlled clinical trial = 0 hits
   c. Meta-analysis = 0 hits
   d. RCT = 0 hits
   e. Review = 0 hits
4. Psychosocial intervention and deliberate self-harm = 332,910 total hits
   a. Clinical trial = 0 hits
   b. Controlled clinical trial = 0 hits
   c. Meta-analysis = 0 hits
   d. RCT = 0 hits
   e. Review = 0 hits

Academic Search Complete:

1. Psychosocial intervention and suicide = 20 total hits
2. Psychosocial intervention and suicide attempt = 6 total hits
3. Psychosocial intervention and suicidal behavior = 14 total hits
4. Psychosocial intervention and deliberate self-harm = 1 total hit

PsychNet:

1. Psychosocial intervention and suicide = 164
   a. Literature review = 23
   b. Systemic review = 1
   c. Meta-analysis = 1
   d. Quantitative studies = 48
   e. Treatment outcome/randomized clinical trial = 1

(continued on next page)

Table I. Continued

2. Psychosocial intervention and suicide attempt = 23
    a. Literature review = 4
    b. Systemic Review = 0
    c. Meta-Analysis = 0
    d. Quantitative Studies = 9
    e. Treatment Outcome/Randomized Clinical Trial = 0
3. Psychosocial intervention and deliberate self-harm = 10
    a. Literature review = 0
    b. Systemic review = 0
    c. Meta-analysis = 0
    d. Quantitative studies = 6
    e. Treatment outcome/randomized clinical trial = 0
4. Psychosocial intervention and suicidal behavior = 68
    a. Literature review = 7
    b. Systemic review = 1
    c. Meta-analysis = 1
    d. Quantitative studies = 25
    e. Treatment outcome/randomized clinical trial = 2

Note. Subcategories related to the Medline search represent the methodological categorization options available for that search engine. Similarly, the subcategories under the PsychNet search represent that search engine's method specification options. No method options were available for Academic Search Complete.

trials, RCTs), by disabling the SmartText option resulting in the identification of only research articles which employed those methodologies rather than identifying any articles containing those words or phrases. Similar steps were followed for the PsychNet search using the preset methodology categories of that database. Methodological search functions were not available for Academic Search Complete. Thus, in addition to the general search results, Table 1 also provides search results obtained from the specific methodological searches when available.

As we conducted these searches and compiled the data, a few aspects became apparent immediately. First and most obvious was the appearance of a considerably large literature base that was easily identified using the term "psychosocial intervention" and various suicidal behavior-related terms. Case in point, within the Medline database, the number of hits ranged from 1,187 for "psychosocial intervention and suicide" to 403,248 hits for the more inclusive search phrase "psychosocial intervention and suicidal behavior." Similarly PsychNet searches ranged in the number of hits from a high of 164 for "psychosocial intervention and suicide" to a low of 23 for "psychosocial intervention and suicide attempt." The range of hits using Academic Search Complete was from 20 for "psychosocial intervention and suicide" to 1 for "psychosocial intervention and deliberate self-harm." Thus, there was considerable variability in the number of "hits" as both a function of search terms and search engines. The large number of hits and the variability across search engines are likely to be in part a function of the lack of specificity with the search term "psychosocial intervention."

Second, and related to the previous point, the initial results of these searches would suggest that we know much more about suicide and psychosocial interventions than might be accurate. Specifically, as we moved from merely identifying incidences in the literature where the various search words appeared to refining the searches as a function of methodological design and rigor using Medline and PsychNet filters, the numbers changed significantly. For example, within the Medline searches, no *randomized control* or *clinical trials* were identified, while PsychNet identified three *treatment outcome/randomized clinical trials* with one under psychosocial intervention and suicide, and two under the broader classification of psychosocial intervention and suicidal behavior. Thus, while it appears that a considerable amount of literature exists in this area, the question of the quality of that literature as it relates to providing a basis for developing interventions for suicidal individuals rests on specifying criteria for "evidence-based" practices.

Defining Evidence-Based

There is clearly controversy regarding the specification of methodological criteria for defining *evidence-based* research. For example, with reference to treatment research, the Evidence-Based Medicine Working Group (1992) suggested that randomization of research participants to conditions and the ability of researchers to account for all participants entering a study at its conclusion (including study dropouts) is the hallmark of evidence-based research. In the field of psychology, approaches to specifying what constitutes *evidence* were spearheaded by Division 12 (Clinical Psychology) of the American Psychological Association and became identified as the empirically validated treatment (EVT) movement (Chambless et al., 1996, 1998) and its related formulation as empirically supported treatments (EST) through Division 17 of the same organization (Wampld, Lichtenberg, & Waehler, 2002). While the EVT and EST approaches differ somewhat in the specification of criteria, there is agreement with the Evidence-Based Working Group that randomization is the key component necessary for strong interpretations with regard to evidence in treatment research. In fact, influential reviews of the literature related to psychosocial interventions for suicidal individuals generally have adopted the randomized controlled trials (RCT) or study as the gold standard for inclusion (e.g., Comtois & Linehan, 2006; Crawford et al., 2007; Hawton et al., 1999; Hepp, Wittmann, Schnyder, & Michel, 2004; Rudd, Joiner, Trotter, Williams, & Cordero, 2009).

Beyond the issues of randomization and control, as alluded to by the Evidence-Based Medicine Working Group (1992) is the matter of diagnosis. While suicide and other nonlethal suicidal behaviors do not represent independent diagnostic categories, the point made by the Working Group in this regard is relevant to the research in suicidology. Specifically, the Working Group indicated that to be methodologically rigorous, treatment studies must include "an appropriate spectrum of mild and severe" (p. 2423) cases of the treatment condition. With regard to the study of psychosocial interventions for suicide then, this would suggest that research studies include participants across a continuum of risk for suicide. Unfortunately, as identified by Linehan (1997) and reiterated by Rudd et al. (2009), the majority of studies in this area have specifically excluded high-risk participants, severally limiting the ability to identify evidence-based interventions for actively suicidal individuals.

Further complicating the issue of inclusion of participants across levels of suicidal risk is the lack of an accepted and systematic classification system for suicidal individuals (Silverman, Berman, Sanddal, O'Carroll, & Joiner, 2007a). Despite persistent efforts aimed at developing a nomenclature for classifying suicidal behaviors across the spectrum (e.g., O'Carroll et al., 1996; Silverman, 2006; Silverman, Berman, Sanddal, O'Carroll, & Joiner, 2007b), there remains little agreement in the field as to what are appropriate criteria for classifying individuals based on cognitive and behavioral indices. In fact, one basic assumption underlying much of the suicide-related research is that information gained from studying individuals who have engaged in nonfatal suicidal behaviors is generalizable in a way that helps us understand those who have died or might die by suicide (e.g., Rogers, Lewis, & Subich, 2002). However, that assumption has been challenged and remains only an assumption in the absence of rigorous empirical research (Rogers, 2003).

Adding to the confusion with regard to classification is the proliferation of numerous terms to describe behaviors associated with suicide. These loosely defined terms include suicidal thoughts, suicidal intentions, suicidal ideation, suicide gestures, parasuicide, deliberate self-harm (DSH), suicide attempts, and suicide completions to name a few. Lacking a systematic classification strategy for suicidal behaviors to differentiate levels of risk, the ability to unambiguously identify evidenced-based psychosocial interventions is severely hampered.

A final consideration in judging research as contributing to an evidence-based body of literature is the issue of outcome criteria which is necessarily tied to a conceptual understanding of suicidal behavior in general. That is, the goal of psychosocial interventions must be the prevention of suicide and nonfatal suicidal behaviors (Rudd et al., 2009). This goal as an outcome variable is intimately tied to a conceptualization of suicidality in terms of being viewed variously as a state-like time-limited phenomenon (as in the case of the crisis intervention model; Rogers & Soyka, 2004) or, as suggested by Comtois and Linehan (2006) a more long-term phenomenon with suicides subsequent to a nonfatal attempt most likely to occur within a 2-year time period. The impact on research methodology here is in identifying appropriate lengths of time for follow-up to judge the effectiveness of psychosocial interventions. For example, Rudd et al. (2009) have suggested that "Without longitudinal tracking after treatment, it will never be known whether *effective* treatments reduce suicide and attempt rates or just delay them for brief periods of time (e.g., 12–18 months)" (p. 340; emphasis added). We would argue that treatments cannot be termed "effective" in the absence of supportive data related to suicides and attempts over longer follow-up periods and that the specification of follow-up time frames should be grounded in relevant theory and/or data. Otherwise, what does it mean to be effective? Thus, a critical issue in the extant psychosocial intervention research is the lack of theoretical or conceptual arguments supporting researchers' choice of time periods for follow-up. Rather than theoretically or empirically derived follow-up time periods, it appears that tracking time frames in the existing body of research are somewhat arbitrarily determined or based on criteria other than researchers' conceptualizations of suicidal behavior in this regard.

In summary, there are a number of important criteria to consider when judging whether psychosocial treatment research outcomes provide support for an interpretation of evidence-based interventions for suicide. The first criterion, similar to many recent reviews of the literature in this area and supported by the Evidence-Based Working Group (1992), is that results must be based on RCT methodology. Second, again supported by the Working Group, studies must include moderate and high-risk suicidal individuals. Here, we would add the fact that those levels of risk or classification of individuals based on their status vis-à-vis suicide should be grounded in a clearly articulated and supportable classification scheme for their identification. Third, since "effectiveness" in this context is related to the prevention of suicide and nonfatal suicidal behaviors, follow-up assessment time frames should be rationally derived from an equally well-articulated theory of suicidality in terms of duration expectations. Although arguments surely can be made for different time frames, Rudd et al. (2009) have suggested that even "Follow-up of 12 to 18 months is not convincing ... but is a step in the right direction" (p. 341).

Rather than duplicate the recent multiple overlapping reviews of the literature on evidence-based psychosocial interventions for suicide that already exist, we next briefly present three prominent reviews of the psychosocial treatment literature in terms of inclusion criteria and conclusions drawn from those reviews (Crawford et al., 2007; Hawton et al., 1999; Hepp et al., 2004). Following this, we summarize the work of Rudd et al. (2009) in their critique of the treatment literature and provide an overview of their suggestions and recommendations regarding approaches necessary to advance efforts in this critical area. Finally, we add to the suggestions offered by Rudd et al. related to advancing research in psychosocial interventions for suicide and other nonfatal suicidal behaviors.

Reviews

Consistent with the identification of randomization and control as the backdrop for evidence-based interpretations, the primary inclusion criterion for the three reviews of psychosocial treatments for suicidal behavior was that the included studies provided random selection into treatment conditions and that those conditions included either treatment as usual or a control condition beyond the targeted intervention. In addition to randomization and control are criteria related to participants, outcome criteria, and follow-up time frames. Table 2 provides a listing of the relevant inclusion and outcome criteria for each of the reviews as well as the number of studies included in each and the range of time for follow-up.

Table 2. Inclusion criteria, number of studies, and outcome follow-up time periods across the reviews

	Crawford et al. (2007)	Hawton et al. (1999)	Hepp et al. (2004)
Inclusion criteria			
Interventions	"Psychosocial"	"Psychosocial" and pharmacological	Psychological and "psychosocial"
Methodology	Randomization Control comparison	Randomization Control comparison	Randomization Control comparison
Participants	Deliberate self-harm	Deliberate self-injury Deliberate self-poisoning	Suicide attempt Deliberate self-harm Self-poisoning
Outcome	Suicide	Repeated self-harm	Attempted suicide Completed suicide
Follow-up time (months)	3–24	3–24	4–24
Number of studies	18	23	25

Beginning chronologically with the Hawton et al. (1999) review, 23 RCT studies were included in their analyses. Conclusions drawn by Hawton and his colleagues were not positive in terms of providing evidence-based support for psychosocial and pharmacological treatments. In fact, their conclusion with regard to preventative efforts was that

> there continues to be insufficient evidence on which to make firm recommendations about the most effective forms of treatment for patients who have recently engaged in DSH. This is a serious situation given the size of the problem of DSH throughout the world and its importance for suicide prevention (p. 8).

From the perspective of these authors, the main limitations of the randomized controlled trials that they considered in their review were insufficient sample sizes and the lack of replication research. By contrast, the review by Hepp et al. (2004) that included 17 of the studies in the Hawton et al. (1999) review and an additional eight studies was a bit more positive in terms of conclusions. While identifying that none of the studies demonstrated a reduction in completed suicide, these authors suggested that five randomized controlled trials (three of which were also included in the Hawton et al. review) resulted in a significant decrease in DSH behaviors. These five trials included Bateman and Fonagy (1999), Guthrie et al. (2001), Linehan, Armstrong, Suarez, Allmon, and Heard (1991), Salkovskis, Atha, and Storer (1990), and Welu (1997). Of course, as suggested by Hawton et al., none of these studies have been replicated and except in the case of the Guthrie et al. study with 119 participants, have suffered from small sample sizes.

Finally, Crawford et al. (2007) reviewed 18 RCT studies, 16 of which were reviewed in the previous two intervention reviews. Unique to this review were the trials reported in

Brown et al. (2005) and Tyrer, Thompson, and Schmidt (2003). Crawford and his colleagues interpreted the results of their meta-analysis by stating that

> Results of this meta-analysis do not provide evidence that additional psychosocial interventions following self-harm have a marked effect on the likelihood of subsequent suicide (p. 11).

They noted, however, that individual RCTs indicated statistically significant reductions in repeated DSH behavior, but that it would be premature to extend those results to infer effectiveness with regard to suicide. Similar to Hawton et al. (1999), Crawford et al. pointed to small sample sizes in the reviewed studies as being a significant limitation to stronger interpretations. Thus, considering the conclusions across these three reviews related to attempts to identify evidence-based psychosocial interventions for suicide and nonfatal suicidal behaviors, it would appear that, at best, only tentative statements can be made related to what is known about effective interventions. Notwithstanding, and taking a less pessimistic perspective, Rudd et al. (2009) provided a critique of this body of literature with a focus on what *can* be learned from the RCT research on psychosocial interventions.

Rudd et al. (2009) provided a critical review of the literature on suicidality and psychosocial treatments that included the reviews in Table 2 as well as some additional literature. In their critique, these authors highlighted the paucity of RCTs and the limited methodological practices of the available RCTs as being a major stumbling block to advancing treatment effectiveness. In terms of methodological issues, they suggested that the exclusion of high-risk participants (i.e., multiple attempts of suicide and individuals who have recently attempted suicide) from many studies makes it difficult to generalize the results as efficacious treatments for reducing suicidal behavior. According to Rudd et al., many of the studies focused on measuring symptoms associated with suicide such as hopelessness, suicidal ideation, and depression rather than focusing on high-risk individuals who are most in need of treatment. Another area of critique noted by these authors was the limited follow-up periods that many studies have utilized as markers for treatment outcomes, suggesting that a 12–18-month follow-up period is a start, but to be sure of the outcome, longer follow-up periods are required.

From a more positive perspective, Rudd et al. (2009) were interested in identifying core elements across studies that may be associated with effective treatments and in determining if those elements shared any common themes. Thus, they focused on efficacy questions regarding appropriate treatment settings, diagnostic criteria, treatment durations, utility of booster sessions, retention rates and compliance, and specific elements of treatments that may be helpful and are as yet unanswered in the current literature. To look at these issues, Rudd and his colleagues focused on the RCT literature using cognitive behavioral treatment (CBT) approaches.

According to the authors, they focused on CBT-based approaches primarily because more support exists that identifies these approaches as successful in reducing rates of suicide attempts compared to other theoretically based treatments (e.g., interpersonal and psychodynamic). Highlighting the CBT-based studies of Brown et al. (2005),

Linehan, Comtois, and Korslund (2004), Linehan et al. (1991), and Salkovkis, Atha, and Storer (1990) which demonstrated reductions in suicide attempt rates, Rudd et al. (2009) identified eight commonalities. These commonalities across the studies include:

1. Being theoretically based and containing a language that is easy to understand.
2. High-risk cases with broad inclusion criteria.
3. Training clinicians well using manualized treatment and providing them with adequate supervision.
4. Treatment focus being specific to suicide rather than other associated symptoms or diagnoses.
5. Plan for compliance and continuity of care.
6. Interventions incorporating education on skill sets such as emotion regulation and problem solving.
7. Emphasis on internal locus of control and personal responsibility.
8. An element of crisis management.

In summary, Rudd et al. suggested that these common elements can be used to guide future RCT studies as well as to inform clinical practice, regardless of the theoretical orientation of the researcher or clinician. They concluded their critique by suggesting that there is a great deal that remains unknown about effective treatments of suicidality; however, integrating these common components into research and treatment protocols can be a step in the right direction.

Beyond the methodological issues of sample size, inclusion and exclusion criteria, and the lack of replication studies identified in the three reviews and the Rudd et al. critique, a consideration of the inclusion criteria listed in Table 2 in conjunction with our previous discussion clearly underscores additional reasons as to why research in this area has not resulted in the identification of clear support for evidence-based psychosocial interventions for suicidal behavior. As we suggested previously, a major issue here is the lack of specificity in the term "psychosocial" and attempts to employ the term in an overly broad and inconsistent manner. For example, even when controlling for date of publication different studies were included across the reviews, some indicating differing perspectives on criteria that constitute a "psychosocial" intervention. We would argue that advances in identifying evidence-based interventions will only accrue when we abandon attempts to artificially lump interventions together using such an inclusive and perhaps illusive category as "psychosocial." As we identified with the Rudd et al. (2009) critique, combining like interventions such as those authors did with CBTs, even though limited in number, allowed for the identification of some specific methodological components that show promise and can be integrated into future research to move the field forward.

A second major issue is the lack of specificity in inclusion criteria related to participants. As applied across the three reviews, the category of deliberate self-harm (deliberate self-injury, deliberate self-poisoning, suicide attempt, etc.) is very problematic as, like "psychosocial," the terminology is overly inclusive. Important here is a consideration that, for example, "deliberate self-harm" behavior may or may not be related to suicidality. Being a broad category, DSH is inclusive of the apparently growing involvement of individuals in what has become to be termed as nonsuicidal self-injurious behaviors (Muehlenkamp, 2006) where distinctions are based on suicidal intent or specific intent to die. Likewise, following the work of Silverman et al. (2007a), suicide attempt behavior can be categorized as with or without intent to die. It would seem reasonable to expect that there might be different treatment responses from research participants as a function of these important distinctions. While different terms have been used across the research in this area, what is important with regard to identifying evidence-based treatments for suicide and nonfatal suicidal behaviors is that future studies move away from broad classification strategies that are overly inclusive and focus specifically on suicidal participants as identified in an empirically or in a theoretically consistent manner that can be replicated.

Finally, it does not seem surprising that the reviews have provided only limited data related to identifying evidence to support suicide-related interventions when considering the variability in follow-up time periods. As indicated in Table 2, those time periods across the reviewed RCTs have ranged from 3 months to 2 years with most studies being around 12 months (Crawford et al., 2007). An important question to ask here is: What is the rationale for selecting those time frames for follow-up? Is the selection of time frames based on an empirical or theoretical distinction between suicidal states as acute versus chronic phenomenon (Conrad et al., 2009; Jobes, Jacoby, Cimbolic, & Hustead, 1997) or are they chosen for logistic or economic reasons? The wide variability in the extant intervention studies in conjunction with other confounds is likely to mask potential treatment effects and serve to hamper the advancement of research in this area.

Conclusion

Although the extant RCT research on psychosocial interventions for suicide and nonfatal suicidal behaviors is limited and has not resulted in the identification of interventions that would meet the criteria to be classified as evidence-based, there seems to be growing consensus with regard to the potential efficacy of cognitive behavioral interventions. Additionally, reviews and critiques of this literature have resulted in the recognition of methodological components of the existing research that can be used to inform and refine future research in this area. Furthermore, in our consideration of the research, we believe it critical that synthesis researchers reconsider the use of the overly inclusive categories of "psychosocial" and "deliberate self-harm" in their work and shift to greater specificity in their inclusion criteria for RCTs in meta-analyses and other reviews.

With regard to individual studies, in addition to considering the suggestions of Rudd et al. (2009) related to the development or delivery of RCT interventions, we believe it important to systematically differentiate between nonsuicidal self-injurious participants and those with suicidal intent as well as to distinguish between participants based on level of intent. As suggested by Rogers and Soyka (2004), the "one size fits all" approach to interventions with suicidal individuals has not proven to be effective.

Finally, we certainly support the conclusion of Rudd and his colleagues' suggestion that follow-up time frames of 12–18 months need to be expanded to draw conclusions on treatment effectiveness and efficacy. However, we believe strongly that, at the least, identification of time frames needs to be derived from an articulated theoretically or empirically based conceptualization of suicidality. That is, time frames should be tied to conceptualizations of suicidality as existing somewhere on a duration timeline from acute to chronic to lifelong. Thus, shorter time frames for follow-up may be appropriate if a supportable argument is made from a time-limited suicidal crisis perspective and the study sample is aptly identified.

In sum, past research and recent reviews of the literature related to psychosocial interventions for suicide have moved the field along considerably. It is time, however, to refine studies in this area from both theoretical and methodological perspectives in ways that will allow researchers to make strong and empirically supported recommendations related to the identification of evidence-based interventions for suicidal individuals.

References

American Association of Suicidology. (2009). Suicide data page: 2006. Retrieved June 19, 2009, from http://www.suicidology.org/web/guest/stats-and-tools/statistics.

Bateman, A., & Fonagy, P. (1999). Effectiveness of partial hospitalization in the treatment of borderline personality disorder: A randomized controlled trail. *American Journal of Psychiatry, 156*, 1563–1569.

Brown, G., Ten Haves, T., Henrique, G., Xie, S., Hollender, J., & Beck, A. (2005). Cognitive therapy for the prevention of suicide attempts: A randomized controlled trial. *Journal of the American Medical Association, 294*, 563 570.

Chambless, D. L. (1996). In defense of dissemination of empirically supported psychological interventions. *Clinical Psychology Science and Practice, 3*, 230–235.

Chambless, D. L., Baker, M. J., Baucom, D. H., Beutler, L. E., Calhoun, K. S., & Daiuto, A. (1998). Update on empirically validated therapies, II. *The Clinical Psychologist, 51*, 3–16.

Comtois, K. A., & Linehan, M. M. (2006). Psychosocial treatments of suicidal behaviors: A practice-friendly review. *Journal of Clinical Psychology: In Session, 62*, 161–170.

Conrad, A. K., Jacoby, A. M., Jobes, D. A., Lineberry, T., Shea, C., Fritsche, K., et al. (2009). A psychometric investigation of the Suicide Status Form with a psychiatric inpatient sample. *Suicide & Life-Threatening Behavior, 39*, 307–320.

Crawford, M. J., Thomas, O., Khan, N., & Kulinskaya, E. (2007). Psychosocial interventions following self-harm: Systematic review of their efficacy in preventing suicide. *British Journal of Psychiatry, 190*, 11–17.

DeLao, D., Bertolote, J., & Lester, D. (2002). Self-directed violence. In E. G. Krugg, L. L. Dahlberg, J. A. Mercy, A. B. Zwi, & R. Lozano (Eds.), *World report on violence and health* (pp. 183–240). Geneva, Switzerland: World Health Organization.

Evidence-Based Medicine Working Group. (1992). Evidence-based medicine: A new approach to teaching the practice of medicine. *Journal of the American Medical Association, 268*, 2420–2425.

Guthrie, E., Navneet, K., Moorey, J., Mackway-Jones, K., Chew-Graham, C., Moorey, J., et al. (2001). Randomized controlled trial of brief psychological intervention after deliberate self poisoning. *British Medical Journal, 323*, 135–138.

Hawton, K. E., Townsend, E., Arensman, E., Gunnell, D., Hazell, P., House, A., et al. (1999). Psychosocial and pharmacological treatments for deliberate self harm. *Cochrane Database of Systematic Reviews, 4*, 1–43.

Hepp, U., Wittmann, L., Schnyder, U., & Michel, K. (2004). Psychological and psychosocial interventions after attempted suicide: An overview of treatment studies. *Crisis, 25*, 108–117.

Jobes, D. A., Jacoby, A. M., Cimbolic, P., & Hustead, L. A. T. (1997). The assessment and treatment of suicidal clients in a university counseling center. *Journal of Counseling Psychology, 44*, 368–377.

Linehan, M. M. (1997). Behavioral treatments of suicidal behaviors: Definitional obfuscation and treatment outcomes. *Annals of the New York Academy of Sciences, 836*, 302–328.

Linehan, M. M., Armstrong, H. E., Suarez, A., Alllmon, D., & Heard, H. L. (1991). Cognitive-behavioral treatment of chronically parasuicidal borderline patients. *Archives of General Psychiatry, 48*, 1060–1064.

Linehan, M. M., Comtois, K. A., & Korslund, K. E. (2004). Dialectical behavior therapy versus nonbehavioral treatment by experts in the community: Clinical outcomes. In J. R. Koum & N. Lindenboim (Chairs). *Advances in the treatment of suicide behavior.* Symposium conducted at the 112th Convention of the American Psychological Association, Honolulu, HI.

Muehlenkamp, J. (2006). Empirically supported treatments and general therapy guidelines for non-suicidal self-injury. *Journal of Mental Health Counseling, 28*, 166–185.

O'Carroll, P. W., Berman, A. L., Maris, R. W., Mosciki, E. K., Tanney, B. L., & Silverman, M. M. (1996). Beyond the Tower of Babel: A nomenclature for suicidology. *Suicide & Life-Threatening Behavior, 26*, 237–252.

Pompili, M., Angeletti, G., De Pisa, E., & Tatarelli, R. (2006). Commentaries: Psychosocial intervention for reducing suicide risk in schizophrenia. In R. Tatarelli, M. Pompili, & P. Girardi (Eds.), *Suicide in schizophrenia*. Hauppauge, NY: Nova Science.

Rogers, J. R. (2003). The anatomy of suicidology: A psychological science perspective on the status of suicide research. *Suicide & Life-Threatening Behavior, 33*, 9–20.

Rogers, J. R., Lewis, M. M., & Subich, L. M. (2002). Validity of the suicide assessment checklist in an emergency crisis center. *Journal of Counseling and Development, 80*, 493–502.

Rogers, J. R., & Soyka, K. M. (2004). "One size fits all": An existential constructivist perspective on the crisis intervention approach with suicidal individuals. *Journal of Contemporary Psychotherapy, 34*, 7–22.

Rudd, M. D., Joiner, T. E., Trotter, D., Williams, B., & Cordero, L. (2009). The psychosocial treatment of suicidal behavior: A critique of what we know (and don't know). In P. M. Kleespies (Ed.), *Behavioral emergencies* (pp. 339–350). Washington, DC: American Psychological Association.

Salkovskis, P. M., Atha, C., & Storer, D. (1990). Cognitive-behavioral problem solving in the treatment of patients who repeatedly attempt suicide: A controlled trail. *British Journal of Psychiatry, 157*, 871–876.

Silverman, M. M. (2006). The language of suicidology. *Suicide & Life-Threatening Behavior, 36*, 519–532.

Silverman, M. M., Berman, A. L., Sanddal, N. D., O'Carroll, P. W., & Joiner, T. E. (2007a). Rebuilding the Tower of Babel: A revised nomenclature for the study of suicide and suicidal behaviors. Part 1: Background, rationale, and methodology. *Suicide & Life-Threatening Behavior, 37*, 264–277.

Silverman, M. M., Berman, A. L., Sanddal, N. D., O'Carroll, P. W., & Joiner, T. E. (2007b). Rebuilding the Tower of Babel: A revised nomenclature for the study of suicide and suicidal behaviors. Part 2: Suicide-related ideations, communications, and behaviors. *Suicide & Life-Threatening Behavior, 37*, 264–277.

Tyrer, P., Thompson, S., & Schmidt, U. (2003). Randomized controlled trial of brief cognitive behavior therapy versus treatment as usual in recurrent deliberate self-harm: The POPMACT study. *Psychological Medicine, 33*, 969–976.

Wampld, B., Lictenburg, J., & Waehler, C. (2002). Principles of empirically supported interventions in counseling psychology. *The Counseling Psychologist, 30*, 197–217.

Welu, T. C. (1977). A follow-up program for suicide attempters: Evaluation of effectiveness. *Suicide & Life-Threatening Behavior, 7*, 17–20.

World Health Organization, Suicide Prevention. (2009). *Suicide prevention: Live your life.* Retrieved from http://www.who.int/mental_health/prevention/suicide/suicideprevent/en/.

About the Authors

James R. Rogers, PhD, is a Professor in the Collaborative Program in Counseling Psychology at the University of Akron, OH, and an Adjunct Professor of Behavioral and Community Health Sciences at the Northeastern Ohio Universities College of Medicine and Pharmacy. In addition to serving as co-training director for the Collaborative Program in Counseling Psychology, Dr. Rogers also serves as the editor of the *Journal of Mental Health Counseling.*

Teri L. Madura is a doctoral candidate in the Collaborative Program in Counseling Psychology at the University of Akron, OH. She has co-authored a previous chapter on suicide and personality and her research interests include suicidology, ethics, and women's issues.

Jennifer L. Hardy is a School Psychologist and doctoral student in the Collaborative Program in Counseling Psychology at the University of Akron, OH. Her research interests include suicidology, ethics, and school-based mental health.

James R. Rogers
Department of Counseling
The University of Akron
27 South Forge Street
Akron, OH 44325-5007
USA
Tel.: +1 330 972 8635
E-mail: jrr1@uakron.edu

Evidence-Based Suicide Prevention by Helplines

A Meta-Analysis

David Lester

Department of Psychology, The Richard Stockton College of New Jersey, Pomona, NJ, USA

It has proven to be difficult to provide evidence that suicide prevention and crisis intervention services have an impact on suicidal behavior in the communities they serve. Typically, these services provide access to crisis intervention counselors by telephone 24 hours a day and 7 days a week. Occasional services may have walk-in clinics available during some hours and offer outreach services, such as shelters in depressed areas of cities and radio-dispatched teams to go out for emergencies in the community. While some suicide prevention centers include the term "crisis intervention" in their name, others label themselves solely as crisis intervention services. Thus, evaluating such services simply by focusing on the mortality of the clients is a rather narrow approach.

It is becoming increasingly important in mental health programs to evaluate the services provided. Partly because funding sources, public and private, are demanding feedback as to how beneficial their money has been for the community, and partly because in the past too many programs made claims for their usefulness that were undocumented or, when documented, found to be unsubstantiated, few programs can exist today without advancing some data to justify their continued funding.

On the other hand, faced with the demand that a program be evaluated, administrators are often hardpressed to find meaningful ways to do so. Inspection of the annual reports of telephone counseling services reveals that the most common way of demonstrating the effectiveness of the service is to present data on its activity. If an agency made contact with N clients, then this is seen as evidence of its usefulness to the community and justification of its continued funding. The astute observer who compares several annual reports will quickly note that the number N varies between 50 and 25,000 among different telephone counseling services, and yet each agency is satisfied with its performance.

A documentation of activity, though of interest, will not do as a measure of effectiveness for several reasons. First, the services rarely if ever have any notion of what the need of the community might be. Although the service may be counseling 100 clients a month, there may be 1,000 or even 10,000 people in the community in need of help. Second, the service may not be counseling those to whom it is directed. Suicide prevention centers counsel large numbers of clients, but the available evidence indicates that they rarely receive calls from the individuals in the community who are about to complete suicide (rather than those who are experiencing suicidal ideation or planning to attempt suicide). Third, there is no indication that those clients counseled received adequate, beneficial counseling. The clients calling the service might conceivably be helped more were there no telephone counseling service to call. Finally, telephone counseling services might be doing harm to the community, for example, by impeding the development of independence in its clients. Therefore, the presentation of data on the volume of activity of the service by itself is insufficient to answer these points. Better methods of evaluation must be used.

Because of the difficulty in evaluating crisis intervention helplines, Lester (1970a, 1970b, 1970c, 1970d), in a series of articles, suggested indirect ways of providing evidence to support the utility of such services, including

1. Counselor-rated improvement of clients.
2. Success in referring clients to face-to-face services.
3. The extent to which high-risk groups in the community have heard of the service.
4. Tracking to see whether completed suicides in the community ever called the service, a task made difficult by the fact that most clients remain anonymous.
5. The efficiency of the service (e.g., how long does it take a caller to get through to a counselor).
6. How well are the contact sheets completed by the counselors.
7. The counseling effectiveness of the counselors.

Thirty years later, Mishara and Daigle (2001) reviewed research exploring the evaluation of crisis intervention services using the criteria of client satisfaction with services, and the results of follow-up, repeated use of the services, and referral success. Mishara and Daigle also suggested the value of evaluating the process of the service provided, including the technical aspects (such as whether the counselor engaged in important aspects of the crisis intervention, Fowler & McGee, 1973) and clinical aspects (such as whether the counselor achieved high levels of empathy, Knickerbocker & McGee, 1973). Mishara and Daigle (1997) moved this type of analysis further by studying actual telephone contacts between clients and counselors, and relating the style of counseling with the outcome. For example, they found that a Rogerian (person-centered) style of counseling resulted in a greater decrease in depression by the end of the call.

In the next few sections, I examine the methods for evaluating suicide prevention services in greater detail. The first step is to evaluate whether the service meets its objectives.

The Objectives of the Service

It is obvious that to evaluate a program, its objectives must be clearly stated. Though obvious, this is rarely the case. Occasionally, the name of the agency implies an objective. A suicide prevention center has the unavoidable implication that, at the least, it will prevent suicide in the community. (That this implication is unavoidable may account for why many suicide prevention centers have reoriented themselves as crisis clinics!) Other services, such as teen hotlines, have no objectives implied in their title.

It would be a useful exercise for a telephone counseling service to try to formulate its idealized objectives, as Suchman (1967) has called them. What changes does the agency hope to effect in its community? The suicide prevention center might reduce the community's suicide rate or its attempted suicide rate; the teen hotline might reduce drug use, illegitimate births, absence from school for emotional reasons, or the incidence of delinquency; a crisis intervention service might reduce admissions to psychiatric facilities, reduce recidivism in former psychiatric clients, or speed up the referral process in which a distressed individual in the community is referred to an appropriate helping agency.

For an agency to be forthright enough to state its idealized objectives is a courageous act, for most likely these objectives may not be reached. (It would be wise, nonetheless, to be aware of the idealized objectives, even though they are not advertised.) The experience of telephone counseling services indicates that they release a flood of responses from the community which indicates a vast amount of emotional distress among members of the community who hitherto had no resources to which to turn. However, there are no data yet that counseling these clients has any general or specific effect on the mental health of the community.

Lesser Objectives

A telephone counseling service can formulate lesser objectives for itself. For example, if a service addresses itself to a particular subgroup of the population, several possibilities are available.

1. The potential clientele can be asked whether they have heard of the service, whether they have used it, and what their image of it is. For example, Motto (1971) found that 80% of a sample of depressed and suicidal clients admitted to a psychiatric unit had heard of the local suicide prevention center, but that only 11% had called it. Evidence from Los Angeles (Weiner, 1969) indicated that only 2% of completed suicides had called the suicide prevention center.
2. Who calls the center? If the center is addressed to a particular clientele, do these people call the service? For example, the typical completed suicide is old, white, and male. The typical caller to the Chicago suicide prevention center was young, black, and female (Maris, 1969).

3. Are the calls coming from the appropriate areas of the community? For example, if the suicide rate is high in a particular locale in the community, does the center receive a high proportion of calls from that locale? In Buffalo, Lester (1971) was able to demonstrate that this was occurring. The monitoring of the areas where calls come from to the agency enables the agency, if it desires, to adjust its advertising and outreach activities accordingly and so provides useful feedback to the agency.

Categories of Evaluation

Aside from the objectives of a program, Suchman (1967) noted that programs can be evaluated in terms of the different types of effects that they have on the community. These categories represent different criteria by which a program may be judged. To date, very little research or evaluation of telephone counseling services has been conducted for any of these criteria. However, it may be informative to list the criteria mentioned by Suchman.

1. *Effort*. What is the quantity and the quality of the activity that takes place and how does this compare to the counseling resources? This, of course, varies from service to service. The Suicide Prevention and Crisis Service in Buffalo served a community of about one million and received some 24,000 client calls a year on its three telephone services (suicide prevention service, teen hotline, and problems-in-living service). The service was staffed by about 75 volunteers. The quality of the service was unknown.
2. *Performance*. What is the effect of the effort put out by the service? Do people receive help from the service? A few studies have attempted to follow up callers to telephone counseling services and assess the impact of the service. For example, Murphy et al. (1969) interviewed a sample of callers to a suicide prevention center who had called on their own behalf and found that only about half had followed through on the advice given to them by the counselor.
3. *Adequacy of performance*. Is the performance of a service sufficient to cope with the community need?
4. *Efficiency*. Could the service provided by the agency be better provided by a different kind of agency or by an agency with a different structure?
5. *Process*. How does the agency produce the results that it does?

Evaluating the Internal Operations

So far, the methods of evaluation discussed have been unsuitable for the majority of telephone counseling services. To evaluate idealized objectives is a gamble. To evaluate lesser objectives is expensive. To evaluate in the areas suggested by Suchman is to break new ground for telephone counseling services, and most services are not equipped to do this.

What can telephone services do to evaluate their services if these alternatives are not feasible?

A number of telephone counseling services that do evaluate their performance focus upon low-level objectives concerned primarily with the internal operation of the agency, the administrative functions, and the performance of the counselors. There are many possibilities here and a number of them are described below.

The Internal Operation of the Agency

1. How long does it take to obtain a counselor at a telephone counseling service? Lester (1970a) called a telephone counseling service at different hours during the week and noted how long it took a counselor to answer the telephone and how often he obtained a busy signal. In this way, a center can identify peak periods of activity and monitor the performance of its counselors. McGee et al. (1973) called different centers in the southeast United States and noted the time that passed until a counselor was obtained. This latter study provided data on the speed with which a center could respond to a call depending upon its system for answering calls: an answering service, use of a local agency such as the fire station, locating the counselors at their homes or in the center, and so forth.
2. The success in referring clients to other resources can be noted by finding out the proportion of referrals who show at these resources. The Suicide Prevention and Crisis Service in Buffalo referred clients to its own crisis clinic, and Lester (1970b) studied the proportion of referrals who showed. Over several months, this varied from 29% to 56%. The success in referring clients can also be noted for each counselor. Following up on this finding, Lester (1970e; Lester & Priebe, 1971) tried to identify from the data on the initial contact sheets (completed by the counselors when a client first called) those characteristics that distinguished shows from no-shows. The shows were older, less likely to be single, and more likely to be calling on the suicide prevention line than on the other lines (teen hotline and problems-in-living line).

   Slaikeu et al. (1973) pursued this issue by carrying out a content analysis of the telephone calls during which shows and no-shows were referred to the crisis clinic. The major finding was that clients who themselves suggested a referral were more likely to show. In this way, it is possible to provide feedback to the counselors as to the factors likely to lead a client to follow through with the referral made for him.
3. The completeness with which client records are kept can be assessed. Do counselors obtain the information from clients that the center requires? Kolker and Katz (1971) found at their suicide prevention center that, if counselors failed to note down the age of the caller, then they were also less likely to collect information necessary to recontact the client if this is necessary (if the client hangs up, if the line inadvertently gets disconnected, or for a follow-up contact).

Whittemore (1970) compared samples of initial contact sheets at different centers and noted that whereas the sex of the client was noted in 99.9% of the calls he checked, the age was not noted for 16.9% of the callers, marital status was unknown for 10.4%, and religion was unknown for over 75%.

4. Whittemore (1970) in his comparison of 10 centers provided data on the kinds of callers and calls that different centers receive. For example, Whittemore found that the proportion of anonymous calls at the 10 centers varied from 18% to 63%. The proportion of calls with no suicidal involvement varied from 43% to 79%. Telephone counseling services can easily collect their own data and compare the data to those from the 10 centers studied by Whittemore.
5. Many centers ask counselors to rate the improvement of the clients as a result of the telephone contact. This rating can provide some data as to how well the counselors feel that they are performing.
6. Although it is obvious that the cost of the service is not necessarily related to the adequacy and quality of the service, the cost per telephone contact can easily be computed and compared with other centers.
7. Motto (1969) devised a set of standards for suicide prevention centers in terms of the adequacy of the administration, staffing, and evaluation of the program, the training and supervision of counselors, consultation resources, and ethical standards. The American Association of Suicidology now has a formal program in place to evaluate crisis intervention services to see whether they meet these standards (www.suicidology.org).

The Adequacy of the Counselor's Performance

A separate and crucial area for evaluation is the adequacy of the counseling provided by the staff of a telephone counseling service. Most centers require some kind of supervision of counselors, and this is, of course, crucially important. However, it is also necessary to devise standardized means of evaluating the effectiveness of counselors. Not all centers can obtain adequate supervisors for counselors, and not all supervisors are competent. The availability of standardized evaluation procedures would enable centers to make additional checks on the competence of their staff and, furthermore, enable centers to compare their performance with that of other centers.

Knickerbocker and McGee (1973) trained judges to make ratings of concreteness, empathy, warmth, and genuineness, as defined by Carkhuff (1969), and then gave them written excerpts from actual conversations between telephone counselors and clients to rate. Interestingly, Knickerbocker and McGee found that lay volunteers obtained higher scores than professional volunteers on these dimensions, but both groups performed at an acceptable level. Applying these to the functioning of a sample of counselors at the Suicide Prevention and Crisis Service in Buffalo, Lester (1970d) found that the only dimension that appeared to be related to whether a client shows or fails to show for an appointment at the center was the dimension of concreteness.

Fowler and McGee (1973) developed a "technical effectiveness" scale that measured the performance of the counselors at the tasks they were supposed to do, including

1. Can the caller be immediately recontacted?
2. Did the counselor ask for or obtain specific information regarding significant others?
3. Were specific problems identified?
4. Did the counselor communicate that he/she is willing to help?
5. Did the counselor develop a structured plan of action or help the caller develop one?
6. Did the caller agree to the action plan?
7. Was it determined whether or not this was a suicide case?
8. Did the counselor ask about a suicide plan?
9. or, if the caller voluntarily disclosed the information, did the counselor inquire for further details?
10. Was it determined if the caller had made prior suicide attempts?

Fowler and McGee had judges make these ratings from recordings of actual telephone calls made by clients and showed that the scale could be employed meaningfully to compare counselors and to monitor the progress of individual counselors over time. Rogers and Subich (1990) have also explored the usefulness of a standardized means of data collection and risk assessment of clients by telephone counselors.

Mishara and Daigle (1992) had observers listen in to actual calls at two suicide prevention centers in Quebec. The observers classified the types of statements made by counselors, finding that the most frequent response was *acceptance*, followed by *orientation investigation* (asking direct questions). The observers also rated changes in the depression level of the client (about 14% of the clients were judged to have become less depressed by the end of the call), changes in the probability of suicidal behavior in the client (27% of the clients were judged to have a lower suicidal risk at the end of the call), and whether the counselor and client reached an agreement (which happened in 68% of the calls).

Others have made simulated crisis calls to telephone counselors. Williamson et al. (1973) devised a series of simulated client calls. In these, an actor calls the counselor (who may or may not be informed that the call is a test call) and presents a rehearsed role. The response of the counselor to this standardized call can then be evaluated.

Bobevski and McLennan (1998) had counselors come into the clinic and handle calls from people they knew to be role-playing. Bobevski and McLennan found that the effectiveness of the counselors, as rated by the callers, was related to the level of the counselors' expertise, the cognitive effort they put into the counseling, the level of emotional involvement with the caller, and their level of anxiety.

Do these simulated calls assess behavior when taking real calls? Garrett et al. (1993) had counselors take a simulated call and then real calls while an evaluator listened in. They found that performance on the simulated call predicted performance on the real calls quite well.

Research to explore which traits predict performance as a telephone counselor would be useful in helping crisis service staff select new counselors. Along these lines,

Tekavcic-Grad and Farberow (1989) asked telephone crisis counselors in Ljubljana (Yugoslavia) and Los Angeles (USA) to list the traits that a good counselor should possess. Both sets of counselors rated motivation to work and being a good listener as the most important traits. However, while the counselors in Los Angeles felt that they possessed the desirable traits for being a good counselor, counselors in Ljubljana did not. Research to identify traits that actually predict good counselor performance would be useful for those involved in the selection and training of telephone counselors.

To explore reasons for the high drop-out rate of telephone counselors (Mahoney & Pechura, 1980), Mishara and Giroux (1993) explored determinants of the stress level experienced by telephone counselors. They found that experience as a counselor, the urgency of the call, and inappropriate coping mechanisms on the part of the counselors contributed to their stress level, and they made recommendations for the selection and training of counselors based on their findings. The adequacy of the training program for telephone counselors can also be evaluated (Tierney, 1991).

Several recent studies have explored how attempted suicides rate the treatment they received at the hospitals to which they went or were taken (Grootenhuis & Papp, 1993; Kocmur & Zavasnik, 1991; Treloar & Pinfold, 1993). For example, Grootenhuis and Papp (1993) found that their sample of suicide attempters wished that they had been treated in a "more human way." It would be of interest to follow up clients of suicide prevention centers to see how they evaluate the service.

Discussion

Traditional crisis counseling is based on the person-centered system of therapy devised by Carl Rogers. Rogers always advocated the importance of formulating goals for counseling and of evaluating whether these goals were met. Rogers and his staff and students at the counseling center, which he established at the University of Chicago, recorded and analyzed interviews with clients, followed up clients to see whether they improved and devised ways of testing whether one method or another was better for producing change in their clients (Kirschenbaum, 1979). For Rogers, research was not incompatible with providing excellent services. Indeed, without research, he could not be sure that the center provided excellent services!

Do Suicide Prevention Services Prevent Suicide?

The critical issue in evaluating the effectiveness of suicide prevention and crisis intervention services is whether they have an impact on suicide. Although it would be of interest to examine whether these services have an impact on nonfatal suicidal behavior (known as attempted suicide, parasuicide, or deliberate self-harm), most communities do not have adequate record keeping to assess the incidence of these nonfatal suicide behaviors and changes in this incidence.

Therefore, research is restricted to an examination of whether these services prevent completed suicide. In an early review of the research on this question, Dew et al. (1987) examined five studies and concluded that there was no overall combined evidence for a preventive impact. However, Dew et al. did not review all of the studies available at that time on this issue. Lester (1997a) provided a complete review of all of the impact studies and combined the results in a meta-analysis. Lester identified 21 published studies on whether suicide prevention centers prevent suicide, but several of these 21 papers were further analyses or reports of the same data sets. There remained only 14 independent studies. Since then three further papers have appeared, and the present chapter includes the results of these studies in the meta-analysis.

The meta-analysis was guided by Rosenthal (1984) who provided formulae for transforming any statistic to a Pearson's correlation. Averaging of correlation coefficients, both within studies and between studies, was done using Fisher's z method (Ferguson, 1976). In some cases, the data from the study were reanalyzed for the present meta-analysis. The studies are of two major types: (1) ecological in which the suicide rates of regions with different numbers of suicide prevention centers are compared and (2) time series in which the association between the number of centers in one region each year (a number that typically grows over time) with the annual suicide rate is studied over time. The ecological studies are of two types: (1) in a given year, the number of suicide prevention centers in each region is compared with the suicide rate of the regions and (2) the number of suicide prevention centers in each region is compared with changes in the suicide rates of those regions over a period of time. The original studies and the results are shown in Table 1. The overall Pearson correlation was −0.09 with 2,562 degrees of freedom, indicating a small, but highly significant, preventive effect from suicide prevention centers on the suicide rate.

Three new studies have appeared since Lester's (1997a) meta-analysis: Leenaars and Lester (2004) reported a follow-up study on Canada, Lester (1997b) reported a study on the five major regions of Great Britain and Ireland, and Lester (2004) reported a time-series study of Scotland. The data from these three studies have been added to Table 1, and the overall average effect recalculated (see Table 1). The resulting average correlation coefficient was −0.09 with 3,068 degrees of freedom, still a small, statistically significant, preventive effect from suicide prevention centers on the suicide rate.

All of these studies were, of course, correlational and do not show cause-and-effect relationships. Furthermore, few of the studies considered other mediating variables on the suicide rates, such as changing socioeconomic conditions and changes in the methods for certifying suicides. For example, Lester (1990) contrasted the impact of the growth of the number of suicide prevention centers in England and Wales, and the detoxification of domestic gas on the suicide rates of the counties. Although Lester did not find any significant impact of either factor, this study illustrates the importance of controlling for other factors. In particular, changes in the accurate certification of suicide play a major role in changing suicide rates in some nations (e.g., Cantor, Leenaars, & Lester, 1997; Lester 2002).

Table 1. A meta-analysis of studies on whether suicide prevention services prevent suicide

	Pearson (*r*)	*df*	Type of study	Nation	Time period
Original meta-analysis					
Bridge et al. (1977)	−0.05	194	B	USA counties	1970–1971
Huang and Lester (1995)	−0.35	15	C	Taiwan	1965–1985
Jennings et al. (1978)	0.08	97	A	English boroughs	1957–1973
Leenaars and Lester (1995)	−0.22	96	A	Canadian provinces	1985–1991
Lester (1974)	−0.11	22	A	USA cities	1960–1969
Lester (1980)/Bagley (1968)	−0.35	54	A	English towns	1957–1964
Lester (1990)	−0.18	18	A	English towns	1958–1967
Lester (1993)	−0.1	405	A	USA states	1970–1980
Lester (1994)	−0.13	90	C	England	1960–1975
Lester et al. (1996)	−0.22	183	C	Japan	1970–1989
Medoff (1984)	−0.11	462	B	USA states	1979
Miller et al. (1984)	−0.05	924	A	USA counties	1968–1972
Riehl et al. (1988)	No data		C	German cities	1945+
Weiner (1969)	−0.31	2	C	USA cities	1955–1967
Average	−0.09	2,562			
New studies					
Leenaars and Lester (2004)	−0.22	216	A	Canadian provinces	1985–1989/ 1994–1998
Lester (1997b)	−0.13	101	C	UK and Ireland	1952–1985
Lester (2005)	0.2	189	C	Scotland	1958–1981
New average	−0.09	3,068			

A, ecological study of changes over time in the regions; B, single year ecological studies; and C, time-series studies on a single region.

The preventive effect of suicide prevention centers on the suicide rate, though small, is encouraging. It is critical that researchers continue to work on this issue using longer time periods, other nations, and more sophisticated research designs so that we can have a more reliable meta-analysis in the future.

References

Bagley, C. (1968). The evaluation of a suicide prevention scheme by an ecological method. *Social Science & Medicine, 2*, 1–4.

Bobevski, I., & McLennan, J. (1998). The telephone counseling interview as a complex, dynamic, decision process. *Journal of Psychology, 132*, 47–60.

Bridge, T., Potkin, S., Zung, W., & Soldo, B. (1977). Suicide prevention centers. *Journal of Nervous and Mental Disease, 164*, 18–24.

Cantor, C. H., Leenaars, A. A., & Lester, D. (1997). Under-reporting of suicide in Ireland 1960–1989. *Archives of Suicide Research, 3*, 5–12.

Carkhuff, R. (1969). *Helping and human relations*. New York: Holt, Rinehart, & Winston.

Dew, M. A., Bromet, E. J., Brent, D., & Greenhouse, J. B. (1987). A quantitative literature review of the effectiveness of suicide prevention centers. *Journal of Consulting and Clinical Psychology, 55*, 239–244.

Ferguson, G. A. (1976). *Statistical analysis in psychology and education*. New York: McGraw-Hill.

Fowler, D. E., & McGee, R. K. (1973). Assessing the performance of telephone crisis workers. In D. Lester & G. W. Brockopp (Eds.), *Crisis intervention and counseling by telephone* (pp. 287–297). Springfield, IL: Charles Thomas.

Garrett, C. R., Teare, J. F., Reed, C. R., Shanahan, D. L., & Coughlin, D. D. (1993). Counselor evaluation. In D. Lester (Ed.), *Suicide '93* (pp. 109–111). Denver, CO: American Association of Suicidology.

Grootenhuis, M. A., & Papp, R. P. (1993). How do suicide attempters evaluate the treatment in a general hospital? *Italian Journal of Suicidology, 3*, 25–28.

Huang, W. C., & Lester, D. (1995). Have suicide prevention centers prevented suicide in Taiwan? *Chinese Journal of Mental Health, 8*(3), 27–29.

Jennings, C., Barraclough, B. M., & Moss, J. R. (1978). Have the Samaritans lowered the suicide rate? *Psychological Medicine, 8*, 413–422.

Kirschenbaum, H. (1979). *On becoming Carl Rogers*. New York: Delacorte.

Knickerbocker, D. A., & McGee, R. K. (1973). Clinical effectiveness of nonprofessional and professional telephone workers in a crisis intervention center. In D. Lester & G. W. Brockopp (Eds.), *Crisis intervention and counseling by telephone* (pp. 298–309). Springfield, IL: Charles Thomas.

Kocmur, M., & Zavasnik, A. (1991). Patients' experience of the therapeutic process in a crisis intervention unit. *Crisis, 12*(1), 69–81.

Kolker, H., & Katz, S. (1971). If you've missed the age you've missed a lot. *Crisis Intervention, 3*, 34–37.

Leenaars, A. A., & Lester, D. (1995). Impact of suicide prevention centers on suicide in Canada. *Crisis, 16*, 39.

Leenaars, A. A., & Lester, D. (2004). The impact of suicide prevention centers on the suicide rate in the Canadian provinces. *Crisis, 25*, 65–68.

Lester, D. (1970a). Steps toward the evaluation of a suicide prevention center: Part one. *Crisis Intervention, 2*(Suppl. 2), 42–45.

Lester, D. (1970b). Steps toward the evaluation of a suicide prevention center: Part two. *Crisis Intervention, 2*(Suppl. 1), 12–18.

Lester, D. (1970c). Steps toward the evaluation of a suicide prevention center: Part three. *Crisis Intervention, 2*(Suppl. 1), 19–21.

Lester, D. (1970d). Steps toward the evaluation of a suicide prevention center: Part four. *Crisis Intervention, 2*(Suppl. 4), 20–22.

Lester, D. (1970e). A comparison of patients who show for appointments and those who do not show. *Crisis Intervention, 2*, 75–76.

Lester, D. (1971). Geographical location of callers to a suicide prevention center. *Psychological Reports, 28*, 421–422.

Lester, D. (1974). Effect of suicide prevention centers on suicide rates in the United States. *Health Services Reports, 89*, 37–39.

Lester, D. (1980). Suicide prevention by the Samaritans. *Social Science & Medicine, 14A*, 85.

Lester, D. (1990). Was gas detoxification or establishment of suicide prevention centers responsible for the decline in the British suicide rate? *Psychological Reports, 66*, 286.

Lester, D. (1993). The effectiveness of suicide prevention centers. *Suicide & Life-Threatening Behavior, 23*, 263–267.

Lester, D. (1994). Evaluating the effectiveness of the Samaritans in England and Wales. *International Journal of Health Sciences, 5*, 73–74.

Lester, D. (1997a). The effectiveness of suicide prevention centers. *Suicide & Life-Threatening Behavior, 27*, 304–310.

Lester, D. (1997b). Effect of suicide prevention centers in Ireland and Great Britain. *Psychological Reports, 81*, 1186.

Lester, D. (2002). The scientific study of suicide requires accurate data. *Crisis, 23*, 133–134.

Lester, D. (2005). The impact of the Samaritan centres on suicide in Scotland. *Psychological Reports, 97*, 587–588.

Lester, D., & Priebe, K. (1971). Patients who show for therapy and those who fail. *Crisis Intervention, 3*, 69–72.

Lester, D., Saito, Y., & Abe, K. (1996). Have suicide prevention centers prevented suicide in Japan? *Archives of Suicide Research, 2*, 125–128.

Mahoney, H., & Pechura, C. (1980). Value and volunteers. *Psychological Reports, 47*, 1007–1012.

Maris, R. (1969). The sociology of suicide prevention. *Social Problems, 17*, 132–149.

McGee, R. K., Richard, W. C., & Bercun, C. (1973). A survey of telephone answering systems in suicide prevention and crisis intervention agencies. In D. Lester & G. W. Brockopp (Eds.), *Crisis intervention and counseling by telephone* (pp. 24–40). Springfield, IL: Charles Thomas.

Medoff, M. H. (1984). An evaluation of the effectiveness of suicide prevention centers. *Journal of Behavioral Economics, 15*(Fall), 43–55.

Miller, H. L., Coombs, D. W., Leeper, J. D., & Barton, S. N. (1984). An analysis of the effects of suicide prevention facilities in the United States. *American Journal of Public Health, 74*, 340–343.

Mishara, B. L., & Daigle, M. (1992). The effectiveness of telephone interventions by suicide prevention workers. *Canada's Mental Health, 40*(3), 24–29.

Mishara, B. L., & Daigle, M. (1997). Effects of different telephone intervention styles with suicidal callers at two suicide prevention centers. *American Journal of Community Psychology, 25*, 861–895.

Mishara, B. L., & Daigle, M. (2001). Helplines and crisis intervention services. In D. Lester (Ed.), *Suicide prevention: Resources for the millennium* (pp. 153–171). Philadelphia: Brunner-Routledge.

Mishara, B. L., & Giroux, G. (1993). The relationship between coping strategies and perceived stress in telephone intervention volunteers at a suicide prevention center. *Suicide & Life-Threatening Behavior, 23*, 221–229.

Motto, J. (1969, March). Development of standards for suicide prevention centers. *Bulletin of Suicidology*, 33–37.

Motto, J. (1971). Evaluation of a suicide prevention center by sampling the population at risk. *Life-Threatening Behavior, 1*, 18–22.

Murphy, G., Wetzel, R., Swallow, C., & McClure, J. (1969). Who calls the suicide prevention center? *American Journal of Psychiatry, 126*, 314–324.

Riehl, T., Marchner, E., & Moller, H. J. (1988). Influence of crisis intervention telephone services ("crisis hotlines") on the suicide rate in 25 German cities. In H. J. Moller, A. Schmidtke, & R. Welz (Eds.), *Current issues of suicidology* (pp. 431–436). New York: Springer-Verlag.

Rogers, J. R., & Subich, L. M. (1990). Reliability analysis of the crisis line suicide risk scale. In D. Lester (Ed.), *Suicide '90* (pp. 224–233). Denver, CO: American Association of Suicidology.

Rosenthal, R. (1984). *Meta-analytic procedures for social research*. Beverly Hills, CA: Sage.

Slaikeu, K., Lester, D., & Tulkin, S. R. (1973). Show versus no show. *Journal of Consulting and Clinical Psychology, 40*, 481–486.

Suchman, E. A. (1967). *Evaluative research*. New York: Russell Sage Foundation.

Tekavcic-Grad, O., & Farberow, N. L. (1989). A cross-cultural comparison of ideal and undesirable qualities of crisis line workers. *Crisis, 10*, 152–163.

Tierney, R. J. (1991). Suicide intervention training evaluation. In D. Lester (Ed.), *Suicide '91* (p. 113). Denver, CO: American Association of Suicidology.

Treloar, A. J., & Pinfold, T. J. (1993). Deliberate self-harm. *Crisis, 14*, 83–89.

Weiner, I. W. (1969). The effectiveness of a suicide prevention program. *Mental Hygiene, 53*, 357–363.

Whittemore, K. (1970). *Ten centers*. Atlanta: Lullwater Press.

Williamson, J. W., Goldberg, E., & Packard, M. (1973). Use of simulated patients in evaluating patient management skills of telephone counselors. In D. Lester & G. W. Brockopp (Eds.), *Crisis intervention and counseling by telephone* (pp. 310–322). Springfield, IL: Charles Thomas.

About the Author

David Lester has doctoral degrees from Cambridge University (UK) in Social and Political Science and Brandeis University (USA) in Psychology. He is Distinguished Professor of Psychology at the Richard Stockton College of New Jersey. He has been President of the International Association for Suicide Prevention, and he has published extensively on suicide, murder, and other issues in thanatology. His recent books include *Katie's Diary: Unlocking the Mystery of a Suicide* (2004), *Suicide and the Holocaust* (2005), *Is there Life after Death?* (2005), *Preventing Suicide: Closing the Exits Revisited* (2009), and *Understanding Suicide: Why We Don't and How We Might* (2010).

David Lester
The Richard Stockton College of New Jersey
PO Box 195
Jimmie Leeds Road
Pomona
NJ 08240-0195
USA
Tel.: +1 609 652 4512
E-mail: lesterd@stockton.edu

Suicide Prevention Programs Through Education in the Community and in the Frame of Healthcare

Konstantinos N. Fountoulakis[1] and Zoltán Rihmer[2]

[1]3rd Department of Psychiatry, Aristotle University of Thessaloniki, Greece
[2]Department of Clinical and Theoretical Mental Health, and Department of Psychiatry and Psychotherapy, Semmelweis University, Faculty of Medicine, Budapest, Hungary

Today, we know that suicide is a complex and multicausal behavior and needs a complex approach to understand and prevent it (Rihmer, Kantor, Rihmer, & Seregi, 2004). It has been reported that at least 25–50% of mood disorder patients attempt suicide at least once in their lifetime (Jamison, 2000; Valtonen et al., 2006). Schizophrenia is also another major cause of suicide with 9–13% of patients dying annually by suicide (Pompili & Lester, 2007).

Major depressive disorder is strongly associated with suicide attempts, accounting for 65–70% of cases; however, bipolar disorder (BD) patients carry the strongest risk for completed suicide (Balazs et al., 2006; Baldessarini, Pompili, & Tondo, 2006; Gray & Otto, 2001), which occurs early and in association with severe depressive or mixed states (Balazs et al., 2006; Baldessarini, Pompili, et al., 2006; Rihmer, 2007b). Risk factors for suicide in BD include agitation, depressive mixed states (including pseudo-unipolar depression) (Akiskal, Benazzi, Perugi, & Rihmer, 2005; Isometsa et al., 1994a, 1994b; Maser et al., 2002; Rihmer & Aksikal, 2006), higher number of prior depressive episodes and suicide attempts (Oquendo, Currier, & Mann, 2006; Rihmer, 2007b; Valtonen et al., 2006), including a rapid cycling course, comorbid anxiety especially panic attacks and generalized anxiety disorder (Frank et al., 2002; Rihmer, 2007b; Simon et al., 2007), personality disorders and substance and alcohol dependence (Comtois, Russo, Roy-Byrne, & Ries, 2004; Oquendo et al., 2007) as well as family history of suicides (Cavazzoni et al., 2007; Hawton, Suton, Haw, Sinclair, & Harriss, 2005; Oquendo et al., 2007). The risk factors for suicide in schizophrenia include young age, male gender, high premorbid expectations, paranoid type, the presence of hopelessness and depression, as well as comorbid alcohol and substance use disorders (Axelsson & Lagerkvist-Briggs, 1992; Fenton, McGlashan, Victor, & Byler, 1997; Pompili & Lester, 2007). It is well documented that the recurrence of suicidal behavior across depressive episodes shows high consistency (Rihmer, 2007a, 2007b; Szanto, Mulsant, et al., 2007;

Valtonen et al., 2005; Williams, Crane, Barnhofer, Van der Does, & Segal, 2006). The fact that the majority of suicide victims die by their first attempt (Isometsa et al., 1994b; Rihmer, 2007b; Rihmer, Belso, & Kiss, 2002) limits the value of the stronger prognostic variable, which is the history of prior suicide attempt (Hawton et al., 2005; Oquendo et al., 2006; Rihmer, 2007b).

Widespread psychoeducation to general public starting at a younger age while at school or targeting specific populations has been proposed as a possible effective strategy to reduce the risk of suicidal behavior. It has been argued that such an education will alert the laypeople toward the problem and facilitate help-seeking by those at risk; at the same time, it will increase the adherence to treatment and boost the process of therapeutic alliance between patients and therapists. A number of such programs have been launched in various countries around the world usually within the frame of broader mental health initiatives or broader suicide prevention strategies, with Finland being the first country to have developed such a program in the mid-1980s, but really implementing the same in 1992. In the US, a similar such program was launched in 1999 and in the UK in 2002 (De Leo & Evans, 2004).

As our knowledge on the diagnosis and treatment of mood disorders, the most common leading cause of suicidal behavior, keeps on developing continuously, a postgraduate training for the general practitioners (GPs) and other healthcare professionals has been proposed as yet another effective strategy for reducing suicide morbidity and mortality, at least among those, who contact the healthcare system (Hegerl, Althaus, Schmidtke, & Niklewski, 2006; Henriksson & Isacsson, 2006; Rihmer & Rutz, 2009; Rihmer, Rutz, & Pihlgren, 1995; Rihmer, Rutz, Pihlgren, & Pestality, 1998; Rutz, Walinder, von Knorring, Rihmer, & Pihlgren, 1997; Szanto, Kalmar, Hendin, Rihmer, & Mann, 2007). This strategy is particularly important because about two thirds of suicide victims have (mostly untreated) major depressive episode at the time of their death (Baldessarini, Pompili, et al., 2006; Isometsa et al., 1994a; Jamison, 2000; Rihmer, 2007b; Rihmer & Akiskal, 2006; Rihmer et al., 2002, 2004; Valtonen et al., 2006) and more than half of them contact their GPs in the last few weeks or months of their life (Rihmer & Rutz, 2009; Rihmer et al., 2002). However, several retrospective and prospective follow-up studies show that successful acute and long-term treatment of unipolar depression and BDs markedly reduces the risk of suicidal behavior even in this high-risk population (Baldessarini, Tondo, et al., 2006; Guzzetta, Tondo, Centorrino, & Baldessarini, 2007; Rihmer, 2007a , 2007b; Rihmer & Akiskal, 2006; Rihmer et al., 2004, 2006; Szanto, Mulsant, et al., 2007; Tondo, Lepri, & Baldessarini, 2008).

Current Approaches to Treatment and Prevention

Community-Based Personal-Focused Educational Programs for Reducing Suicidal Behavior

As a starting point, it is important to know the public opinion and attitude before trying to develop and assess a psychoeducational program. All papers reporting on this problem suggest that mental health and illness are conceived by the general public as the product of cultural and socioeconomic factors (Kalish, Reynolds, & Farberow, 1974), and mainly in relation to stress and marital problems, domestic violence, and poverty (Kermode et al., 2007; Mofidi, Ghazinour, Salander-Renberg, & Richter, 2008). However even professionals at key positions (gatekeepers) such as teachers seem to have limited knowledge on suicide despite the fact that they are alert to detect suicidal intentions (MacDonald, 2004). Two thirds of the people feel sympathetic toward those who lost a relative from suicide, but almost one third has mixed and undetermined feelings. Even worse, a small minority of around 2% hold a negative attitude. Undetermined feelings were more frequently found among the young poorly educated males without prior experience of these events in their environment and bearing some degree of depression, while inappropriate feelings were found in those people who were marked by similar characteristics but by a much more severe depressive affect. Also around 16% of the general population held an indifferent stance (Minamizono, Motohashi, Yamaji, & Kaneko, 2008).

There was a large debate as to whether talking openly on the topic of suicide would prove to be beneficial or harmful. Many clinicians believe the fact that when patients talk on their suicidal thoughts to each other, these thoughts tend to transmit from one patient to another and thus increases the risk of suicide. Research suggests no evidence of the iatrogenic effects of suicide screening programs (Gould et al., 2005). This fact suggests that educating the youth should not be considered as dangerous even when it pertains to emotionally vulnerable youth (Shaffer et al., 1990). On the other hand, there is a prevailing opinion that the school has the responsibility to impart health education. In the same wavelength, there is the concept of a general duty to care for pupils, their parents, and the community. These factors led to school-based educational programs for suicide prevention aiming at potential "helpers," based on the knowledge that peers are a primary support for troubled adolescents. However, the evaluation of these programs failed to provide any solid evidence for effectiveness, even at the level of increased awareness or acceptance (Hazell & King, 1996).

The literature includes the description of several community-based mainly person-targeted psychoeducational programs on suicide prevention:

1. SOS is a school-based prevention program that has been developed by Screening for Mental Health, Inc., a nonprofit organization in Wellesley, Massachusetts. The program focuses on two of the most prominent risk factors for suicidal behavior: underlying mental illness, particularly depression, and problematic use of alcohol. This program also stresses on the fact that suicide is not a normal reaction to stress or emotional upset, that specific signs and symptoms could serve as alarming mechanisms, and that suicide constitutes a state of emergency with specific actions and steps that should be followed (Aseltine, James, Schilling, & Glanovsky, 2007).
2. The model adopted by the Province of Alberta, Canada was based on interrelated programs pertaining to outreach, education and training, research, and fund-raising (Boldt, 1985).

3. The Zuni Life Skills Development Program was a high-school-based suicide prevention intervention program (Lafromboise & Lewis, 2008).
4. A more tribally diverse, culturally informed model was the American Indian Life Skills Development Curriculum (Lafromboise & Lewis, 2008).
5. The Youth Emergency Services model incorporated a workshop training of school and community professionals, so that they could identify young persons at the highest risk, education on the prevention of suicide, risk factors, and interventions, for both adolescents and parents, a partnership with the local hotline to facilitate community screening and referral to appropriate crisis services for families and youths, collaboration with a large primary care provider network to streamline the after-hours crisis referral process, using the hotline; and the use of a website to inform individuals about services and resources (McArt, Shulman, & Gajary, 1999).
6. A gatekeeper model developed for youth in the African American churches included the training of lay helpers and clergy to recognize the risk and protective factors for depression and suicide, to make referrals to appropriate community mental health resources, and to deliver a curriculum on community education (Molock, Matlin, Barksdale, Puri, & Lyles, 2008).
7. A community-based program in the state of Kentucky, US, the Stop Youth Suicide Campaign, was launched in October 2000 and included more than 30 local agencies. It included public education, education of medical care providers, school teachers, school counselors, youth service center personnel, and many other entities that deal with adolescents. This program used face-to-face encounters, website, video, and other forms of media education (Omar, 2005).
8. The suicide prevention program for the elderly in the Japanese small town of Nagawamachi Aomori developed a screener for depression and educational programs to address how to recognize the symptoms of depression and to develop a community network for the elderly to communicate with locals and support each other. This program also focused on a social schema to produce a society that respects "being" and not just "doing" (Ono, 2004).
9. A 3-hour multimedia community education program on depression and suicide in later life, designed for families, older adults, and service providers, provides information and teaches the skills needed to recognize and respond to depression and suicidal behavior in the elderly (Pratt, Schmall, Wilson, & Benthin, 1991).
10. An element of the National Training Initiative in Injury and Violence Prevention, the PREVENT (preventing violence through education, networking, and technical assistance) program included suicide prevention and began in late 2003 to train those practitioners who were involved in addressing violence against women, sexual violence, child maltreatment, youth violence, and suicide in varied community settings, to address multiple types of violence by encouraging a more widespread use of the evidence-based approaches to primary prevention. The program used a combination of varied types of face-to-face training and distance learning coupled with opportunities for networking and technical assistance,

and ultimately intended to stimulate and facilitate changes in individual, organizational, and cultural awareness and practices fostering primary prevention of violence (Runyan et al., 2005; Schmall & Pratt, 1993; Staal, 2001).

11. The Winter Comforts are all designed to increase knowledge about and skills for responding to three common mental health concerns in later life: loss/grief, depression/suicide, and alcohol abuse (Schmall & Pratt, 1993).
12. The US Air Force developed a formalized program of community awareness and education based on suicidal risk detection, assessment, and support facilitation (Staal, 2001).
13. The Australian government after extensive consultation with the Aboriginal community developed a range of culturally appropriate interventions on suicide prevention, focusing on community gatekeeper training workshops (Capp, Deane, & Lambert, 2001).
14. The cooperation between a community teaching hospital and a neighborhood Intermediate School on health promoting education in an urban setting had received the Council of Supervisors and Administrators Education Program Award for 1987 in New York City. Among the targets was suicide prevention through a series of health education events designed to provide needed information (Weiner, Cantara, Kuo, & Lione, 1988).
15. A statewide initiative in a northeastern US state aiming at developing regional critical incident stress management teams among colleges and universities was structured and intended to improve each member college or the university's capacity to respond comprehensively and effectively to critical incidents that affect its community, including suicide (Wiesen & Lischer, 2006).
16. MindMatters is an innovative, national mental health promotion program that provides a framework for imparting education on mental health in Australian schools, aiming at facilitating practice by adopting whole-school approaches; developing mental health education resources, curriculum, and professional development programs that are appropriate for a wide range of schools, a wide category of students, and a wide gamut of learning areas; incorporating trial guidelines on mental health and suicide prevention; and encouraging the development of partnerships between schools, parents, and community support agencies to promote the mental well-being of young people (Wyn, Cahill, Holdsworth, Rowling, & Carson, 2000).
17. A 7-year implementation of intervention including group activity, psychoeducation, and self-assessment of depression screening with follow-up by GPs and a 10-year implementation of public education in Japan (Oyama, Fujita, Goto, Shibuya, & Sakashita, 2006).
18. The Multisite Intervention Study on Suicidal Behaviours (SUPRE-MISS), launched by the WHO in 2000, evaluated an innovative intervention in a large randomized controlled trial that brought together the elements of information, education, and practical advice from brief interventions with the maintenance of long-term follow-up contact on a regular basis (Flaischmann et al., 2008).

Healthcare-Based Educational Programs for Reducing Suicidal Behavior

The four major healthcare-based educational programs, which showed that postgraduate training of GPs and other healthcare workers, particularly in combination with public education, could reduce the rate of completed and attempted suicides in the area that was served by the trained doctors are as follows:

1. The pioneering Gotland Study performed in the early 1980s in the last century (Rihmer et al., 1995; Rutz et al., 1997).
2. The Nuremberg Alliance Against Depression (NAAD) project performed in Germany between 2000 and 2002 (Hegerl et al., 2006).
3. The Swedish Jämtland study performed between 1995 and 2002 (Henriksson & Isacsson, 2006).
4. The Hungarian GP depression-management educational program between 2000 and 2005 implemented in a region of Kiskunhalas where the baseline suicide rate was twice the national average (Szanto, Kalmar, et al., 2007).

Sources of Research Evidence

A systematic review of the literature on the efficacy of psychoeducational interventions aimed at the general public and the education of doctors in reducing the risk for attempting or committing suicide has not been done so far. Thus, a thorough search of the MEDLINE was done and the relevant papers identified.

Evidence for Efficacy of Current Approaches

Community-Based Personal-Focused Educational Programs for Reducing Suicidal Behavior

The few papers assessing interventions report that community education intervention programs increase some specific indices such as gatekeepers' skills, general awareness for the public, coping with depression, hospital admissions for attempted suicide (Allen, 1976; Aseltine & DeMartino, 2004; Aseltine et al., 2007; Bhugra & Hicks, 2004; Capp et al., 2001; Cross, Matthieu, Cerel, & Knox, 2007; Deykin, Hsieh, Joshi, & McNamarra, 1986; Gask, Dixon, Morriss, Appleby, & Green, 2006; Goldney & Fisher, 2008; Kalafat & Elias, 1994; Matthieu, Cross, Batres, Flora, & Knox, 2008; Meilman & Hall, 2006; Portzky & van Heeringen, 2006; Shaffer, Garland, Vieland, Underwood, & Busner, 1991; Slaven & Kisely, 2002; Spirito, Overholser, Ashworth, Morgan, & Benedict-Drew, 1988; Thompson, Eggert, & Herting, 2000; Vieland, Whittle, Garland, Hicks, & Shaffer, 1991) or increase medical and psychological help-seeking (Klein et al., 2001); but it is doubtful that they reduce suicide itself (Deykin et al., 1986; Goldney & Fisher, 2008) or even worse, the results are reported to be negative (Goldney, Fisher, Wilson, & Cheok, 2002; Vieland et al., 1991; Weaver, 1995). There has been only on exception so far; this related to a program with proven efficacy that took place in Japan where the elderly individuals aged 65 years or above were evaluated and the municipalities affected by this intervention compared with the municipalities acting as controls. This program included a 7-year implementation of depression screening with follow-up by GPs and a 10-year implementation of public education (Oyama, Fujita, et al., 2006; Oyama, Goto, Fujita, Shibuya, & Sakashita, 2006; Oyama, Koida, Sakashita, & Kudo, 2004; Oyama et al., 2005).

The assessment of data from the region of Yasuzuka (with a population of 4,940; elderly suicide rate for women, 275/100,000; elderly suicide rate for men, 323/100,000) suggests that there was a 64% reduction in the risk for women in the intervention area, whereas no significant change was noticed in the risk for men in area and either men or women in the referent municipalities (Oyama, Fujita, et al., 2006). In the Matsudai town (population 6,015; suicide rate for males 290.6/100,000 and that for females 361.3/100,000), the female risk of completing suicide in the intervention area was reduced by 70%, whereas no change in the risk for males in the intervention area nor for males or females in the reference area, which was the Kawanishi town (population 9,425; elderly suicide rate for males 212.2/100,000 and that for females 151.9/100,000) (Oyama, Goto, et al., 2006). In the rural town of Joboji (population 7,010), the results suggest that for both males and females the risk was reduced to almost 25% more than a regional historical trend, with a better response for females than for males (Oyama et al., 2004). In the Yuri town (population 6,817; elderly suicide rate 291.4/100,000) in comparison to the control town of Chokai (population 8,136; elderly suicide rate 216.5/100,000), the risk for elderly females in Yuri completing suicide was reduced by 76%, whereas there was no change in the risks for Yuri's elderly males and both Chokai's elderly males and females (Oyama et al., 2005). The reduction of suicide risk in all the intervention areas was greater than the historical trend.

The WHO organized brief intervention and contact (BIC) study for 1867 suicide attempters seen at the emergency care departments in the five participating countries (Brazil, India, Sri Lanka, Islamic Republic of Iran, and China) showed that a brief individual intervention before discharge and regular contact with the suicide attempters (eight contacts during the 18-month follow-up) resulted in significantly less completed suicides (0.2%) in the BIC group (n = 872) than in the treatment-as-usual group (n = 827, 2.2%, $p < .001$) (Flaischmann et al., 2008).

Healthcare-Based Educational Programs for Reducing Suicidal Behavior

The results of the Swedish Gotland Study showed that 2 years after the 2-day postgraduate educational program on the diagnosis and treatment of depression for the GPs in 1983, the suicide rate of Gotland decreased by 60%, the prescription of antidepressants increased from 50% to 80% of Swedish average, and the utilization of nonspecific medications (benzodiazepines and antipsychotics) decreased by 25% compared to the Swedish average.

The number of referrals to psychiatry for depressive disorders decreased by 50% and the inpatient care for depression as well as the number of days on sick leave because of depression also decreased by 75% and 50%, respectively. All these changes were in contrast to the earlier trends on Gotland and/or contemporary trends in the rest of Sweden (Rutz et al., 1997). Most importantly, the rate of depressive suicides among all suicides decreased significantly after the program (42–16%, $p < .01$), indicating that the decline in suicide mortality after the education resulted directly from a robust decrease in depressive suicides, particularly among those who used violent suicide methods (Rihmer et al., 1995). However, the decline in depressive suicides after the training was almost entirely the result of a decrease in female depressive suicides, whereas male suicidality was almost unchanged. Few suicidal males were known to the local medical services, although many of them were known to the police and social welfare services. However, the overall favorable effect of the education faded in a few years and repeated education in 1993 and 1995 again led to another marked decrease in suicides, again mainly in females (Rutz et al., 1997). As the well-known seasonality of suicides seems to be the consequence of the seasonal nature of depression-related suicides, the significantly decreased seasonality of suicides on Gotland after the GP training (Rihmer et al., 1998) also supports the specific effect of the depression training on suicide mortality.

The NAAD, a 2-year intervention program, was performed in Nuremberg (440,000 inhabitants) at four levels: (a) training GPs, (b) a public relations campaign, (c) cooperation with community facilitators (teachers, priests, and local media), and (d) support for the self-help activities and for high-risk groups (depressed patients, suicide attempters and their relatives). The results showed that compared to control region (Würzburg, 290,000 inhabitants), a significant reduction in the frequency of all suicidal acts (suicides and suicide attempts combined) was observed in the intervention region during the 2-year intervention period (2002 versus 2000, Nuremberg: 24% reduction, Würzburg: 7% increase, $p < .004$). The reduction in all suicidal acts was most pronounced for violent methods. However, as regards only completed suicides there was no significant difference in the decline of suicide rate between the intervention and control region (Hegerl et al., 2006).

Evaluating the effects of continuing medical education program (eight seminars between 1995 and 2002) for the GPs on depression in Jämtland county, Sweden (136,000 inhabitants), the authors found that compared to the preintervention period (1970–1994) the mean suicide rate of the Jämtland county decreased by 36% in the intervention period (1995–2002); whereas the mean suicide rate of Sweden decreased "only" by 30% during the same time. The use of antidepressants in Jämtland county increased from 25% below the Swedish average to the same level. In line with the greater reduction of suicide rate in Jämtland county, the use of antidepressants increased by 161% in this county whereas the same figure for the whole of Sweden was "only" 108% (Henriksson & Isacsson, 2006).

As for the Hungarian GP depression-management educational program, in the intervention region (region of Kiskunhalas, 73,000 inhabitants) the 5-year preintervention (1996–2000) and postintervention (2001–2005) mean annual suicide rates per 1 million population were 59.7 and 49.9 (16% decrease). In the local control region (Kiskunfélegyháza, 54,000 inhabitants), the same figures were 50.4 and 45.1, respectively (11% decrease). Despite the fact that this difference is mathematically not significant, the difference shows in the expected direction and is in good agreement with the finding that the raise in antidepressant prescription and the rate of antidepressant-treated persons increased significantly more in the intervention than in the control region. Further, the decrease in annual suicide rate was significantly greater in the intervention region (9.8/100,000) compared with the county minus intervention region (6.9/100,000) and compared with whole of Hungary (4.5/100,000) (Szanto, Kalmar, et al., 2007).

Although the four major healthcare-based educational programs, discussed above, were performed in different time frames and used somewhat different research designs, the main results show in the same direction, indicating that better care of psychiatric (and particularly depressive) patients is one important contributing factor in declining suicide rates of the areas served by trained GPs and other healthcare workers.

Improving and Optimizing Current Practice

Some papers deal with the problem of psychoeducation of the general public in a theoretical way. The general agreement is that plain but increased professional contact by itself is not related to increased mental health literacy in a general or suicide in a specific manner. It has been argued that more specific psychoeducational programs are required (Goldney et al., 2002). Some authors insist that there are persuasive data on the fact that suicide prevention is possible using broad community and professional education programs, as well as by the optimum management of mental disorders (Goldney, 2005; Rihmer & Rutz, 2009). However, broad community-based psychoeducational interventions fail to reach the target groups; instead, they reach all the others (Goldney & Fisher, 2008). Little evidence if any has emerged to support the efficacy of some traditional approaches to suicide prevention, such as school-based suicide educational programs and telephone hotlines. On the other hand, it is broadly believed that there are effective selective and universally applicable interventions for important known risk factors for depression and suicidal behavior, both in the frame of primary care (Hegerl et al., 2006; Henriksson & Isacsson, 2006; Rihmer & Rutz, 2009; Rihmer et al., 1995; Rutz et al., 1997; Szanto, Kalmar, et al., 2007) and in psychiatric settings (Baldessarini, Tondo, et al., 2006; Guzzetta et al., 2007; Rihmer, 2007a; Tondo et al., 2008). Youth suicide prevention strategies in Australia have generally employed traditional approaches that focus on clinical interventions for self-harmers, restricting access to lethal means, providing services to high-risk groups, and enhancing GP responses (Burns & Patton, 2000). The seminal review of trends and outcomes for suicide suggests that if any, the results of broad mental health programs aiming at suicide reduction are not so marked as they could be or isolated and masked by other strong parallel changes in the socio-political-economic environment (De Leo & Evans, 2004).

The social and cultural environment and psychosocial factors such as younger age, being divorced or widowed, and experiencing adverse life situations seem to relate with increased suicidal ideation and higher prevalence of attempts and suicide completion, particularly among patients with untreated major mood disorders (Baldessarini, Pompili, et al., 2006; Hawton et al., 2005; Oquendo et al., 2006; Rihmer, 2007b; Rihmer et al., 2002). Recognition of early warning signs and easy access to health services could also play an important role (Hegerl et al., 2006; Rihmer & Rutz, 2009). This is the likely conclusion we arrive at from the research on the declining suicidal rates during the past two decades throughout Europe, the US, and Canada. Data show that the most pronounced decrease took place in countries with traditionally high suicide rates and the decline was greater for women. It seems that better recognition of major depression as well as availability of treatment with antidepressants and mood stabilizers could be one of the major underlying factors (Rihmer & Akiskal, 2006). It is also possible that contemporary suicide attempters suffer from more severe forms of depression in comparison to attempters in the past, maybe suggesting that the overall intervention is so far at least partially effective (Henriques, Brown, Berk, & Beck, 2004). What is impressive is the fact that in spite of frequent medical contacts before the suicide event, only a small minority of depressive suicide victims had received appropriate antidepressant pharmacotherapy, and this observation is particularly strong as regards primary care (Isometsa et al., 1994a; Rihmer, 2007b; Rihmer & Rutz, 2009; Rihmer et al., 2002). It is almost certain, although relevant data do not exist, that psychosocial treatment is also frequently inadequately administered.

However, improved primary care education in isolation does not have any significant long-term effect on suicide mortality; on the other hand, only complex educational and organizational interventions that incorporate continuous clinical education and enhanced role of psychologists, nurses, social workers, and gatekeepers as well as high level of integration between primary and secondary care are beneficial. Finally, it should also be noted that because healthcare workers can help only those who contact them, a combination of healthcare-based approaches and community-based public health educational programs provides the best results (Rihmer et al., 2004; Wasserman & Durkee, 2009).

Potential Problems, Costs, and Resources

The research on the outcome of interventions is poor and underdeveloped. In essence, there are only few data on the outcome of psychosocial therapy (Rucci et al., 2002; Williams et al., 2008) on suicidal behavior, whereas the results on the pharmacological prevention of suicidal behavior, particularly among those with unipolar depression and BDs, are promising (Baldessarini, Tondo, et al., 2006; Guzzetta et al., 2007; Rihmer, 2007a; Rihmer & Akiskal, 2006; Tondo et al., 2008). Although our knowledge on the recognition and management of suicidal persons has improved substantially in the last decade, the main problem in everyday clinical practice remain underdiagnosis and undertreatment of mood disorders both with pharmacotherapy and with psychotherapeutical interventions. Misdiagnosis of depressive episode of BD as unipolar depression leading to inadequate acute and long-term treatment is still quite common. However, it has been shown that antidepressant monotherapy (unprotected by mood stabilizers) could worsen the short-term and long-term courses of illness and could increase the risk of suicidal behavior (Akiskal et al., 2005; Rihmer, 2007b; Rihmer & Akiskal, 2006). It is important to undertake focused research particularly on the issue of community-based educational programs to determine whether any of these complex and resource consuming programs do work or not and to what extent. This will demand significant investment in resources, but it will give the necessary answers that are currently lacking.

Further Reading

Isacsson, G., Holmgren, A., Ösby, U., & Ahlner, J. (2009). Decrease in suicide among the individuals treated with antidepressants: A controlled study of antidepressants in suicide, Sweden 1995–2005. *Acta Psychiatrica Scandinavica, 120*, 37–44.

Kapusta, N. D., Niederkrotenthaler, T., Etzersdorfer, E., Voracek, M., Dervic, K., Jandl-Jager, E., et al. (2009). Influence of psychotherapist density and antidepressant sales on suicide rates. *Acta Psychiatrica Scandinavica, 119*, 236–242.

Tatarelli, R., Pompili, M., & Girardi, P. (Eds.). (2007). *Suicide in psychiatric disorders*. New York: Nova Science.

Tondo, L., Albert, M. J., & Baldessarini, R. J. (2006). Suicide rates in relation to health care access in the United States: An ecological study. *Journal of Clinical Psychiatry, 67,* 517–523.

Wasserman, D., & Wasserman, C. (Eds.). (2009). *Oxford textbook of suicidology and suicide prevention*. New York: Oxford University Press.

References

Akiskal, H. S., Benazzi, F., Perugi, G., & Rihmer, Z. (2005). Agitated "unipolar" depression re-conceptualized as a depressive mixed state: Implications for the antidepressant-suicide controversy. *Journal of Affective Disorders, 85*, 245–258.

Allen, N. H. (1976). The health educator as a suicidologist. *Suicide & Life-Threatening Behavior, 6*, 195–201.

Aseltine, R. H. Jr., & DeMartino, R. (2004). An outcome evaluation of the SOS suicide prevention program. *American Journal of Public Health, 94*, 446–451.

Aseltine, R. H. Jr., James, A., Schilling, E. A., & Glanovsky, J. (2007). Evaluating the SOS suicide prevention program: A replication and extension. *BMC Public Health, 7*, 161.

Axelsson, R., & Lagerkvist-Briggs, M. (1992). Factors predicting suicide in psychotic patients. *European Archives of Psychiatry and Clinical Neuroscience, 241*(5), 259–266.

Balazs, J., Benazzi, F., Rihmer, Z., Rihmer, A., Akiskal, K. K., & Akiskal, H. S. (2006). The close link between suicide attempts and mixed (bipolar) depression: Implications for suicide prevention. *Journal of Affective Disorders, 91*, 133–138.

Baldessarini, R. J., Pompili, M., & Tondo, L. (2006). Suicide in bipolar disorder: Risks and management. *CNS Spectrums, 11*, 465–471.

Baldessarini, R. J., Tondo, L., Davis, P., Pompili, M., Goodwin, F. K., & Hennen, J. (2006). Decreased risk of suicides and attempts during long-term lithium treatment: A meta-analytic review. *Bipolar Disorders, 8*, 625–639.

Bhugra, D., & Hicks, M. H. (2004). Effect of an educational pamphlet on help-seeking attitudes for depression among British South Asian women. *Psychiatric Services, 55*, 827–829.

Boldt, M. (1985). Towards the development of a systematic approach to suicide prevention: The Alberta model. *Canadian Mental Health Association, 33*(2), 2–4.

Burns, J. M., & Patton, G. C. (2000). Preventive interventions for youth suicide: A risk factor-based approach. *Australian and New Zealand Journal of Psychiatry, 34*, 388–407.

Capp, K., Deane, F. P., & Lambert, G. (2001). Suicide prevention in aboriginal communities: Application of community gatekeeper training. *Australian and New Zealand Journal of Psychiatry, 25*, 315–321.

Cavazzoni, P., Grof, P., Duffy, A., Grof, E., Muller-Oerlinghausen, B., Berghofer, A., et al. (2007). Heterogeneity of the risk of suicidal behavior in bipolar-spectrum disorders. *Bipolar Disorders, 9*, 377–385.

Comtois, K. A., Russo, J. E., Roy-Byrne, P., & Ries, R. K. (2004). Clinicians' assessments of bipolar disorder and substance abuse as predictors of suicidal behavior in acutely hospitalized psychiatric inpatients. *Biological Psychiatry, 56*, 757–763.

Cross, W., Matthieu, M. M., Cerel, J., & Knox, K. L. (2007). Proximate outcomes of gatekeeper training for suicide prevention in the workplace. *Suicide & Life-Threatening Behavior, 37*, 659–670.

De Leo, D., & Evans, R. (2004). *International suicide rates and prevention strategies*. Göttingen, Germany: Hogrefe & Huber.

Deykin, E. Y., Hsieh, C. C., Joshi, N., & McNamarra, J. J. (1986). Adolescent suicidal and self-destructive behavior. Results of an intervention study. *Journal of Adolescent Health Care, 7*(2), 88–95.

Fenton, W. S., McGlashan, T. H., Victor, B. J., & Blyler, C. R. (1997). Symptoms, subtype, and suicidality in patients with schizophrenia spectrum disorders. *American Journal of Psychiatry, 154*, 199–204.

Flaischmann, A., Bertolote, J. M., Wasserman, D., Bolhari, D. J., Botega, N. J., de Silva, D., et al. (2008). Effectiveness of brief intervention and contact for suicide attempters: A randomized controlled trial in five countries. *Bulletin of the WHO, 86*, 703–709.

Frank, E., Cyranowski, J. M., Rucci, P., Shear, M. K., Fagiolini, A., Thase, M. E., et al. (2002). Clinical significance of lifetime panic spectrum symptoms in the treatment of patients with bipolar I disorder. *Archives of General Psychiatry, 59*, 905–911.

Gask, L., Dixon, C., Morriss, R., Appleby, L., & Green, G. (2006). Evaluating STORM skills training for managing people at risk of suicide. *Journal of Advanced Nursing, 54*, 739–750.

Goldney, R. D. (2005). Suicide prevention: A pragmatic review of recent studies. *Crisis, 26*, 128–140.

Goldney, R. D., & Fisher, L. J. (2008). Have broad-based community and professional education programs influenced mental health literacy and treatment seeking of those with major depression and suicidal ideation? *Suicide & Life-Threatening Behavior, 38*, 129–142.

Goldney, R. D., Fisher, L. J., Wilson, D. H., & Cheok, F. (2002). Mental health literacy of those with major depression and suicidal ideation: An impediment to help seeking. *Suicide & Life-Threatening Behavior, 32*, 394–403.

Gould, M. S., Marrocco, F. A., Kleinman, M., Thomas, J. G., Mostkoff, K., Cote, J., et al. (2005). Evaluating iatrogenic risk of youth suicide screening programs: A randomized controlled trial. *Journal of the American Medical Association, 293*, 1635–1643.

Gray, S. M., & Otto, M. W. (2001). Psychosocial approaches to suicide prevention: Applications to patients with bipolar disorder. *Journal of Clinical Psychiatry, 62*(Suppl. 25), 56–64.

Guzzetta, F., Tondo, L., Centorrino, F., & Baldessarini, R. J. (2007). Lithium treatment reduces suicide risk in recurrent major depressive disorder. *Journal of Clinical Psychiatry, 68*, 380–383.

Hawton, K., Sutton, L., Haw, C., Sinclair, J., & Harriss, L. (2005). Suicide and attempted suicide in bipolar disorder: A systematic review of risk factors. *Journal of Clinical Psychiatry, 66*, 693–704.

Hazell, P., & King, R. (1996). Arguments for and against teaching suicide prevention in schools. *Australian and New Zealand Journal of Psychiatry, 30*, 633–642.

Hegerl, U., Althaus, D., Schmidtke, A., & Niklewski, G. (2006). The alliance against depression: 2-year evaluation of a community-based intervention to reduce suicidality. *Psychological Medicine, 36*, 1225–1233.

Henriksson, S., & Isacsson, G. (2006). Increased antidepressant use and fewer suicides in Jämtland county, Sweden, after a primary care educational programme on the treatment of depression. *Acta Psychiatrica Scandinavica, 114*, 159–167.

Henriques, G. R., Brown, G. K., Berk, M. S., & Beck, A. T. (2004). Marked increases in psychopathology found in a 30-year cohort comparison of suicide attempters. *Psychological Medicine, 34*, 833–841.

Isometsa, E. T., Henriksson, M. M., Aro, H. M., Heikkinen, M. E., Kuoppasalmi, K. I., & Lonnqvist, J. K. (1994a). Suicide in psychotic major depression. *Journal of Affective Disorders, 31*, 187–191.

Isometsa, E. T., Henriksson, M. M., Aro, H. M., Heikkinen, M. E., Kuoppasalmi, K. I., & Lonnqvist, J. K. (1994b). Suicide in major depression. *American Journal of Psychiatry, 151*, 530–536.

Jamison, K. R. (2000). Suicide and bipolar disorder. *Journal of Clinical Psychiatry, 61*(Suppl. 9), 47–51.

Kalafat, J., & Elias, M. (1994). An evaluation of a school-based suicide awareness intervention. *Suicide & Life-Threatening Behavior, 24*, 224–233.

Kalish, R. A., Reynolds, D. K., & Farberow, N. L. (1974). Community attitudes toward suicide. *Community Mental Health Journal, 10*, 301–308.

Kermode, M., Herrman, H., Arole, R., White, J., Premkumar, R., & Patel, V. (2007). Empowerment of women and mental health promotion: A qualitative study in rural Maharashtra, India. *BMC Public Health, 7*, 225.

Klein, J. D., Allan, M. J., Elster, A. B., Stevens, D., Cox, C., Hedberg, V. A., et al. (2001). Improving adolescent preventive care in community health centers. *Pediatrics, 107*, 318–327.

Lafromboise, T. D., & Lewis, H. A. (2008). The Zuni life skills development program: A school/community-based suicide prevention intervention. *Suicide & Life-Threatening Behavior, 38*, 343–353.

MacDonald, M. G. (2004). Teachers' knowledge of facts and myths about suicide. *Psychological Reports, 95*, 651–656.

Maser, J. D., Akiskal, H. S., Schettler, P., Scheftner, W., Mueller, T., Endicott, J., et al. (2002). Can temperament identify affectively ill patients who engage in lethal or near-lethal suicidal behavior? A 14-year prospective study. *Suicide & Life-Threatening Behavior, 32*, 10–32.

Matthieu, M. M., Cross, W., Batres, A. R., Flora, C. M., & Knox, K. L. (2008). Evaluation of gatekeeper training for suicide prevention in veterans. *Archives of Suicide Research, 12*, 148–154.

McArt, E. W., Shulman, D. A., & Gajary, E. (1999). Developing an educational workshop on teen depression and suicide: A proactive community intervention. *Child Welfare, 78*, 793–806.

Meilman, P. W., & Hall, T. M. (2006). Aftermath of tragic events: The development and use of community support meetings on a university campus. *Journal of American College Health, 54*, 382–384.

Minamizono, S., Motohashi, Y., Yamaji, M., & Kaneko, Y. (2008). Attitudes towards those bereaved by a suicide: A population-based, cross-sectional study in rural Japan. *BMC Public Health, 8*, 334.

Mofidi, N., Ghazinour, M., Salander-Renberg, E., & Richter, J. (2008). Attitudes towards suicide among Kurdish people in Iran. *Social Psychiatry and Psychiatric Epidemiology, 43*, 291–298.

Molock, S. D., Matlin, S., Barksdale, C., Puri, R., & Lyles, J. (2008). Developing suicide prevention programs for African American youth in African American churches. *Suicide & Life-Threatening Behavior, 38*, 323–333.

Omar, H. A. (2005). A model program for youth suicide prevention. *International Journal of Adolescence Medicine and Health, 17*, 275–278.

Ono, Y. (2004). Suicide prevention program for the elderly: The experience in Japan. *Keio Journal of Medicine, 53*, 1–6.

Oquendo, M. A., Bongiovi-Garcia, M. E., Galfalvy, H., Goldberg, P. H., Grunebaum, M. F., Burke, A. K., et al. (2007). Sex differences in clinical predictors of suicidal acts after major depression: A prospective study. *American Journal of Psychiatry, 164*, 134–141.

Oquendo, M. A., Currier, D., & Mann, J. J. (2006). Prospective studies of suicidal behavior in major depressive and bipolar disorders: What is the evidence for predictive risk factors? *Acta Psychiatrica Scandinavica, 114*, 151–158.

Oyama, H., Fujita, M., Goto, M., Shibuya, H., & Sakashita, T. (2006). Outcomes of community-based screening for depression and suicide prevention among Japanese elders. *Gerontologist, 46*, 821–826.

Oyama, H., Goto, M., Fujita, M., Shibuya, H., & Sakashita, T. (2006). Preventing elderly suicide through primary care by community-based screening for depression in rural Japan. *Crisis, 27*, 58–65.

Oyama, H., Koida, J., Sakashita, T., & Kudo, K. (2004). Community-based prevention for suicide in elderly by depression screening and follow-up. *Community Mental Health Journal, 40*, 249–263.

Oyama, H., Watanabe, N., Ono, Y., Sakashita, T., Takenoshita, Y., Taguchi, M., et al. (2005). Community-based suicide prevention through group activity for the elderly successfully reduced the high suicide rate for females. *Psychiatry and Clinical Neurosciences, 59*, 337–344.

Pompili, M., & Lester, D. (2007). Suicide risk in schizophrenia. In R. Tatarelli, M. Pompili, & P. Girardi (Eds.), *Suicide in psychiatric disorders* (pp. 315–332). New York, NY: Nova.

Portzky, G., & van Heeringen, K. (2006). Suicide prevention in adolescents: A controlled study of the effectiveness of a school-based psycho-educational program. *Journal of Child Psychology and Psychiatry, 47*, 910–918.

Pratt, C. C., Schmall, V. L., Wilson, W., & Benthin, A. (1991). A model community education program on depression and suicide in later life. *Gerontologist, 31*, 692–695.

Rihmer, Z. (2007a). Pharmacological prevention of suicide in bipolar patients – A realizable target. *Journal of Affective Disorders, 103*, 1–3.

Rihmer, Z. (2007b). Suicide risk in mood disorders. *Current Opinion in Psychiatry, 20*, 17–22.

Rihmer, Z., & Akiskal, H. (2006). Do antidepressants t(h)reat(en) depressives? Toward a clinically judicious formulation of the antidepressant-suicidality FDA advisory in light of declining national suicide statistics from many countries. *Journal of Affective Disorders, 94*, 3–13.

Rihmer, Z., Belso, N., & Kiss, K. (2002). Strategies for suicide prevention. *Current Opinion in Psychiatry, 15*, 83–87.

Rihmer, Z., Kantor, Z., Rihmer, A., & Seregi, K. (2004). Suicide prevention strategies – A brief review. *Neuropsychopharmacologia Hungarica, 6*, 195–199.

Rihmer, Z., & Rutz, W. (2009). Treatment of attempted suicide and suicidal patients in primary care. In D. Wasserman & C. Wasserman (Eds.), *Oxford textbook of suicide and suicide prevention* (pp. 463–470). New York, NY: Oxford University Press.

Rihmer, Z., Rutz, W., & Pihlgren, H. (1995). Depression and suicide on Gotland. An intensive study of all suicides before and after a depression-training programme for general practitioners. *Journal of Affective Disorders, 35*, 147–152.

Rihmer, Z., Rutz, W., Pihlgren, H., & Pestality, P. (1998). Decreasing seasonality in suicide may indicate lowering rate of depressive suicides in the population. *Journal of Psychiatry Research, 81*, 233–240.

Rucci, P., Frank, E., Kostelnik, B., Fagiolini, A., Mallinger, A. G., Swartz, H. A., et al. (2002). Suicide attempts in patients with bipolar I disorder during acute and maintenance phases of intensive treatment with pharmacotherapy and adjunctive psychotherapy. *American Journal of Psychiatry, 159*, 1160–1164.

Runyan, C. W., Gunther-Mohr, C., Orton, S., Umble, K., Martin, S. L., & Coyne-Beasley, T. (2005). PREVENT: A program of the national training initiative on injury and violence prevention. *American Journal of Preventive Medicine, 29*(Suppl. 2), 252–258.

Rutz, W., Walinder, J., von Knorring, L., Rihmer, Z., & Pihlgren, H. (1997). Prevention of depression and suicide by education and medication: Impact on male suicidality. An update from the Gotland study. *International Journal of Psychiatry in Clinical Practice, 1*, 39–46.

Schmall, V. L., & Pratt, C. C. (1993). Community education on mental health in later life: Findings from an evaluation of a series of three model programs. *Journal of Mental Health Administration, 20*, 190–200.

Shaffer, D., Garland, A., Vieland, V., Underwood, M., & Busner, C. (1991). The impact of curriculum-based suicide prevention programs for teenagers. *Journal of American Academy of Child and Adolescent Psychiatry, 30*, 588–596.

Shaffer, D., Vieland, V., Garland, A., Rojas, M., Underwood, M., & Busner, C. (1990). Adolescent suicide attempters. Response to suicide-prevention programs. *Journal of the American Medical Association, 264*, 3151–3155.

Simon, N. M., Pollack, M. H., Ostacher, M. J., Zalta, A. K., Chow, C. W., Fischmann, D., et al. (2007). Understanding the link between anxiety symptoms and suicidal ideation and behaviors in outpatients with bipolar disorder. *Journal of Affective Disorders, 97*, 91–99.

Slaven, J., & Kisely, S. (2002). The Esperance primary prevention of suicide project. *Australian and New Zealand Journal of Psychiatry, 36*, 617–621.

Spirito, A., Overholser, J., Ashworth, S., Morgan, J., & Benedict-Drew, C. (1988). Evaluation of a suicide awareness curriculum for high school students. *Journal of American Academy of Child and Adolescent Psychiatry, 27*, 705–711.

Staal, M. A. (2001). The assessment and prevention of suicide for the 21st century: The Air Force's community awareness training model. *Military Medicine, 166*, 195–198.

Szanto, K., Kalmar, S., Hendin, H., Rihmer, Z., & Mann, J. J. (2007). A suicide prevention program in a region with a very high suicide rate. *Archives of General Psychiatry, 64*, 914–920.

Szanto, K., Mulsant, B. H., Houck, P. R., Dew, M. A., Dombrowski, A., Pollock, B. G., et al. (2007). Emergence, persistence, and resolution of suicidal ideation during treatment of depression in old age. *Journal of Affective Disorders, 98*, 153–161.

Thompson, E. A., Eggert, L. L., & Herting, J. R. (2000). Mediating effects of an indicated prevention program for reducing youth depression and suicide risk behaviors. *Suicide & Life-Threatening Behavior, 30*, 252–271.

Tondo, L., Lepri, B., & Baldessarini, R. J. (2008). Suicidal status during antidepressant treatment in 789 Sardinian patients with major affective disorder. *Acta Psychiatrica Scandinavica, 118*, 106–115.

Valtonen, H., Suominen, K., Mantere, O., Leppamaki, S., Arvilommi, P., & Isometsa, E. T. (2005). Suicidal ideation and attempts in bipolar I and II disorders. *Journal of Clinical Psychiatry, 66*, 1456–1462.

Valtonen, H. M., Suominen, K., Mantere, O., Leppamaki, S., Arvilommi, P., & Isometsa, E. T. (2006). Prospective study of risk factors for attempted suicide among patients with bipolar disorder. *Bipolar Disorders, 8*, 576–585.

Vieland, V., Whittle, B., Garland, A., Hicks, R., & Shaffer, D. (1991). The impact of curriculum-based suicide prevention programs for teenagers: An 18-month follow-up. *Journal of American Academy of Child and Adolescent Psychiatry, 30*, 811–815.

Wasserman, D., & Durkee, T. (2009). Strategies in suicide prevention. In D. Wasserman & C. Wasserman (Eds.), *Oxford textbook of suicide and suicide prevention* (pp. 381–384). New York, NY: Oxford University Press.

Weaver, A. J. (1995). Has there been a failure to prepare and support parish-based clergy in their role as frontline community mental health workers: A review. *Journal of Pastoral Care, 49*, 129–147.

Weiner, P. D., Cantara, J. D., Kuo, N. H., & Lione, J. (1988). A partnership in health education between a neighborhood school and a community hospital. *Journal of Community Health, 13*, 184–194.

Wiesen, F. E., & Lischer, D. K. (2006). College crisis intervention: An initiative to develop regional campus critical incident stress management teams. *International Journal of Emergency Mental Health, 8*, 183–187.

Williams, J. M., Alatiq, Y., Crane, C., Barnhofer, T., Fennell, M. J., Duggan, D. S., et al. (2008). Mindfulness-based cognitive therapy (MBCT) in bipolar disorder: Preliminary evaluation of immediate effects on between-episode functioning. *Journal of Affective Disorders, 107*, 275–279.

Williams, J. M., Crane, C., Barnhofer, T., Van der Does, A. J., & Segal, Z. V. (2006). Recurrence of suicidal ideation across depressive episodes. *Journal of Affective Disorders, 91*, 189–194.

Wyn, J., Cahill, H., Holdsworth, R., Rowling, L., & Carson, S. (2000). MindMatters, a whole-school approach promoting mental health and wellbeing. *Australian and New Zealand Journal of Psychiatry, 34*, 594–601.

About the Authors

Konstantinos N. Fountoulakis, MD, PhD, is Assistant Professor of Psychiatry at Aristotle University of Thessaloniki, AHEPA University Hospital, in Thessaloniki, Greece. Dr. Fountoulakis received his medical degree (1989), performed his residency in psychiatry (1998), and earned his PhD in Psychiatry (1999) at the Aristotle University of Thessaloniki. His areas of clinical and research interest are general psychiatry, biological psychiatry, psychopharmacology, mood disorders, schizophrenia, and personality disorders. He chairs the ISNP and the Neuropsychological and Psychometric Instruments Section of the Greek Psychiatric Association, and since 2008 he is Co-Chairman of the Private Practice Section of the World Psychiatric Association. In 2009 he was appointed member of the Greek Ministry of Health Committee for the Administrative, Economic, and Scientific Supervision of the Mental Health Units of the deinstitutionalization project. Dr. Fountoulakis is Editor-in-Chief of *Annals of General Psychiatry* and is Section Editor of *Current Opinion in Psychiatry.* He has co-authored more than 250 papers delivered to congresses and more than 100 of them are published in international journals such as the *Lancet, Biological Psychiatry, International Journal of Neuropsychopharmacology, Journal of Affective Disorders, Schizophrenia Research, Psychiatry Research, Bipolar Disorders, Annals of General Hospital Psychiatry,* and the *British Journal of Psychiatry.* He authored or co-authored a number of chapters in books including the mood disorders chapter for the Wiki project of the World Psychiatric Association (WPA). He has received a number of national and international research awards.

Professor Zoltán Rihmer, MD, PhD, DSc, received his medical diploma in 1971. Since then he has been working at the National Institute for Psychiatry and Neurology, Budapest, Hungary. Since 2007 he is Professor of Psychiatry at the Department of Psychiatry and Psychotherapy and the Scientific Director at the Department of Clinical and Theoretical Mental Health at the Semmelweis University, Faculty of Medicine, in Budapest. Dr. Rihmer has three special examinations: psychiatry (1976), neurology (1979), and clinical pharmacology (1990). He received his PhD at the Hungarian Academy of Sciences in 1993, and his DSc in 2004. His special interest is in the clinical and biological aspects of mood and anxiety disorders with particular regard to prediction of treatment response and prevention of suicide. He has published more than 350 scientific articles/book chapters (more than 180 in English) and four books. He received the Brickell Suicide Research Award of the Department of Child and Adolescent Psychiatry, Columbia University, NY, and the Life Achievement Award of the Hungarian Psychiatric Association. He is National Clinical Audit Lead in Psychiatry of Hungary. Professor Rihmer is a member of several Hungarian and international scientific boards and associations, including the editorial board of the *Journal of Affective Disorders*, the *International Journal of Psychiatry in Clinical Practice*, *Neuropsychobiology*, and the *World Journal of Biological Psychiatry*. He is also a member of the Executive Committee of the European College of Neuropsychopharmacology.

Konstantinos N. Fountoulakis
6, Odysseos Street (1st Parodos Ampelonon Street)
55535 Pylaia Thessaloniki
Greece
Tel.: +30 2310 435702
Fax: +30 2310 266570
E-mail: kfount@med.auth.gr

Evidence-Based Interventions for Preventing Suicide in Youths

Maurizio Pompili,[1,2] Marco Innamorati,[3] Paolo Girardi,[1]
Roberto Tatarelli,[1] and David Lester[4]

[1]Department of Neurosciences, Mental Health and Sensory Functions, Suicide Prevention Center, Sant'Andrea Hospital, Sapienza University of Rome, Italy
[2]McLean Hospital, Harvard Medical School, Boston, MA, USA
[3]Università Europea di Roma, Italy
[4]Department of Psychology, The Richard Stockton College, Pomona, NJ, USA

Suicide among young people is one of the most serious public health problems. According to the National Center for Health Statistics, the suicide rate for those youths aged 15–24 years has more than tripled since 1950, and suicide is now the second or third leading cause of death in this age group. Recent studies indicate that the incidence of suicide attempts among adolescents may exceed 10% annually. The roles of caregivers and schools (as well as colleges and universities) are important in the assessment, management, and prevention of suicidal behavior in children and youth.

Adolescence is a time when dramatic biological, cognitive, social, and emotional changes take place. Among the various problems that emerge during this period, suicide among young people, especially among adolescent boys, has become a major source of concern in many countries (Cantor & Neulinger, 2000). Overall, suicide ranks as the third leading cause of death in the 15 to 24-year-old age group. Although the actual base rate of adolescent suicide is still relatively low (approximately 7.9 adolescents per 100,000 per year in the United States take their life [National Center for Health Statistics, 1996]), it is of great concern that the rates of adolescent suicide have increased rapidly over the past four decades (Cantor et al., 1996; World Health Organization, 1982). Recent data reported in the US suggest that the suicide rate for 15- to 19-year-olds is six times that for 10- to 14-year-olds (Anderson & Smith, 2003). During 2001, 4,382 American youths between the ages of 15 and 24 years committed suicide. According to Peters, Kochenek, and Murphy (1998), the suicide rates for youths between the ages of 15 and 19 years rose 245% between 1956 and 1994.

Gould, Greenberg, Velting, and Shaffer (2003) reviewed two plausible explanations for the escalation in adolescent suicide rates during the 1960s, 1970s, and 1980s: (1) a greater exposure of adolescents to drugs and alcohol, and (2) the increased availability of firearms. Further investigation is needed because there has not been an appreciable decline in drug and alcohol abuse by adolescents to correspond with a more recent decline in the adolescent suicide rates. Additionally, the recent decrease in the availability of firearms has not resulted in a corresponding decrease in using firearms as a method of adolescent suicide. As regards the recent decline in the suicide rates, a plausible explanation attributed to this development is the surge in antidepressants being prescribed for adolescents (Gibbons et al., 2007; Gould et al., 2003).

The high rates of nonlethal suicide attempts are also disconcerting. Several studies on large general populations report that the suicide attempt rates range from 7% to 16% among the adolescents (Adcock, Nagy, & Simpson, 1991; Kandel, Raveis, & Davies, 1991; Lewinsohn, Rohde, & Seeley, 1996; Reynolds & Mazza, 1992; Shaffer et al., 1990; Windle, Miller-Tutzauer, & Domenico, 1992). These studies show clear gender differences, with approximately 4–10% of boys and 10–20% of girls reporting a history of suicide attempts. While female adolescents are two to four times more likely to attempt suicide, males are far more likely than their female counterparts to complete suicide (King, 1997).

Young males represent one of the most challenging groups to access for implementing the suicide-prevention strategies. A greater understanding of the pathways that lead young people to take their lives is important for ensuring that suicide-prevention strategies and health service delivery are as effective as possible. Rotheram-Borus, Walker, and Ferns (1996) observed that almost one quarter of all suicide attempts took place within 1 month of using health services, a fact that stressed the importance of screening for suicidality at intake. Ironically, however, once patients are identified, it is unknown whether specific treatment approaches would prove effective or not, both within specific diagnostic entities and across the diverse range of psychological states that the suicidal adolescents present (Beautrais, Joyce, & Mulder, 1998). When a treatment plan is instituted, it should address the psychopathology that places the individual at risk (Links, Balchand, Dawe, & Watson, 1999).

One valuable approach to understanding the dynamics of suicide has been the use of psychological autopsies (Hawton et al., 1998). Based on the interviews conducted with the relatives of the deceased and on the evidence from medical, criminal, and social service records, psychological autopsy studies suggest that more than 90% of youth suicides are associated with mental health disorders, with high rates of comorbid mental health, addictive and physical disorders (Brent, Baugher, Bridge, Chen, & Chiappetta, 1999; Runeson & Beskow, 1991; Shaffer et al., 1996). Gould, Fisher, Parides, Flory, and Shaffer (1996) conducted a case-control, psychological autopsy study of 120 youth suicides (101 of whom were aged between 15 and 19 years), which was specifically designed for systematically examining the environmental, social, and family characteristics. They found that psychosocial factors significantly increase the risk of suicide among children and adolescents, independent of any psychiatric disorder present. The overall effect size of psychosocial factors on increasing the risk of suicide in adolescents was found to be comparable to that of diagnostic variables. The most notable psychosocial risks for adolescents were poor communication with their father, a father with a history of troubles with the police, a family history of suicidal behavior, disciplinary crises, recent losses (for males), and school or work problems.

Regardless of age, ethnicity, or gender, firearms are the most common and lethal method of committing suicide in the US, and this is also true in the case of adolescents (Shaffer & Pfeffer, 2001; Shenassa, Catlin, & Buka, 2003). Hanging is the second most common method of suicide in adolescents, followed by an overdose of medication in female adolescents and carbon monoxide poisoning in male adolescents (Brent et al., 1999). Jumping from a high place is also common in male adolescent suicides, whereas asphyxiation and carbon monoxide poisoning are also common in female adolescent suicides (Brent et al., 1999).

There is a body of literature examining the cultural meanings of suicidal behavior that may help explain these gender differences. For example, studies of American college students suggest that nonfatal suicide attempts are viewed as more "feminine" and less potent, and that they are interpreted as a cry for help, a behavior that is expected more of women (Linehan, 1973; Suter, 1976). Other surveys of college students identified a perception of female suicide as wrong, foolish, and weak, and less permissible than male suicide. In the United States, cultural scripts of gender and suicidal behavior are likely to influence adolescents' decisions about suicidal behavior (Canetto, 1997). Adolescents are quite sensitive and responsive to cultural messages, even more so than the adults, given the fact that they are in the midst of defining their identities. Thus, the influence of "gender-appropriate" suicidal behavior may be significant and requires further evaluation.

Looking at the methods adopted for committing suicide, a decline in suicide by overdosing with medications may be related to the introduction of less toxic antidepressant medications such as selective serotonin reuptake inhibitors (SSRIs) (although some authors have argued that the use of antidepressant drugs in pediatric patients is associated with a modestly increased risk of suicidality [Hammad, Laughren, & Racoosin, 2006]). The use of more lethal methods of suicide by girls in recent years may be a product of changes in the cultural patterns that allow girls, and women in general, to hold similar roles as their male counterparts.

It is important to note that several studies have attempted to characterize the different types of suicides among young people, but with conflicting results. An early study of nonfatal overdoses by 50 adolescents identified a group of adolescents with chronic behavioral problems who were more likely to express a greater intent to die and who had higher rates of repetition at a 1-year follow-up as compared with their peers who did not have behavioral disturbances (Hawton, Osborn, O'Grady, & Cole, 1982). A study of suicides in those under 15 years by Beautrais (2001) also identified behavioral problems in a group of young people living away from their parents, with relatively low levels of mental illness, high rates of social welfare involvement, severe family difficulties, and multiple lifestyle changes. Sankey and Lawrence (2005) classified the self-inflicted deaths of 187 adolescents aged 12–17 years in New South Wales (Australia) into three groups. The majority of them (66%) had enduring difficulties both at home and in school. Behavioral disorders and depression were the most common forms of mental health problems that were experienced by this group of adolescents. Stressful life events accounted for 14% of the deaths, and 15% were a result of experimentation, with half of these deaths due to using either drugs or alcohol. In a psychological autopsy study of suicide deaths of 19 young people in Belgium (Portzky, Audenaert, & van Heeringen, 2005b), the authors identified a subset of young people who had no previous behavioral or emotional difficulties, but who completed suicide following the development of an adjustment disorder (Portzky, Audenaert, & van Heeringen, 2005a).

A case-control psychological autopsy study by Shaffer et al. (1996) examined 120 consecutive suicides (mean age 16 years) in an ethnically diverse area of the United States. They found that 90% of the youths suffered from at least one DSM-III psychiatric disorder and 70% suffered from two or more disorders. The most common disorders were mood disorders (61%), disruptive disorders (50%), and substance abuse disorders (35%). The prevalence of psychiatric diagnoses in the suicides increased with age, except for adjustment disorder, with depressed mood and disruptive disorders more common in the younger male and female suicides, respectively. Substance abuse was found significantly more often in males than in females and was present in about two thirds of the 18–19-year-old male suicides. Although disruptive disorders were prevalent for both sexes, their effect on risk became statistically insignificant when adjusted for other significant risk factors (previous attempt, mood disorder, and substance abuse disorder). Two-thirds of the youths who committed suicide carried at least one of the three risk factors. For males, a previous suicide attempt, mood disorder, and substance abuse disorder significantly increased the risk of suicide with ORs of 19.4 (95% CI: 2.3–162.1), 7.8 (95% CI: 2.6–23.2), and 5.8 (95% CI: 1.6–20.6), respectively. For females, having made a previous attempt and having a mood disorder (OR: 20.8, 95% CI: 1.4–320) were identified as the significant risk factors. Youths who committed suicide were significantly more likely to have received psychiatric treatment in the 3 months prior to their death, but fewer than 10% had been treated with antidepressants or had undergone treatment for substance abuse.

Brent et al. (1999) conducted a study of 140 consecutive suicides aged 13–19 years and found similar significant psychopathologic risk factors. In age-stratified, case-control comparisons, they found that the presence of any psychiatric disorder resulted in a much greater risk for suicide in the older adolescents (16–19 years) as compared to the younger adolescents (13–15 years). Parent-child conflict was more frequent which resulted in a higher risk for suicide among the younger adolescents (13–15 years). Other particularly significant risk factors cited for the younger age group were mood disorder, presence of a firearm at home, and a previous suicide attempt. A lifetime history of physical abuse conferred an immensely increased risk for suicide, with odds ratios as high as 49.3 (95% CI: 6.4–377.3) for males. Other risk factors for males that reached statistical significance were psychopathology in a first-degree relative, conflict with parents, conflict in a romantic relationship, loss of a romantic relationship, living in a nonintact family, legal or disciplinary problems, and a firearm at home. For girls, loss of a romantic relationship, legal or disciplinary problems, physical abuse, and a firearm at home were statistically significant risk factors for completed suicide.

Methods

We performed careful MedLine and PsycINFO searches from 1980 to 2008. The following search terms were used: "adolescents," suicid* (which comprises suicide, suicidal, suicidality, and other suicide-related terms), risk factors, and prevention. In addition, each category was cross-referenced with the others using the MeSH (Medical Subjects Headings) method. The search limitations were used for selecting meta-analyses, controlled trials, and other quantitative studies. The selection of papers that are suitable for this study allowed the inclusion of only those articles that were published in the English peer-reviewed journals. Included were those studies that added an original contribution to the literature. We also searched the TRIP database.

Results

Risk and Protective Factors, and Warning Signs

Clinicians must remember that emotional problems in children and adolescents can be both serious and long-lasting, and may frequently lead to consequences such as poor academic achievement, social isolation, school failure, hazardous and risk-taking behaviors (e.g., drug or alcohol misuse and promiscuity), health problems, and suicidal behaviors.

The literature identified several risk and protective factors. However, it must be remembered that these factors are not necessarily present in each and every case and may vary from one country to another, depending on cultural, political, and economic features (World Health Organization, 2000).

Risk factors may be categorized in several classes:

1. Cultural and sociodemographic factors, such as low socioeconomic status, poor education, and unemployment in the family. Minorities may be assigned to this group, because they often experience emotional problems, linguistic difficulties, and limited social networks. Children and adolescents who lack cultural roots have marked identity problems and lack a model for conflict resolution. In some stressful situations, they may resort to self-destructive behavior such as suicidal behavior (Matschnig, Fruhwald, & Frottier, 2006).
2. Family patterns and negative life events during childhood. Destructive family patterns and traumatic events in early childhood affect young people's lives thereafter, especially when they have been unable to cope with the trauma (Crawford, Thomas, Khan, & Kulinskaya, 2007). Aspects of family dysfunction and instability, and negative life events that are often found in suicidal children and adolescents include parental psychopathology (Tarrier, Taylor, & Gooding, 2008), alcohol and substance abuse disorders, a family history of suicidal

behaviors, a history of neglect, physical and sexual abuse, and family rigidity. Evidence suggests that young suicidal people often come from families with more than one problem, and the risks are cumulative.
3. Cognitive style and personality, such as anger or aggressive behavior, impulsivity, irritability, rigid thinking and coping patterns, poor problem solving, and uncertainty pertaining to gender identity or sexual orientation.
4. Psychiatric disorders. Suicidal behavior is overrepresented in children and adolescents with depressive disorders, anxiety disorders, substance abuse disorders, and psychotic disorders.
5. Current negative life events, for example, victimization (Epstein & Spirito, 2009).

Adolescents spend most of their daytime at school, and hence school staff must be educated to notice any warning signs of suicide. Common signs of distress that should be checked by the school staff are as follows (Beautrais, Coggan, Fergusson, & Rivers, 1997):

1. Unexpected poor academic performance or failure, extreme disappointment at being rejected for a course or abrupt changes in attendance, such as increased absences, tardiness, or truancy.
2. Ideas and themes of depression, death, and suicide, such as reading selections, written essays, conversation, and artwork containing themes of depression, death, and suicide; statements or suggestions that they would not be missed if they were gone; collecting and discussing information on suicide methods; giving away the prized possessions (possibly with some elevation in mood); and previous direct or indirect suicide threats or attempts.
3. Change in mood, such as withdrawal, sudden tearfulness, and remarks that indicate profound unhappiness, despair, hopelessness, and helplessness; anger at self, irritability, moodiness and aggressiveness; lack of interest in surroundings and activities, and marked emotional instability; and involvement in high-risk activities.
4. Grief about a significant loss; stress due to recent disintegration of their family; a recent death or suicide in the family; loss of a friend through death or suicide; and a break up with a boyfriend or a girlfriend.
5. Withdrawal from relationships; a change in relationships with friends and classmates; loss of interest in extracurricular activities; dropping out of sports and other clubs; and beginning to spend long periods of time in solitude.
6. Physical symptoms with emotional causes; eating disorders; physical complaints; and reduced self-care.
7. High-risk behaviors; increased use of alcohol and drugs; dangerous driving; and risky sex (Epstein & Spirito, 2009).

Clinicians should also evaluate protective factors. Some of the protective factors are the opposite of the risk factors, such as good family patterns, good social skills, social integration, and support from relevant people. Other protective factors that are relevant for the prevention of suicide are reasons for living and religious beliefs.

Principles of Treatment and Prevention

A continuum of services including emergency response, primary prevention, and secondary prevention are necessary for treating children and adolescents with suicidal behavior (Steele & Doey, 2007). Hospitalization is necessary when the youth has several risk factors and limited community support. Day treatment programs may be preferred when the adolescent faces emotional and environmental stressors, and needs more time to be stabilized (Shaffer & Pfeffer, 2001). However, there is no sound evidence that either hospitalization or day treatment is effective in reducing the rates of suicidal ideation, attempted suicide, or completed suicide among adolescents (Gould et al., 2003). On the other hand, the benefits of outpatient therapy must be weighed against the lower rates of compliance (Steele & Doey, 2007).

Beautrais et al. (1997) suggested that the single most important factor in the prevention of suicide is to address the causes of mental health and personal adjustment problems in young people. Efforts aimed at the prevention of suicide should be taken within the context of health education programs and cultural development processes that promote a safe and healthy environment, increase self-esteem, and address adolescent difficulties. In general, efforts should be made to address and manage the difficulties faced by young people coming from adverse childhood backgrounds who have multiple problems of personal adjustment (including disorders such as depression, alcohol and drug abuse, and conduct).

School-Based Suicide-Prevention Strategies

Given the fact that in many countries and regions most of the adolescents attend school, this appears to be an excellent place for developing preventive programs for suicide. School-based prevention strategies have included universal programs, targeted programs, screening for suicidal youth, and postvention programs.

Before initiating a suicide-prevention program, it is necessary to establish policies and procedures focused on such issues as how to respond effectively to a student who may be indicating suicidal ideation or threats, how to respond to the aftermath of a suicide attempt or a death by suicide, and the various roles school personnel may play in preventing, intervening, and coping with a student who may be suicidal (Table 1). These policies increase the likelihood that a school-based suicide-prevention program would be effectively implemented and maintained (Lazear, Roggenbaum, & Blase, 2003).

A qualitative review by Guo and Harstall (2002) included 10 studies (three of them randomized controlled trials, RCTs) focused mainly on high school students 12–19 years old. These school-based suicide-prevention programs conducted for adolescents varied considerably in objectives, focus, target population, and delivery modes. The duration

Table 1. Myths and Facts about adolescent suicide. Adapted from Lazear, Roggenbaum, and Blase (2003)

Myth	Fact
Adolescent suicide is decreasing.	Since the 1950s, the US suicide rate for adolescents has more than tripled (K. A. King, 1999). From 1980 to 1992, the suicide rate for 15–19 year olds and 10–14 year olds increased 28% and 120%.
Most teenagers will not reveal that they are suicidal.	Most teens will reveal that they are suicidal. They prefer to discuss suicidal thoughts with a peer rather than a school staff member (Zenere & Lazarus, 1997).
Adolescents who talk about suicide do not attempt or commit suicide.	Adolescents who make threats of suicide should be taken seriously and provided the help that they need (Kirk, 1993).
Educating teens about suicide leads to increased suicidal behavior.	Directly asking an adolescent if he or she is thinking about suicide displays care and concern, and may aid in clearly determining whether or not an adolescent is considering suicide. Research shows that when issues concerning suicide are taught in a sensitive and educational manner, students demonstrate significant gains in knowledge about the warning signs of suicide and develop more positive attitudes toward help-seeking behaviors with troubled teens (Gould et al., 2003; Kalafat & Elias, 1994).
Parents are often aware of their child's suicidal behavior.	Studies have shown that as much as 86% of parents were unaware of their child's suicidal behavior (Zenere & Lazarus, 1997).
Most adolescents who attempt suicide fully intend to die.	Most suicidal adolescents are torn between wanting to end their psychological pain through death and wanting to continue living, though only in a more hopeful environment. Such ambivalence is communicated to others through verbal statements and behavior changes in 80% of suicidal youths (K. A. King, 1999).
Because female adolescents complete suicide at a lower rate than male adolescents, their attempts should not be taken seriously.	One of the most powerful predictors of completed suicide is a prior suicide attempt, regardless of sex of the attempter.
The only one who can help a suicidal adolescent is a counsellor or a mental health professional.	Most adolescents who are contemplating suicide are not presently seeing a mental health professional. They are mostly like to approach a family member, peer or school professional for help.

of programs ranged from one 1½-hour session to 180 sessions of 55 minutes each. The prevention programs were usually delivered by school staff (teachers, school nurses, or counselors) or by social workers with previous training. The programs studied in the trials were grouped into the following four categories, with the first two categories showing evidence of some added benefit:

1. Three suicide-prevention programs for adolescents at high risk that focused on skills training and social support appeared to be effective in reducing the risk factors (such as depression, hopelessness, stress, anxiety, and anger) and enhancing the protective factors (such as personal control, problem-solving skills, self-esteem, and network support).
2. Two suicide-prevention programs that focused on behavioral change and coping strategies in the general school population demonstrated lowered suicidal tendencies, improved ego identity, and improved coping ability.
3. Four studies evaluated curriculum-based suicide education programs in the general school population. One study with a relatively large sample size demonstrated an improvement in knowledge about helping resources, but found only a slight change in adolescents' attitudes toward suicide. No long-term effect on suicidal behavior was demonstrated.
4. One study evaluated a postvention program, but did not demonstrate any benefit.

For school-based suicide-prevention programs, one of the major methodological limitations was that some studies did not establish the validity and the reliability of the outcome measurement tools. In addition, different tools were used to measure the same outcomes. Therefore, the results from these studies are difficult to compare, and the soundness of conclusions based on these studies may be questioned (Guo & Harstall, 2002).

Children and adolescents in distress or at risk of suicide are often hypersensitive to other people's style of communication. This is because often they have lacked trustful relationships with their families and peers during their upbringing and, therefore, have experienced an absence of interest, respect, or even love. The suicidal student's hypersensitivity is apparent in both verbal and nonverbal communications. Here, the body language plays as large a role as verbal communication. Adults should not be discouraged by distressed and/or suicidal children's or adolescents' reluctance to speak to them. Instead, they should remember that this attitude of avoidance is often a sign of distrust of adults. Suicidal children and adolescents also display marked ambivalence about whether to accept or to reject the help that is offered to them and about whether to live or die. This ambivalence has evident repercussions on the suicidal young person's behavior, which can show rapid changes from help-seeking to rejection and may easily be misinterpreted by others.

In 2000, the Australian Institute of Family Studies evaluated the National Youth Suicide Prevention Strategy (Mitchell, 2000). The technical report assessed the programs funded under the National Youth Suicide Prevention Strategy, which were based in schools or which were focused on issues for schools. The National Youth Suicide Prevention Strategy funded two major projects targeting secondary schools (MindMatters and Educating for Life [Educating for Life: A guide for a school-based response to preventing self-harm and suicide]). A number of other projects also included strategies targeting schools. These projects mostly used schools as a forum for recruiting parents into parenting programs. The two projects, MindMatters and Educating for Life, have emphasized the importance of a whole-school approach to suicide prevention. The whole-school approach involves directing attention to all aspects of the school environment to ensure that policies, procedures, and activities throughout the whole school are consistent with the aims of making a place that nurtures and promotes the mental health and well-being of young people. The whole-school approach used by these projects is based on the Health Promoting Schools Framework that emphasizes three main areas of activity: curriculum, school ethos, and community partnerships.

However, first, MindMatters consortium members opined that some schools struggled to understand the concept of a whole-school approach to mental health promotion. The idea that a whole-school approach includes everyone in the school community including staff, parents, students, and community groups was noted as particularly difficult for some schools to grasp. Second, MindMatters consortium members observed that schools that had a very hierarchical approach to decision-making found it harder to understand and to develop the whole-school model. Similarly, schools that were organized strongly along departmental lines tended to have poorer communication between staff and found it more difficult to understand and adopt a whole-school approach.

Moreover, professional development and support provided by MindMatters was focused primarily on the curriculum component of the project. Schools and project team members felt that other aspects of the whole-school approach (such as changing school ethos and developing partnerships) did not receive adequate attention in the professional development and support provided by the project team, and that this was a major factor in these aspects of the approach not being implemented as comprehensively as the curriculum component.

Strategic planning was one of the central strategies employed by the project team to encourage schools to adopt a whole-school approach. All pilot schools were encouraged to conduct an audit of policies and activities already taking place in the school that were related to mental health promotion or suicide prevention and to think about how these could be built upon or modified. Schools varied in the extent to which they embraced and utilized the strategic planning exercise. Active participation in the strategic planning process tended to be associated with implementation of more of the components of the whole-school approach. Some schools included broad consultation with staff and students in their strategic planning process, and this was identified as particularly beneficial. Involvement of teaching staff was thought to be enhanced as a result of the site visits made by the MindMatters team members. A number of schools noted that the visits provided a focus, a visible event that acted as a vehicle for publicizing the project as something positive happening within the school.

The MindMatters Project developed a set of curriculum units in four main topic areas: (enhancing resilience, dealing with bullying, understanding mental illness, and loss and grief). As a result of the evaluation of the project, Mitchell (2000) found that a few changes were observed in students' knowledge of and attitudes toward mental health issues.

A major problem in the design faced during the evaluation of the curriculum component of MindMatters was that the schools varied substantially in which parts of the curriculum they chose to try. However, there was some information regarding which aspects of the program worked well. First of all, the interactive teaching methods were identified as one of the aspects of the curriculum that worked particularly well. The evaluation report of the project does not define exactly what is meant by interactive teaching methods, but it is noted that the curriculum materials included many activities that involved the active participation of students. It was observed that most of the teachers did not use the interactive teaching methods that were advocated in the project curriculum because several teachers found the suggestion of using interactive teaching techniques quite threatening and doubted their ability to maintain control of the students. However, when they had tried the methods themselves or adjusted the curriculum materials to address these classroom management concerns, these teachers became advocates of the approaches used.

Matching the curriculum to the intended age group was another aspect that worked well. For example, MindMatters developed the different curriculum units with specific age groups in mind. Most of the schools used the curriculum units with the intended age groups, but others chose to try the curriculum with other age groups. Some of the teachers who used the curriculum with younger students provided a negative feedback, commenting that the educational level of the materials was pitched too high. The evaluators of MindMatters observed that these comments tended to come from schools that had used the curriculum with age groups other than the ones intended by MindMatters.

Teachers in a number of schools noted that they attempted to adapt the materials to the particular needs of their students. The major ways in which teachers adapted the resources included: the target age group of the students, cultural sensitivity for indigenous communities, the length of lessons, and the teaching style. However, some teachers who reported their need to modify the resources said that this was very difficult for them, mainly due to them having limited time for this task. Again, several schools considered that sensitivity to cultural diversity and social issues may have had a positive impact on the effectiveness of the project.

The project devoted a considerable amount of activity to the professional development of teachers who, it was hoped, would implement the curriculum. It was observed that professional development was critically important to the capability of schools to properly implement the curriculum. Several members of the MindMatters consortium noted that the way in which schools structured their curriculum timetable influenced their ability to use the curriculum effectively.

Developing school organization, ethos, and environment was one of the three main strategies emphasized by the MindMatters Project. The main strategy used by the project to stimulate activity in the area of school organization, ethos, and environment was to ask schools to conduct an audit of the current activities and policies that were consistent with making the school a mental health promoting environment and to think about how these could be built upon or modified. Following this audit, the schools were encouraged to develop a strategic plan that identified priority issues and strategies that could be employed to address these. The evaluators of MindMatters noted that a number of schools were very unsure about how to proceed with the audit and strategic plan, and could have benefited from clearer guidance. Schools used different processes to conduct their audits and complete their strategic plans.

The evaluators of MindMatters noted that most of the schools found the audit and strategic planning processes to be useful, but they were more productive when they involved broad consultation with staff and students. Broad consultation was viewed as ensuring that the planning process was based on accurate knowledge of what is happening in the school and provided an opportunity to build an awareness and increase the commitment to and involvement in the project. Further, the physical strategic plan document may be less important than the process of consultation and building consensus around a vision for the school. It was noted that an organizational structure that encouraged collaboration and communication between staff and also active staff involvement in decision-making was more conducive to the successful implementation of several aspects of the project. However, several schools lacked this orientation, and many teachers felt very disempowered.

Curriculum-Based Programs on Education and Awareness About Suicide

One type of preventive program that was evaluated during the last decade dealt with education and awareness about suicide. Programs of education about suicide are generally focused on dispelling the myths, increasing the correct knowledge about adolescent suicide, and encouraging the attitude of seeking help when necessary. However, the results on the effectiveness of curriculum-based programs to promote awareness are mixed (Aseltine & DeMartino, 2004; Ciffone, 1993; Kalafat & Elias, 1994; Kalafat & Gagliano, 1996; Silbert & Berry, 1991), with some studies reporting no benefits at all or potentially dangerous results (Kalafat & Elias, 1994; Overholser, Hemstreet, Spirito, & Vyse, 1989; Shaffer, Garland, Vieland, Underwood, & Busner, 1991; Shaffer et al., 1990; Vieland, Whittle, Garland, Hicks, & Shaffer, 1991). Thus, there is not yet enough information to adequately determine their effectiveness (Gould et al., 2003; Guo & Harstall, 2002).

Because of their potentially dangerous outcomes, Beautrais et al. (1997) recommended that school-based suicide-prevention programs aimed at increasing the awareness among youth about suicide should be undertaken. Lazear et al. (2003) suggested that a curriculum approach focused on destigmatizing suicide, which presents suicide as a reaction to the common stressors of adolescence, may be harmful because an approach of this type normalizes the behavior and reduces the protective taboos, especially when the intervention is extremely brief (often only one session lasting for a duration of 2–4 hours). The authors recommended using a model that identifies suicide as a complicated, abnormal reaction to a number of overwhelming factors. Programs should also emphasize the association between suicide and mental illness, and "oneshot" approaches with students have to be avoided. Furthermore, schools that wish to adopt a curriculum on suicide as a preventive method should use this approach in conjunction with other preventive strategies such as gatekeeper training, screening, establishing community links, and imparting skills training.

The authors have pointed out that schools should not avoid adopting this approach due to a lurking fear that talking about suicide and teaching the students various points about suicide will only provide the students with ideas on and methods of suicidal behaviors, because this opinion is simply not true.

School programs that have used education and awareness about suicide include a program such as the Signs of Suicide (SOS; Aseltine & DeMartino, 2004). This is a 2-day secondary school-based intervention program during which the students are screened for depression and suicide risk, and referred for professional help as indicated. Students also view a video that teaches them how to recognize the signs of depression and suicide in other people. They are also taught the fact that the appropriate response to these signs is to acknowledge them, let the person know you care, and tell a responsible adult (either with the person or on that person's behalf). Students also participate in guided classroom discussions about suicide and depression.

In the attempt to provide a reference for the evidence-based practice in the prevention of suicide in general, and among youths in particular, the Best Practices Registry (BPR) for suicide prevention has been established. It is a collaboration between the Suicide Prevention Resource Center and the American Foundation for Suicide Prevention. The registry looks at the strength of and limitations for the SOS program and assesses its readiness for dissemination using criteria of 2½ on a 0–4 scale.

In the RCTs involving more than 6,000 students from five high schools, SOS participants were approximately 40% less likely than comparable students who did not participate in the intervention program to report attempting suicide in the next 3 months. In one evaluation, 3.6% of intervention participants reported suicide attempts, compared with 5.4% of control students. In the RCTs, SOS participants demonstrated greater knowledge about depression and suicide after participating in the intervention than comparable high school students who had not taken part. In one evaluation, the intervention achieved a small effect size on knowledge (Cohen's $d = 0.35$). SOS participants had more desirable attitudes on depression and suicide after participating in the intervention than comparable high school students. The intervention also achieved a small effect size on attitudes (Cohen's $d = 0.25$ and 0.37 in each of the two evaluations that looked at this outcome).

In 2007, the researchers published a replication study (Aseltine, James, Schilling, & Glanovsky, 2007). Students (4,133) from nine high schools in Columbus (Georgia), western Massachusetts, and Hartford (Connecticut) were randomly assigned to intervention and control groups during the 2001–2002 and 2002–2003 school years. The results indicated that exposure to the SOS program was associated with significantly fewer self-reported suicide attempts. The youths in the treatment group were approximately 40% less likely to report a suicide attempt in the next 3 months compared with the youths in the control group. This equates to a 3-month rate of suicide attempts in the SOS group of 3.0% compared to 4.6% among controls. Furthermore, exposure of students to the SOS program resulted in acquiring greater knowledge about depression and suicide, and more adaptive attitudes toward these problems, although the effects were modest in magnitude. In contrast, the effects of the SOS program on suicidal ideation and help-seeking behavior were not statistically significant. There were some differences in the outcomes by students' demographic characteristics.

Skills-Based School Programs

Another preventive tactic for educating students focuses on appropriate social skills, problem-solving strategies, coping skills, and help-seeking skills. The rationale behind this method lies in the fact that adolescents with deficits in these skills are more prone to suicide. Social skills, problem-solving strategies, and coping skills could be directly taught through lessons or indirectly by incorporating these skills into the existing classes. There has been some evidence to suggest that skills-based training school programs could reduce suicidal behavior and improve the students' attitudes, emotions, and coping skills (Klingman & Hochdorf, 1993; Orbach & Bar-Joseph, 1993; Zenere & Lazarus, 1997).

Some studies have specifically focused on skills training and social support programs with a view to helping students at high risk for school failure or dropout (Eggert, Thompson, Herting, & Nicholas, 1995; Randell, Eggert, & Pike, 2001; Thompson, Eggert, & Herting, 2000; Thompson, Eggert, Randell, & Pike, 2001) and have demonstrated enhanced protective factors and reduced risk factors following the "active" interventions, compared with "intervention as usual," which did not increase the protective factors (Gould et al., 2003). Randell and colleagues noted the superiority of skills-based interventions in reducing depression and enhancing perceived family support, but the decrease in suicidal behaviors did not differ from "intervention as usual." The improvement in self-efficacy, personal control, and problem-solving was specific to the skills-training component (Randell et al., 2001).

In another study, group leader support was found to be critical for building a positive peer-group culture. Higher levels of depression at baseline predicted lower levels of personal control at follow-up, suggesting that strategies to address the existing depression are important for enhancing the adolescent's personal control (Thompson et al., 2000). Interventions in which suicide education is incorporated within a life-skills approach show more consistent evidence of effect, but the effect on the suicide-specific behavior remains uncertain (Burns & Patton, 2000).

Wilcox et al. (2008) investigated the impact later in young adulthood on suicidal ideation and attempts of universal preventive interventions in two first- and second-grade classrooms. The design was epidemiologically based, with randomization at the school and classroom levels, and balancing of children across classrooms. The trial involved a cohort of first-grade children in 19 schools and 41 classrooms with intervention during first and second grades. A replication was implemented with the next cohort of first-grade children with the same teachers, but with little mentoring or monitoring. The first program, the good behavior game (GBG) (Barrish, Saunders, & Wolf, 1969), is a classroom team-based behavior management strategy that promotes good behavior by rewarding the teams that do not exceed maladaptive behavior standards as set by the teacher. The goal of the GBG is to create an integrated classroom social system that is supportive of all children being able to learn with little aggressive, disruptive behavior. The methods involve helping teachers to define unacceptable behaviors clearly and to socialize children with the regulation of a teammate's behavior through a process of team contingent reinforcement and mutual self-interest. In the second program, "mastery learning," intervention teachers received an enhanced reading curriculum that they implemented in the context of a system-wide curriculum. This program may reduce suicidality because of the role that mastery plays in self-esteem, depression, and suicidal thoughts.

The results supported the hypothesis that first graders assigned to GBG classrooms experienced a lower incidence of suicidality throughout childhood, adolescence, and into young adulthood compared to controls, with half the reported lifetime rates of suicidal ideation and attempts compared to their matched controls. For suicidal ideation, the beneficial effect of the GBG program effect was consistent, regardless of whether baseline covariates were included or not. The program's impact on suicide attempts was less definitive once the authors controlled for gender and baseline depressive symptoms. The beneficial impact of the program was consistent for both genders, who showed similar relative risks. However, no statistically significant impact on outcomes was found for the mastery learning program. The absence of positive findings for the mastery learning program suggests that the effect of the GBG program was specific to this program and cannot be attributed to added attention in the GBG classrooms.

Programs that have utilized social skills training include CAST (Coping and Support Training) (Eggert, Thompson, Randell, & Pike, 2002; Randell et al., 2001; Thompson et al., 2001). CAST is a program that is intended to decrease suicidal behavior, depression, and drug use in high-risk 14- to 19-year-old youths who screen positive for suicidal risk. The CAST program is a second step-type program used in conjunction with C-CARE (Counselors – Care, Assess, Respond, Empower). The CAST program begins with an interview assessment session. Students potentially at risk for suicidal behavior are included in a small-group intervention delivered 2 times per week over a 6-week period of time using the following structure: (1) 6–8 students per group; (2) 1-hour sessions including an inaugural session and a valedictory function; (3) 10 skills-training sessions targeting three overall goals – increased mood management (depression and anger), improved school performance, and decreased drug use. Sessions focus on group support, goal setting and monitoring, self-esteem, decision-making skills, better management of anger and depression, "school smarts," control of drug use with relapse prevention, and self-recognition of progress through the program. Each session helps the youths apply newly acquired skills and increase the support that they receive from family and other trusted adults. Detailed lesson plans specify the type of motivational preparation, teaching, skills practice, and coaching activities appropriate for at-risk youth. Every session ends with "Lifework" assignments that call for the youths to practice the skills taught during the sessions with a specific person in their school, home, or peer-group environment; and (4) the sessions are handled by trained, master's-level high school teachers, counselors, or nurses with adequate academic experience.

When used together, C-CARE and CAST have been shown to be effective in decreasing the suicidal risk, depression, hopelessness, stress, and anger, and in increasing the self-esteem and the ability to use social support. The Best Practices Registry for suicide prevention assessed its readiness for dissemination rating as 3½ on a 0–4 scale.

In a clinical RCT that compared CAST participants with the usual-care youths who were also at suicide risk (a 30-minute one-on-one session with a school counselor or nurse), CAST participants showed significantly greater declines relative to the usual-care youths in two of the four suicide risk factors: declines in both positive attitudes toward suicide and suicidal ideation. The rates of decline in these suicidal behaviors were most pronounced in the first 4 weeks after baseline assessment ($p < .05$). A slight rebound occurred in positive attitudes toward suicide at 10 weeks, but reductions were sustained at the 9-month follow-up ($p < .05$). For suicidal ideation, the initial declines were maintained throughout the 9 months of follow-up ($p < .05$).

Reconnecting Youth is a school-based suicide-prevention program that targets young people in grades 9–12 who show signs of poor school achievement, display potential for school dropout, and suicide risk (Eggert & Nicholas, 2004; Eggert, Thompson, Herting, & Randell, 2001; Eggert et al., 1995; Thompson et al., 2000). Reconnecting Youth teaches the necessary skills to build resiliency with respect to risk factors and to moderate early signs of substance abuse and depression/aggression. The program is one semester-long and is divided into five modules: (1) getting started, (2) self-esteem enhancement, (3) decision-making, (4) personal control, and (5) interpersonal communication. The class integrates small-group work and life-skills training models to enhance personal and social protective factors for high-risk youth.

A three-group, repeated measures design was used to examine the effects of Reconnecting Youth program. Students (n = 106) in grades 9–12 were randomly assigned to one of the two treatment conditions or a control group. The analysis supported the program's central hypothesis that teacher and peer-group support, facilitated through the Reconnecting Youth class, increased personal control, which in turn decreased the behaviors associated with suicide risk. In addition, Reconnecting Youth appears to contribute to decreased drug use and depression, risk factors associated with suicide, and to increased school achievement. While the Reconnecting Youth program was studied in six urban schools, it has been implemented in a variety of schools in both urban and suburban settings representing a cross-section of ethnic enrollments.

Gatekeeper-Training Programs

Gatekeeper training is an essential component of any suicide-prevention program. The United Nations (United Nations Department for Policy Coordination and Sustainable Development, 1996), after reviewing numerous articles on general methods of suicide prevention, has recommended that gatekeeper training be considered while implementing an effective strategy to prevent suicide (Beautrais et al., 2007; Gould & Kramer, 2001; Mann et al., 2005). Gatekeeper training teaches specific groups of people how to identify those people who are at high risk for suicide and then to refer them for undergoing treatment. In general, gatekeepers are people who have primary contact with those who are at risk for suicide and could identify them by recognizing the suicide risk factors. The function of gatekeeping is seen as an attempt to make informal channels of help more effective rather than to build or to superimpose formal channels through social engineering.

Historically, gatekeepers have been divided into two main groups, defined as either designated and emergent (Isaac et al., 2009; Ramsay, Cooke, & Lang, 1990). The designated group comprises people who have been trained and are designated as helping professionals (e.g., those who work in the fields of medicine, social work, nursing, and psychology). The emergent group comprises of community members who may not have been formally trained to intervene with someone who is at risk for suicide, but who emerge as potential gatekeepers as recognized by those with suicidal intent. Because schools provide a valuable window of observation where young people at risk could be identified, the school staff should be encouraged to share this responsibility by taking part in regular and ongoing training that includes: increasing knowledge of the symptoms of distress and risk of suicide, increasing staff members' confidence and competence to refer and support distressed young people, increasing staff members' willingness, and increasing competence to work in these situations (Beautrais et al., 1997).

The gatekeeper training usually consists of imparting training to any adult who interacts with or observes the students to be able to identify any student who may be at risk for suicide, determine the level of risk, know where to refer a potentially at-risk student, know how to contact these referral sources, and what school policies are in place that relate to suicidal crisis situations. Although teachers are expected to act as gatekeepers and know how to identify a student who is potentially at risk for suicidal actions, they should be informed that they are not meant to take on an additional role as a mental health counselor, but are simply meant to act as a watchful eye and "sound the alarm" (Lazear et al., 2003). However, usually teachers do not have the requisite confidence when assigned the task of recognizing an adolescent at risk (King, Price, Telljohann, & Wahl, 1999).

Isaac et al. (2009) performed a systematic review of gatekeeper training as a preventive intervention for suicide. The authors found that the highest level of evidence for gatekeeper-training programs was level 1B (i.e., RCTs). The authors examined two main outcomes when reporting the use of gatekeeper training: (1) the impact of the training in increasing knowledge, changing attitudes, and imparting skills to the trainee and (2) the effect on the suicide rate.

Gatekeeper-training programs have been studied by school counselors, educators, and peer helpers with positive effects on knowledge, skills, and attitudes (Centers for Disease Control and Prevention, 1992; Garland & Zigler, 1993; Gould & Kramer, 2001; King & Smith, 2000; Wyman et al., 2008). Recently, Wyman et al. (2008) performed a group-based randomized trial with 32 schools that examined the impact of Question, Persuade, Refer (QPR) training on a stratified random sample of 249 staff with a 1-year average follow-up. To test the impact of the QPR program, the authors introduced and contrasted two models of gatekeeper-training effects in a population: gatekeeper surveillance and gatekeeper communication.

The training was for a duration of 1½ hours covering the following themes: rates of youth suicide; warning signs and risk factors for suicide; procedures for asking a student about suicide; persuading a student to get help; and referring a student for help. Consistent with QPR training recommendations, the training reviewed local rates of student suicidal behavior and the district protocol for responding to suicidal students. The training was conducted by one of the eight staff from the district's Prevention/Intervention Center who had received QPR instructor and triage training (12–16 hours). The training was co-led by a counselor in each school who received instructor training (6–8 hours) and who served as the primary source for referrals in that school. The training was completed in an average of 2.7 sessions per school, with an average of 28 staff per session. The staff were invited for a 30-minute booster session several months after the training. Refresher sessions were completed in an average of 1.8 sessions. Refresher training took place an average of 282 days after the initial training.

The authors found a consistent positive impact on staff knowledge and appraisals, whereas the impact on behaviors was concentrated among those staff members in certain job classes and in those communicating with distressed youths about suicide at baseline. At a 1-year follow-up, the authors found a moderate, positive training condition effect on knowledge and very large positive effects on perceived preparedness, self-evaluated knowledge, efficacy, and access to services. With respect to knowledge, training had a medium-size effect on increasing participants' accuracy to identify warning signs and risk factors for youth suicide and to recommend intervention behaviors. Staff entering the study with closer communication with students about emotional distress asked more students about suicide after training. Gatekeeper training has also been examined in a peer gatekeeper program, with similar effects on skills, attitudes, and knowledge as in the studies of educators (Stuart, Waalen, & Haelstromm, 2003).

Isaac et al. (2009) noted that, despite numerous studies showing an increase in skills, attitudes, and knowledge generally, there is a dearth of studies dealing with the effectiveness of school-based gatekeeper programs in decreasing the rates of suicidal ideation, suicide attempts, or deaths by suicide. The authors concluded that gatekeeper training holds promise as part of a multifaceted strategy to combat suicide. It has been proven to positively affect the skills, attitudes, and knowledge of people who undertake the training in many settings. Although research is limited in demonstrating an effect on suicide rates and suicidal ideation, it has been seen in many circles as an extremely promising initiative to prevent suicide.

Peer Support Groups

Research suggests that peer gatekeeper training may be useful in preventing adolescent suicide because up to 40% of male peers and 60% of female peers know someone who has attempted suicide, but only 25% have confided in an adult (Kalafat & Elias, 1995). Some researchers suggested that schools should train the students to recognize potentially suicidal peers and, in addition, provide an opportunity for vulnerable students to meet with other students in a comfortable group climate. Peers may help youths at risk to develop more appropriate coping skills, reduce feelings of isolation, and ameliorate substance abuse and other early risk factors while enhancing important protective factors (White & Jodoin, 1998). Some of the existing programs that use peers focus on the peers listening for and reporting any possible warning signs, while others involve the peers in counseling responsibilities (Gould et al., 2003).

Gatekeeper training has been examined in a peer gatekeeper program, with similar effects on skills, attitudes, and knowledge as in the studies of educators (Stuart et al., 2003). However, negative side effects have not been adequately examined (Gould et al., 2003), and there is some concern with the peers being involved in counseling suicidal youth because of the potential risks posed to the nonsuicidal peer (Steele & Doey, 2007). Lazear et al. (2003) suggest that schools have to use these programs in conjunction with screening programs to identify students at risk. Also, schools should not use peer support programs as a substitute for professional counseling or therapy.

Educating Parents and Community Members

Gatekeeper programs can also be directed to parents and community members. The approach is based on the hypothesis that parental psychiatric disorder and dysfunction are more prevalent in the families of suicidal adolescents and that connectedness with adults may minimize the impact of environmental risk factors.

Recently, King et al. (2006) investigated the efficacy of the Youth-Nominated Support Team – Version 1 (YST-1), a psychoeducational social network intervention, with 289 suicidal, psychiatrically hospitalized adolescents. Adolescents were randomly assigned either to treatment-as-usual plus YST-1 or to treatment-as-usual only. Assessments were completed pre- and postintervention (6 months). YST-1 was designed to supplement routine care for suicidal adolescents following psychiatric hospitalization, providing psychoeducation for support persons whom youths nominate from within and outside their family, and facilitating the supportive weekly contact of these support persons with the suicidal adolescent. However, the hypothesis that the program would be effective in reducing suicidality did not receive support, although gender effects were evident, with adolescent girls reporting greater effects from the program.

Although it may not be the responsibility of schools to train community members, schools should make sure that there are established agreements between the school and crisis services. Only when these links are in place could a perceptive and educated staff member make an effective referral for a student potentially at risk. These links also increase the likelihood that students will receive clear, consistent messages about suicide, which research has shown to increase a student's feeling of competence. Schools should also provide information to parents about warning signs, risk factors, protective factors, community resources, and what to do following a suicidal crisis. Research has found that when schools communicate with and involve parents in the school activities and programs, parents are more likely to cooperate with the school and help the school maintain these programs (Carlyon, Carlyon, & McCarthy, 1998; Marx & Northrop, 1995).

In 2000, the Australian Institute of Family Studies conducted an evaluation of the National Youth Suicide Prevention Strategy (Mitchell, 2000) that had funded seven parenting projects. Together, they formed the National Parenting Initiative. The results from the meta-analysis of parenting projects fell into four major themes: (1) effective strategies for recruiting and engaging parents; (2) interventions that are effective in enhancing parenting skills, knowledge, and confidence; (3) increasing well-being and reducing risk factors for young people; and (4) sustaining and disseminating effective parenting programs.

Recruiting Parents – Universal Strategies

Three of the projects focused primarily on the task of disseminating programs that had been previously developed and identifying effective strategies for recruiting parents. These projects explored issues of recruitment and engagement for parents in a range of settings and socioeconomic areas and with different levels of need. The results indicate that a variety of strategies are required, both universal and selective, and that different approaches are sometimes required when attempting to ensure the participation of parents who could be considered to be socioeconomically disadvantaged or who are experiencing problems with their adolescents.

Results obtained from the Resourceful Adolescent Program for Parents (RAP-P), a program developed for the urban setting which focused mainly on the school setting for recruitment efforts, indicated that the RAP-P should increase its focus by first targeting parents with children facing the transition to high school and, secondly, by training school-based staff to deliver the program as part of the school's usual services. The transition to high school appears to be an important window of opportunity for the delivery of these programs because parents often experience high levels of anticipatory anxiety at this time about their child's entry into adolescence. Consultation with urban parents about the issue of engagement indicated that parent group-based modes of program delivery are only partially successful in engaging parents. It was suggested that a more flexible mode of delivery was needed, in particular a video, so that the program could be available to the large proportion of parents who would not attend parent groups. RAP-P used two different strategies for recruiting parents to the program: recruitment through the general community using mass media including radio, television, and newspapers, and a strategy that involved targeting whole schools. Both strategies were found to be effective in recruiting and engaging parents. However, community recruitment strategy may be more effective in targeting the socioeconomically disadvantaged parents. No information was provided about the extent to which the universal targeting approach was successful in recruiting parents who were experiencing difficulties with their adolescents.

Recruiting Parents – Selective Strategies

These programs targeted those families who were experiencing difficulties with their children. These projects mainly focused on Australian minorities such as Aboriginal people. In this case, the programs emphasized the importance of addressing the historical and political factors that continue to impact family well-being for Aboriginal people and involved key members of the target group, using as personnel members of the same ethnic group.

Enhancing Parenting Skills, Knowledge, and Confidence

Only one of the Strategy's parenting projects, Program for Parents, included comprehensive and rigorous evaluation of the impact of the parenting intervention on parents. The results indicated that the Program for Parents was effective in increasing parents' confidence and satisfaction, and decreasing parental depression compared to a control group. Also, qualitative evaluation of the Family Wellbeing Course and the Home-Start Program indicated that course participants experienced increased confidence and knowledge, and reduced stress. First, the major characteristic of the programs was that almost all of the parenting programs placed central importance on building parents' self-esteem by encouraging awareness of and building on their strengths. It was argued that programs that focus on remediating skill deficits could have the effect of reducing parental confidence. A second feature of the programs was that meeting parents' needs for friendship, support, and positive regard was critical to their ability to parent effectively. A third feature of the programs that seemed important in the effectiveness of the training was the structured use of a group-based approach to parenting skills training. A fourth feature of the programs showed how improvements in parent communication and family relationships were believed to be mediated through changes in parental perceptions of their adolescents. The program curriculum encourages parents to move from negative interpretations of adolescent behavior toward seeing many adolescent behaviors as normative. A fifth feature of the program showed that home visits was a primary prevention tactic and early intervention program that provided flexible support to socially isolated new mothers. Finally, universal targeting may also be important for the effectiveness of group-based parenting programs. One of the projects indicated that there was a strong advantage in including parents with a range of abilities in the parent groups.

Increasing Well-Being and Reducing Risk Factors for Young People

Only one of the group of parenting projects included the evaluation of outcomes for young people. In this program, adolescents in the control school sample showed a trend toward increased self-harm, delinquency, and substance use, and decreased family attachment. In contrast, these negative trends were not observed in the experimental school group. Most of the programs that were assessed emphasized cognitive behavioral and systems theory. Improvements were believed to be mediated through changes in the parents' perceptions of their adolescents.

The results supported the view that, when programs are implemented within a school system, positive effects may extend beyond the minority of families who participate directly in the program. The cognitive reframing approach is designed to move parents away from authoritarian and permissive parenting styles toward authoritative styles, which may be associated with improvement in adolescent behavior. The results of the Program for Parents evaluation suggested that the school-based program may have exerted a preventive effect on the development of delinquency and substance use that is usually observed to increase in prevalence in young people during grades 7 and 8. The results are consistent with the hypothesis that the whole-school context for program delivery had the effect of enhancing the impact of the program on adolescent behavior. The rationale for targeting the whole-school population was to maximize parental exposure to the program and to permit informal dissemination of the educational messages and strategies advocated in the program. Another factor contributing to effectiveness of the preventive program may be the fact that the parenting programs were run in conjunction with programs targeting children and adolescents.

Disseminating Effective Parenting Programs

Three projects in this group of programs concentrated on the task of expanding the reach of programs. The main strategy employed in the dissemination of the parenting programs was to provide training to professionals for delivering these programs. Evaluation of the training provided by these projects suggests that it substantially enhanced the effective delivery of these programs on a wider basis. The features of the programs involved in their effectiveness and diffusion included a systematic documentation of program curricula in manuals (the projects relied on a wide variety of media to promote the programs to both parents and to service providers), ongoing support, and coordination provided to program workers or staff who delivered the programs. The roles of local/regional coordinators included: marketing the program to appropriate agencies; coordinating referrals to the program; organizing programs; supporting group leaders; liaising with other local/regional and national/state level coordinators pertaining to support needs in training, consultation, and evaluation; and writing funding submissions. The roles of state/territory or national coordinators included: liaising with and providing support for local/regional coordinators; providing consultation for leaders who were involved in running their own programs; providing ongoing training and support for program leaders; and performing ongoing evaluation and program development.

Furthermore, several of the projects suggested that locally or community-based support structures are vital to the maintenance of these programs. Community-based support structures appear to be particularly critical to the uptake and maintenance of programs targeting rural-remote and indigenous communities. Results of the evaluations of all the projects also indicated that agencies from a variety of sectors need to be involved if parenting programs are to be implemented effectively on a wide scale. The involvement of schools is particularly helpful in recruiting parents to programs. Parenting programs may also be more effective in engaging parents and achieving outcomes if they are run in parallel with programs for adolescents and children. Project managers and a number of evaluators of projects identified ongoing funding as essential to the maintenance and dissemination of programs of this nature. Significant cost inefficiencies are reported to result from dependence on short-term project funding to sustain parenting programs.

Parent education programs may be combined with preventive programs directed to restrict access to potentially lethal weapons (Lazear et al., 2003). In fact, restricting access to means of suicide, especially firearms, has been shown to be an effective method for decreasing the likelihood of adolescent suicide (Bridges, 2004; Johnson & Coyne-Beasley, 2009; Nordentoft, 2007). The Adolescent Health Committee of the Canadian Paediatric Society (2005) has published guidelines about youth and firearms. The committee recommended that: (1) physicians should routinely inquire about the presence of a firearm in the home and inform parents of the risks of home ownership if one is present; (2) physicians have an obligation to share this information with parents until such time that an effective approach to anticipatory guidance relating to the prevention of firearm injuries is established; (3) physicians should recommend the removal of the firearm from home in cases where there are risk factors for adolescent suicide; (4) firearm safety interventions that include education and environmental interventions – such as the provision of trigger locks and gun safes – would likely be more effective than an education-only program; and (5) childhood firearm safety education cannot be recommended at present because currently available programs have not been shown to result in behavioral change in children, and this education may have unintended negative effects, such as reduced parental vigilance.

However, the research investigating parents' attitudes about physician counseling on firearm dangers has noted mixed results. Webster, Wilson, Duggan, and Pakula (1992) found that 17% of gun-owning parents would be willing to remove a firearm from the home if their physician recommended it, and 84% would be willing to follow advice about storing firearms safely. However, two studies (Grossman et al., 2000; Oatis, Fenn Buderer, Cummings, & Fleitz, 1999) that evaluated the effectiveness of office-based counseling alone in improving gun storage habits showed no improvement in the gun storage habits after the counseling. In a more successful intervention, Brent, Baugher, Birmaher, Kolko, and Bridge (2000) gave parents information about the risks of a firearm at home and recommended the removal of a firearm from homes of adolescents diagnosed with depression. Twenty-seven percentage of the families did remove the firearm from home.

Family physicians play key roles in the community and may have a major role in assessing and treating suicidal youth since most of these youths report that they are most likely to consult their family physician when distressed (Davidson & Manion, 1993). However, one study found that almost 80% of adolescents who had attempted suicide were not recognized as suicidal by their primary care physician (Clark, 1993). Thus, it is necessary to train primary care physicians in the recognition and management of suicidal youth. A study conducted in Sweden indicated that a 2-day training course for primary practitioners on how to evaluate mood disorders and suicidality brought about a reduction in the number of suicides and suicide attempts (among female patients), after the training (Rutz, von Knorring, & Walinder, 1992). However, ongoing repetition of educational programs was needed to maintain gains (Steele & Doey, 2007).

Screening

Screening is a prevention strategy that is intended to identify students who are potentially at risk for suicide through interviews and self-report questionnaires. Several early intervention programs used schools as the main setting for identifying and/or intervening with adolescents. Screening tools typically consist of asking students directly about whether they are experiencing symptoms associated with depression, currently or previously had suicidal ideation or had attempted suicide, and assessing the presence of risk factors for suicide.

Screening can be done in two ways (Lazear et al., 2003). The first way is a broad approach, that seeks to identify students potentially at risk for suicide by screening all students in the school. However, surveys of both high school principals and school psychologists reveal that they view school-wide student screening programs as less acceptable than curriculum-based in-service programs for staff (Eckert, Miller, DuPaul, & Riley-Tillman, 2003; Miller, Eckert, DuPaul, & White, 1999). Insufficient staffing and budgets, scheduling issues, legal concerns, and potential negative responses of administrators, parents, and students are potential "real-world" barriers to program adoption and implementation (Hayden & Lauer, 2000).

Focused screening, on the other hand, would utilize screening in combination with other methods for identifying students at risk for suicidal actions, such as using gatekeepers or peers. Once identified and referred by gatekeepers or peers, those students potentially at risk would be screened and subsequently evaluated by a mental health professional. The underlying rationale behind these programs is that, since suicide is a low incidence event, prevention may be more effective and efficient if only those students who are potentially at risk for suicide are identified and referred.

Lazear et al. (2003) noted that, since suicidality fluctuates in adolescents, repeated screening must be done to measure the changes in suicidality and to avoid missing a student who is not suicidal at one time, but becomes suicidal over time. Also, screening may identify as many as 10% of the adolescents at school as being at risk, creating a costly need to follow up those identified as at risk for suicide. Lastly, in order for schools to initiate a screening session, they must have cooperation and consent from parents. However, research has found that parental consent runs close to only 50%, which means that schools may only be able to screen half of the at-risk students, thereby possibly missing students potentially at risk before screening even begins.

It is important that schools use screening tools that have been evaluated as effective methods for identifying students potentially at risk for suicide. Screening is just one component of a suicide-prevention program. Schools should not rely solely on screening to effectively address adolescent suicide. An effective program is a comprehensive program.

Hallfors et al. (2006) evaluated the feasibility of an adolescent suicide screening measure designed for use in public schools. The researchers recruited students in grades 9–11 from high schools in a large city in the southwestern (site A) and Pacific coast (site B) regions of the United States. All students were participants in a RCT assessing the effectiveness of the Reconnecting Youth prevention program. A random sample of students who were identified as being at high risk (they were in both the upper 25% distribution in terms of absences and the lower 50% distribution in terms of grade point average or they had been referred by a teacher) were invited to take part in the study. Those who agreed to participate completed a baseline questionnaire. Forty-seven percentage of the 1,995 high-risk students eligible to be included in the study completed the questionnaire. Subsequently, a sample of "typical" students were randomly selected to establish "normative behaviors" in the schools and districts. Students were distributed an audio-computer-assisted self-interviewing format of the High School Questionnaire (Eggert, Thompson, Herting, & Nicholas, 1994; Eggert, Thompson, Herting, Nicholas, & Dicker, 1994), a questionnaire assessing school deviance and school connectedness, peer bonding, family support, emotional issues such as self-esteem, stress, anxiety, hopelessness and personal control, high-risk behaviors, substance use, suicide, and several demographic variables. Items assessing suicide were part of the Suicide Risk Screen (Thompson & Eggert, 1999), a screening instrument focusing on sets of rank-ordered criteria based on confirmed suicide risk factors (e.g., suicidal ideation, depression, previous suicide attempts, indirect/direct threats of suicide, and drug misuse).

The results suggested that there was a great need to address suicide-related mental health problems in large urban high schools. Overall, 29% of the participants were rated as at risk for suicide. In further analyses, about half of the students identified were deemed at high risk on the basis of high levels of depression, suicidal ideation, or suicidal behavior. The authors believed that the low specificity resulted in too many false positives for the instrument to be practical in schools, and so they recommended testing a simplified instrument that identifies only students who have attempted suicide in the past year, who have high current levels of suicidal ideation, or who have high current levels of depression and exhibit any degree of suicidal ideation. This instrument identified approximately 11% of urban high school youths for assessment, offering high school officials an important opportunity to identify young people at the greatest levels of need and to target scarce health resources.

Beside these problems associated with the screening instrument itself, the authors indicated some other problems faced while implementing their screening. First of all, the school personnel were reluctant to participate in the training that was offered, and often declined. Most of them believed they had sufficient professional training, but, on the basis of the researchers' experience, training on a standard assessment protocol should be provided to all the involved staff. Second, budget shortages may leave schools unable to take on a screening program alone. Another problem was school readiness. Appropriate personnel were available in most of schools to conduct follow-up interviews, and most of them supported and expressed great interest in doing so. Nevertheless, not all staff and administrators were enthusiastic. Excessive staff turnover and changes in administrative personnel could further hamper a successful implementation. In each of the two districts investigated, the authors found that only a few schools were able to comply with the protocols and act as partners in evaluating the program. Finally, the authors recommend identifying schools that are both stable and innovative and limiting feasibility research to such schools. After sufficient testing and refinement, the program could then be tested in other schools.

An evidence-based screening program is the CARE (Care, Assess, Respond, Empower; formerly called Counselors CARE (Eggert et al., 1995, 2002; Randell et al., 2001; Thompson et al., 2001). CARE is a high school-based suicide-prevention program targeting high-risk youth. CARE includes a 2-hour, one-on-one computer-assisted suicide assessment interview followed by a 2-hour motivational counseling and social support intervention. The counseling session is designed to deliver empathy and support, provide a safe context for sharing personal information, and reinforce positive coping skills and help-seeking behaviors. CARE expedites access to help by connecting each high-risk youth to a school-based caseworker or a favorite teacher and establishing contact with a parent or guardian chosen by the youth. The program also includes a follow-up reassessment of broad suicide risk and protective factors and a booster motivational counseling session 9 weeks after the initial counseling session. The CARE program is typically delivered by school or advanced-practice nurses, counselors, psychologists, or social workers who have completed the CARE implementation training program and certification process.

In the first study (Eggert et al., 1995), suicide risk factors decreased by at least 25% from baseline to 5- and 10-month follow-up assessments in more than 85% of the youths exposed to the CARE program ($p < .001$). At baseline, CARE participants scored significantly higher on suicide risk factors relative to a control group of "typical" youth, and this difference was associated with a large effect size (Cohen's $d = 1.28$). At the 10-month follow-up, CARE participants showed reduced suicide risk factors, bringing them closer to the typical youth, and the effect size for this group difference was reduced from large to medium (Cohen's $d = 0.57$). Male and female CARE participants were equally likely to report decreases in suicide risk behaviors and suicidal ideation over the 10-month follow-up period.

CARE participants' reduction in suicide risk factors was replicated with a specific decrease in suicidal ideation ($p < .05$) in a second study that compared CARE participants with a usual-care control group of suicidal youth over a 9-month follow-up period (Eggert et al., 2002; Randell et al., 2001; Thompson et al., 2001). The control condition involved procedures simulating those typically used by school personnel to respond to youths who show suicidal behavior. As in the earlier study, the findings did not vary by gender. In the first study, hopelessness levels decreased by at least 25% in more than 60% of the CARE participants (both females and males) from baseline through 10 months of follow-up ($p < .001$). This improvement in feelings of hopelessness was replicated in the second study that compared CARE participants with a usual-care control group of suicidal youth. Growth curve analyses showed greater rates of decline in hopelessness for CARE youth compared with controls at 10 weeks ($p < .01$) and 9 months ($p < .05$). With regard to mean levels of hopelessness, controlling for baseline levels, the reported hopelessness of CARE participants was lower at both the 10-week ($p < .004$) and 9-month follow-up assessments ($p < .05$) relative to the usual-care participants. According to the Best Practices Registry for suicide-prevention readiness for dissemination ratings by criteria, the CARE program received an overall rating of 2.2.

Another evidence-based program is the Columbia TeenScreen Program (Scott et al., 2009; Shaffer et al., 2004). This program is committed to using screening tools to identify and arrange treatment for youths who are suffering from depression and other undiagnosed mental illnesses and those who are at risk for suicide. The ultimate goal of this program is to make mental health screening accepted and routinely implemented in school settings. The measures used are the Voice DISC (Diagnostic Interview Schedule for Children). This computerized diagnostic interview uses DSM-IV criteria to assess more than 30 different psychiatric disorders found in children and adolescents. The TeenScreen, a paper and pencil prescreen, is used before the DISC to identify those who require further assessment and those who do not. Other prescreens, such as the Beck Depression Inventory, the Columbia Depression Scale, and the DISC Predictive Scales, can be used instead of the TeenScreen.

Two studies (Scott et al., 2009; Shaffer et al., 1996) examined the efficacy of this program and found that the program efficiently and effectively identified many adolescents who were at high risk for suicidal behaviors yet were not known to others. Hence, these students would presumably never receive treatment because they would have not been recognized as needing help. On the readiness for dissemination ratings by criteria, the TeenScreen received an overall rating of 3.8.

Pena and Caine (2006), in a comprehensive review of suicide screening programs, proposed seven validated screening instruments with good psychometrics that assess suicidal ideation and attempts: Columbia Suicide Screen, Risk of Suicide Questionnaire, Suicidal Ideation Questionnaire, Suicidal Ideation Questionnaire JR, Diagnostic Predictive Scales, Suicide Risk Screen, and Suicide Probability Scale. In high school settings, the Columbia Suicide Screen, the Suicidal Ideation Questionnaire, and the Suicidal Ideation Questionnaire JR tend to yield a large number of false positives. The two most commonly used instruments are the Suicide Risk Screen and the Suicidal Ideation Questionnaire (Joe & Bryant, 2007). The Suicidal Ideation Questionnaire is used as an instrument to assess current suicidal ideation in adolescents. The 30-item version is meant for students in grades 10–12, whereas the Suicidal Ideation Questionnaire JR is a shorter, 15-item questionnaire created for grades 7–9 (Gutierrez, Watkins, & Collura, 2004). Both versions of the Suicidal Ideation Questionnaire have good internal consistencies, ranging from .93 to .97.

Postvention

It is not enough for a suicide-prevention program to implement and maintain "before the fact" prevention elements, designed for preventing a suicidal event from occurring, but a program must also have an established method of responding to a suicidal crisis (Lazear et al., 2003). By having postvention guidelines in place, schools can provide a more timely, effective, and appropriate response to a suicidal crisis. Postvention programs are intended to provide a timely and proper response to a suicidal crisis (suicidal threat, attempt, or death by suicide), and programs may reduce potential copycat suicides (Leenaars & Wenckstern, 1990). When a parent or a sibling commits suicide, the bereaved child is at risk for anxiety disorders including posttraumatic stress disorder, mood disorders, and suicidal ideation in the months immediately following the suicide (Brent, Moritz, Bridge, Perper, & Canobbio, 1996; Pfeffer et al., 1997).

However, long-term support and services are also necessary. Three years after a suicide, adolescent friends who felt they had knowledge of the impending suicide and failed to prevent it are most likely to continue to suffer from major depression and posttraumatic stress disorder (Brent et al., 1996). The goals of the intervention are to decrease the likelihood of other adolescents identifying with the suicidal behavior of the deceased as a coping strategy in dealing with adversity, and to promote grief and mourning, decreasing the adolescent's sense of guilt, trauma, and social isolation (Pfeffer, 1997). This treatment can be given in individual meetings, at group sessions with other teenagers, or in conjunction with parents who need help to support the adaptive capacities of their children and adolescents (Shaffer & Pfeffer, 2001).

A postvention plan should (Beautrais et al., 1997)

- prepare staff for the impact of suicidal behavior such that they are confident about being able to offer an appropriate response;
- facilitate a quick, coordinated, and direct response in the event of an incident;
- allocate specific roles to staff which they can familiarize themselves with before the event;
- develop appropriate links with community resources before they are required and assist in their quick and smooth implementation when needed;
- allow for the needs of all members of the school community (including students, administrators, teachers, and parents) to be carefully considered and appropriate actions planned.

Beautrais et al. (1997) indicated some principles in the development of a postvention plan:

1. Each school should develop its own response plan before a traumatic incident (since there will be no time to develop a plan when an incident occurs).
2. The response plan should involve all sectors of the school and specify the coordination mechanisms. To be effective, a postvention plan should include all staff and make provision to include students, parents, and support agencies from outside the school, as appropriate.
3. The relevant community resources should be identified.
4. The conditions under which the response plan should be implemented must be clearly specified and understood by key staff.
5. The implementation of the plan should allow key staff to be contacted and prepared before they have to respond to other staff, students, and the community. Staff need to avoid being unprepared to deal with students' concerns or to identify students who require assistance.
6. The plan should ensure that the response is conducted in a manner which avoids glorifying the suicide victim(s) and which minimizes sensationalism.
7. Students who have a history of emotional distress and risk of suicide should be identified and should have at least one screening interview with a competent staff member.
8. A timely flow of accurate, appropriate information should be provided to the media.
9. Elements in the school environment that might increase the likelihood of further suicides or suicide attempts should be identified and changed.
10. The plan should be reviewed and evaluated.

In postvention, it is appropriate for all students to be able to discuss the following issues: (1) suicide is not a good choice; (2) suicide is a permanent solution to what are generally temporary problems; and (3) help is available. During discussions with students, staff must watch carefully for those students whose reactions to the suicide seem inappropriate. Inappropriate reactions might be that the death was heroic or that suicide was a good choice. A desire to die in order to be with the victim is also an inappropriate reaction. If students show these reactions, then the discussion should be brought to an end and further help sought. These students may need to be assessed for suicide risk (Beautrais et al., 1997).

Other recommendations include the following. Encourage students to be together. Tell the parents and caregivers that there has been a student death. Ensure that the parents and caregivers of all the young people who are particularly at risk are told that the school is concerned about their safety. Encourage these parents and caregivers to keep their young people safe by knowing where they are, whom they are with, and what they are doing. Encourage parents and caregivers to talk to their young people in supportive and caring ways. Recognize that some parents and caregivers may have difficulty in accepting that their young person is at risk.

The postvention team should ensure that counseling staff have sufficient resources and backup internally and external to the school setting. From within the school, it may be appropriate to free up some staff members through the use of relief, temporary staff, thereby increasing the capability of the school to work with students using staff familiar to the students. The support and backup must include appropriate professional supervision during and after the incident.

Final Recommendations

These guidelines are adapted from the World Health Organization report "Preventing suicide a resource for teachers and other school staff" (World Health Organization, 2000).

Strengthening the Mental Health of School Teachers and Other School Staff

First of all, it is essential to secure the well-being and balance of teachers, and other school staff. For them, the workplace may be rejecting, aggressive, and sometimes even violent. Therefore, they need information that enhances their understanding and proposes adequate reactions to their own, to students' and to colleagues' mental strain and possible mental illness. They should also have access to support and, if necessary, treatment.

Strengthening Students' Self-Esteem

Positive self-esteem protects children and adolescents against mental distress and despondency, and enables them to cope adequately with difficult and stressful life situations. To foster positive self-esteem in children and adolescents, a variety of techniques can be used. Some recommended approaches follow:

- Positive life experiences that will help to forge a positive identity in the young should be accentuated. Positive past experiences increase young people's chances of greater future self-confidence.
- Children and adolescents should not be constantly pressured to do more and better.

- It is not enough for adults to say they love the child; the child must feel loved. There is a big difference between being loved and feeling loved.
- Children should not only be accepted, but also cherished, as they are. They must feel special just because they exist.

Whereas sympathy impedes self-esteem, empathy fosters it because judgment is set aside. Autonomy and mastery are building blocks in the development of positive self-esteem in early childhood. Children's and adolescents' achievement of self-esteem is dependent on their development of physical, social, and vocational skills. For high self-esteem, the teenager needs to establish final independence from family and age-mates; be able to relate to the opposite sex; prepare for an occupation for self-support; and establish a workable and meaningful philosophy of life.

Introducing training in life skills, first using visiting experts and later as part of the regular curriculum, is an effective strategy. The program should convey knowledge to peers on how to be supportive and, if necessary, seek adult help. The education system should also enhance the development and consolidation of every student's sense of identity. Promoting the stability and continuity of students' schooling is another important aim.

Promoting Emotional Expression

Children and adolescents should be taught to take their own feelings seriously and encouraged to confide in parents and other adults, such as teachers, school doctors or nurses, friends, athletic coaches, and religious advisers.

Preventing Bullying and Violence at School

Specific skills should be available in the education system to prevent bullying and violence in and around the school premises in order to create a safe environment free of intolerance.

Providing Information About Care Services

The availability of specific services should be ensured by widely publicizing the telephone numbers of, for example, crisis and emergency helplines, and psychiatric emergency services, and making them accessible to young people. Intervention should be available when a suicide risk is identified. In most cases, children and adolescents in distress and/or at risk of suicidal behavior also experience communication problems. Consequently, it is important to establish a dialog with distressed and/or suicidal adolescents.

Communication

The first step in suicide prevention is invariably trustful communication. During the development of the suicidal process, mutual communication between suicidal young people and those around them is crucially important. Lack of communication and the broken network that ensues result in

- Silence and increased tension in the relationship. The adult's fear of provoking the child or adolescent into committing a suicidal act by discussing his or her suicidal thoughts and messages is often the reason for the silence and absence of dialog.

- Obvious ambivalence. Understandably, adults' confrontation with a child or adolescent suicidal communication brings their own psychological conflicts to the fore. The psychological strain of an encounter with a distressed and/or suicidal child or adolescent is usually great and involves a wide range of emotional reactions. In some cases, the unsolved emotional problems of adults who are in contact with suicidal children and adolescents may come to the surface. Such problems may be accentuated among school staff, whose ambivalence – wanting, but simultaneously being unwilling or unable, to help the suicidal student – may result in avoidance of dialog.
- Direct or indirect aggression. Adults' discomfort is sometimes so great that their ultimate reaction to the child or adolescent who is in distress or suicidal is one of verbal or nonverbal aggression.
- It is important to understand that the teacher is not alone in this communication process, and learning how to achieve good communication is, therefore, fundamental. The dialog should be created in and adapted to each situation. Dialog implies, first and foremost, recognition of children's and adolescents' identity and also their need for help.

Improving School Staff's Skills

This may be done by means of special training courses aimed at improving communication between distressed and/or suicidal students and their teachers, and enhancing awareness and understanding of suicide risk. Training all school staff in the capacity to talk among themselves and with the students about life and death issues, improving their skills in identifying distress, depression, and suicidal behavior, and increasing their knowledge about available support are crucial means of suicide prevention. Clear goals and precise limits as defined in manuals on suicide prevention are important tools in this work.

Referral to Professionals

A prompt, authoritative, and decisive intervention (i.e., taking the suicidal young person to a general practitioner, a child psychiatrist, or an emergency department) can be lifesaving. To be effective, youth health services need to be perceived as approachable, attractive, and nonstigmatizing. Distressed and/or suicidal students should be actively and personally referred by school staff and received by a team composed of doctors, nurses, social workers, and legal representatives whose task is to protect the child's rights. This active transfer of the student to the health care system prevents her or him from dropping out during the referral process, which might happen if the referral is conducted only by correspondence.

Removing Means of Suicide from Distressed and Suicidal Children's and Adolescents' Proximity

Various forms of supervision and removal or locking up of dangerous medicines, guns, firearms, pesticides, explosives, knives, and so forth in schools, parental homes, and other premises are very important life-saving measures. Since these measures alone are not enough to prevent suicide in the long run, psychological support should be offered at the same time.

Informing School Staff and Schoolmates

Schools need to have emergency plans on how to inform school staff, especially teachers, and also fellow pupils and parents, when suicide has been attempted or committed at school, the aim being to prevent a cluster of suicides. The contagion effect results from suicidal children's and adolescents' tendency to identify with destructive solutions adopted by people who have attempted or committed suicide.

Despite research on suicide among youths, little is known about the interplay of factors that precipitate completed suicide. Each suicide represents a lost life, lost talents, lost creativity, lost contributions made to society, and a lost son or daughter. Suicide is the result of a complex interaction of causal factors, including mental illness, poverty, substance abuse, social isolation, losses, relational difficulties, and school problems. Caretakers should pay particular attention to these features, including poor academic achievement, social isolation and failure to complete high school, self-medication with drugs or alcohol, promiscuity, involvement in the criminal justice system, lack of vocational success, inability to live independently, health problems, and suicidal ideation.

Suicide can be prevented. Parents can play a major role in facilitating talk about the issue of psychological pain and suicide, but schools should also be a place where parents, teachers, and others involved in the health and education of children can build effective suicide preventive strategies for adolescents.

Conclusion

Many preventive strategies have been implemented for reducing suicidal behavior in adolescents. However, few methodologically sound research studies are available to indicate the best programs to be used. Daniel and Goldston (2009) suggest that, given the heterogeneity among adolescent suicide attempters, it is unlikely that a "one size fits for all" approach to treatment will prove effective for suicidal youth. Given the fact that multiple developmental contexts are associated with adolescent suicidal behavior, it may be that interventions that affect multiple contexts of at-risk behaviors (e.g., family, peer, and academic contexts) may yield more generalizable and sustainable effects than interventions that are not sensitive to the developmental contexts and nuances of adolescence.

References

Adcock, A. G., Nagy, S., & Simpson, J. A. (1991). Selected risk factors in adolescent suicide attempts. *Adolescence, 26*(104), 817–828.

Adolescent Health Committee of the Canadian Paediatric Society. (2005). Youth and firearms in Canada. *Paediatrics & Child Health, 10*, 473–477.

Anderson, R. N., & Smith, B. L. (2003). Deaths: Leading causes for 2001. *National Vital Statistics Report, 52*(9), 1–85.

Aseltine, R. H., Jr., & DeMartino, R. (2004). An outcome evaluation of the SOS suicide prevention program. *American Journal of Public Health, 94*(3), 446–451.

Aseltine, R. H., Jr., James, A., Schilling, E. A., & Glanovsky, J. (2007). Evaluating the SOS suicide prevention program: A replication and extension. *BMC Public Health, 7*, 161.

Barrish, H. H., Saunders, M., & Wolf, M. M. (1969). Good behavior game: Effects of individual contingencies for group consequences on disruptive behavior in a classroom. *Journal of Applied Behavior Analysis, 2*(2), 119–124.

Beautrais, A. L. (2001). Child and young adolescent suicide in New Zealand. *Australian and New Zealand Journal of Psychiatry, 35*(5), 647–653.

Beautrais, A. L., Coggan, C. A., Fergusson, D. M., & Rivers, L. (1997). *The prevention, recognition and management of young people at risk of suicide: Development of guidelines for schools.* Wellington: National Advisory Committee on Health and Disability.

Beautrais, A. L., Fergusson, D., Coggan, C., Collings, C., Doughty, C., Ellis, P., et al. (2007). Effective strategies for suicide prevention in New Zealand: A review of the evidence. *The New Zealand Medical Journal, 120*(1251), U2459.

Beautrais, A. L., Joyce, P. R., & Mulder, R. T. (1998). Psychiatric contacts among youths aged 13 through 24 years who have made serious suicide attempts. *Journal of the American Academy of Child and Adolescent Psychiatry, 37*(5), 504–511.

Brent, D. A., Baugher, M., Birmaher, B., Kolko, D. J., & Bridge, J. (2000). Compliance with recommendations to remove firearms in families participating in a clinical trial for adolescent depression. *Journal of the American Academy of Child and Adolescent Psychiatry, 39*(10), 1220–1226.

Brent, D. A., Baugher, M., Bridge, J., Chen, T., & Chiappetta, L. (1999). Age- and sex-related risk factors for adolescent suicide. *Journal of the American Academy of Child and Adolescent Psychiatry, 38*(12), 1497–1505.

Brent, D. A., Moritz, G., Bridge, J., Perper, J., & Canobbio, R. (1996). Long-term impact of exposure to suicide: A three-year controlled follow-up. *Journal of the American Academy of Child and Adolescent Psychiatry, 35*(5), 646–653.

Bridges, F. S. (2004). Gun control law (Bill C-17), suicide, and homicide in Canada. *Psychological Reports, 94*(3 Pt 1), 819–826.

Burns, J. M., & Patton, G. C. (2000). Preventive interventions for youth suicide: A risk factor-based approach. *Australian and New Zealand Journal of Psychiatry, 34*(3), 388–407.

Canetto, S. S. (1997). Meanings of gender and suicidal behavior during adolescence. *Suicide & Life-Threatening Behavior, 27*(4), 339–351.

Cantor, C., Leenaars, A. A., Lester, D., Slater, P. J., Wolanowski, A. M., & O'Toole, B. (1996). Suicide trends in eight predominantly English-speaking countries 1960–1989. *Social Psychiatry and Psychiatric Epidemiology, 31*(6), 364–373.

Cantor, C., & Neulinger, K. (2000). The epidemiology of suicide and attempted suicide among young Australians. *Australian and New Zealand Journal of Psychiatry, 34*(3), 370–387.

Carlyon, P., Carlyon, W., & McCarthy, A. R. (1998). Family and community involvement in school health. In E. Marx, S. F. Wooley, & D. Northrop (Eds.), *Health is academic: A guide to coordinated school health programs* (pp. 67–95). New York: Teachers College Press.

Centers for Disease Control and Prevention. (1992). *Youth suicide prevention programs: A resource guide*. Atlanta: Centers for Disease Control.

Ciffone, J. (1993). Suicide prevention: A classroom presentation to adolescents. *Social Work, 38*(2), 197–203

Clark, D. (1993). Suicidal behaviour in childhood and adolescence: Recent studies and clinical implications. *Psychiatric Annals, 23*, 271–283.

Crawford, M. J., Thomas, O., Khan, N., & Kulinskaya, E. (2007). Psychosocial interventions following self-harm: Systematic review of their efficacy in preventing suicide. *British Journal of Psychiatry, 190*, 11–17.

Daniel, S. S., & Goldston, D. B. (2009). Interventions for suicidal youth: A review of the literature and developmental considerations. *Suicide & Life-Threatening Behavior, 39*(3), 252–268.

Davidson, S., & Manion, I. G. (1993). *Canadian youth mental health and illness survey: Survey overview interview schedule and demographic cross tabulations*. Ottawa: Canadian Psychiatric Association.

Eckert, T. L., Miller, D. N., DuPaul, G. J., & Riley-Tillman, T. (2003). Adolescent suicide prevention: School psychologists' acceptability of school-based programs. *School Psychology Review, 32*(1), 57–76.

Eggert, L. L., & Nicholas, L. J. (2004). *Reconnecting youth: A peer group approach to building life skills* (2nd ed.). Bloomington: National Educational Service.

Eggert, L. L., Thompson, E. A., Herting, J. R., & Nicholas, L. J. (1994). Prevention research program: Reconnecting at-risk youth. *Issues in Mental Health Nursing, 15*(2), 107–135.

Eggert, L. L., Thompson, E. A., Herting, J. R., & Nicholas, L. J. (1995). Reducing suicide potential among high-risk youth: Tests of a school-based prevention program. *Suicide & Life-Threatening Behavior, 25*(2), 276–296.

Eggert, L. L., Thompson, E. A., Herting, J. R., Nicholas, L. J., & Dicker, B. G. (1994). Preventing adolescent drug abuse and high school dropout through an intensive school-based social network development program. *American Journal of Health Promotion, 8*(3), 202–215.

Eggert, L. L., Thompson, E. A., Herting, J. R., & Randell, B. P. (2001). Reconnecting youth to prevent drug abuse, school dropout, and suicidal behaviors among high-risk youth. In E. E. Wagner & H. B. Waldron (Eds.), *Innovations in adolescent substance abuse intervention* (pp. 51–84). Oxford: Elsevier Science.

Eggert, L. L., Thompson, E. A., Randell, B. P., & Pike, K. C. (2002). Preliminary effects of brief school-based prevention approaches for reducing youth suicide-risk behaviors, depression, and drug involvement. *Journal of Child and Adolescent Psychiatric Nursing, 15*(2), 48–64.

Epstein, J. A., & Spirito, A. (2009). Risk factors for suicidality among a nationally representative sample of high school students. *Suicide & Life-Threatening Behavior, 39*(3), 241–251.

Garland, A. F., & Zigler, E. (1993). Adolescent suicide prevention: Current research and social policy implications. *American Psychologist, 48*(2), 169–182.

Gibbons, R. D., Brown, C. H., Hur, K., Marcus, S. M., Bhaumik, D. K., Erkens, J. A., et al. (2007). Early evidence on the effects of regulators' suicidality warnings on SSRI prescriptions and suicide in children and adolescents. *The American Journal of Psychiatry, 164*(9), 1356–1363.

Gould, M. S., Fisher, P., Parides, M., Flory, M., & Shaffer, D. (1996). Psychosocial risk factors of child and adolescent completed suicide. *Archives of General Psychiatry, 53*(12), 1155–1162.

Gould, M. S., Greenberg, T., Velting, D. M., & Shaffer, D. (2003). Youth suicide risk and preventive interventions: A review of the past 10 years. *Journal of the American Academy of Child and Adolescent Psychiatry, 42*(4), 386–405.

Gould, M. S., & Kramer, R. A. (2001). Youth suicide prevention. *Suicide & Life-Threatening Behavior, 31*(Suppl.), 6–31.

Grossman, D. C., Cummings, P., Koepsell, T. D., Marshall, J., D'Ambrosio, L., Thompson, R. S., et al. (2000). Firearm safety counseling in primary care pediatrics: A randomized, controlled trial. *Pediatrics, 106*(1 Pt 1), 22–26.

Guo, G., & Harstall, C. (2002). *Efficacy of suicide prevention programs for children and youth. HTA 26: Series A* [Health technology assessment]. Edmonton: Alberta Heritage Foundation for Medical Research.

Gutierrez, P. M., Watkins, R., & Collura, D. (2004). Suicide risk screening in an urban high school. *Suicide & Life-Threatening Behavior, 34*(4), 421–428.

Hallfors, D., Brodish, P. H., Khatapoush, S., Sanchez, V., Cho, H., & Steckler, A. (2006). Feasibility of screening adolescents for suicide risk in "real-world" high school settings. *American Journal of Public Health, 96*(2), 282–287.

Hammad, T. A., Laughren, T., & Racoosin, J. (2006). Suicidality in pediatric patients treated with antidepressant drugs. *Archives of General Psychiatry, 63*(3), 332–339.

Hawton, A., Osborn, M., O'Grady, J., & Cole, D. (1982). Classification of adolescents who take overdoses. *British Journal of Psychiatry, 140*, 124–131.

Hawton, K., Arensman, E., Townsend, E., Bremner, S., Feldman, E., Goldney, R., et al. (1998). Deliberate self harm: Systematic review of efficacy of psychosocial and pharmacological treatments in preventing repetition. *British Medical Journal, 317*(7156), 441–447.

Hayden, D. C., & Lauer, P. (2000). Prevalence of suicide programs in schools and roadblocks to implementation. *Suicide & Life-Threatening Behavior, 30*(3), 239–251.

Isaac, M., Elias, B., Katz, L. Y., Belik, S. L., Deane, F. P., Enns, M. W., et al. (2009). Gatekeeper training as a preventative intervention for suicide: A systematic review. *Canadian Journal of Psychiatry, 54*(4), 260–268.

Joe, S., & Bryant, H. (2007). Evidence-based suicide prevention screening in schools. *Children & Schools, 29*, 219–227.

Johnson, R. M., & Coyne-Beasley, T. (2009 Oct). Lethal means reduction: What have we learned? *Current Opinion in Pediatrics, 21*(5), 635–640.

Kalafat, J., & Elias, M. (1994). An evaluation of a school-based suicide awareness intervention. *Suicide & Life-Threatening Behavior, 24*(3), 224–233.

Kalafat, J., & Elias, M. J. (1995). Suicide prevention in an educational context: Broad and narrow foci. *Suicide & Life-Threatening Behavior, 25*(1), 123–133.

Kalafat, J., & Gagliano, C. (1996). The use of simulations to assess the impact of an adolescent suicide response curriculum. *Suicide & Life-Threatening Behavior, 26*(4), 359–364.

Kandel, D. B., Raveis, V. H., & Davies, M. (1991). Suicidal ideation in adolescence: Depression, substance use, and other risk factors. *Journal of Youth and Adolescence, 20*, 289–308.

King, C. A. (1997). Suicidal behavior in adolescence. In E. W. Maris, M. W. Silverman, & S. S. Canetto (Eds.), *Review of suicidology* (pp. 61–95). New York: Guilford.

King, K. A. (1999). Fifteen prevalent myths about adolescent suicide. *Journal of School Health, 69*, 159–161.

King, C. A., Kramer, A., Preuss, L., Kerr, D. C., Weisse, L., & Venkataraman, S. (2006). Youth-nominated support team for suicidal adolescents (version 1): A randomized controlled trial. *Journal of Consulting and Clinical Psychology, 74*(1), 199–206.

King, K. A., Price, J. H., Telljohann, S. K., & Wahl, J. (1999). High school health teachers' perceived self-efficacy in identifying students at risk for suicide. *The Journal of School Health, 69*(5), 202–207.

King, K. A., & Smith, J. (2000). Project SOAR: A training program to increase school counselors' knowledge and confidence regarding suicide prevention and intervention. *The Journal of School Health, 70*(10), 402–407.

Kirk, W. G. (1993). *Adolescent suicide: A school based approach to assessment and intervention*. Champain: Research Press.

Klingman, A., & Hochdorf, Z. (1993). Coping with distress and self harm: The impact of a primary prevention program among adolescents. *Journal of Adolescence, 16*(2), 121–140.

Lazear, K., Roggenbaum, S., & Blase, K. (2003). *Youth suicide prevention school-based guide – Overview*. Tampa: Department of Child and Family Studies, Division of State and Local Support, Louis de la Parte Florida Mental Health Institute, University of South Florida.

Leenaars, A. A., & Wenckstern, S. (1990). *Suicide prevention in the schools*. New York: Hemisphere Publishing.

Lewinsohn, P. M., Rohde, P., & Seeley, J. R. (1996). Adolescent suicidal ideation and attempts: Prevalence, risk factors, and clinical implications. *Clinical Psychology: Science and Practice, 3*, 25–46.

Linehan, M. M. (1973). Suicide and attempted suicide: Study of perceived sex differences. *Perceptual and Motor Skills, 37*(1), 31–34.

Links, P. S., Balchand, K., Dawe, I., & Watson, W. J. (1999). Preventing recurrent suicidal behaviour. *Canadian Family Physician* [Medecin de Famille Canadien], *45*, 2656–2660.

Mann, J. J., Apter, A., Bertolote, J., Beautrais, A., Currier, D., Haas, A., et al. (2005). Suicide prevention strategies: A systematic review. *Journal of the American Medical Association, 294*(16), 2064–2074.

Marx, E., & Northrop, D. (1995). *Educating for health: A guide for implementing a comprehensive approach to school health education*. Newton: Education Development Center.

Matschnig, T., Fruhwald, S., & Frottier, P. (2006). Suicide behind bars – An international review. *Psychiatrische Praxis, 33*(1), 6–13.

Miller, D. N., Eckert, T. L., DuPaul, G. J., & White, G. P. (1999). Adolescent suicide prevention: Acceptability of school-based programs among secondary school principals. *Suicide & Life-Threatening Behavior, 29*(1), 72–85.

Mitchell, P. (2000). *Primary prevention and early intervention. Evaluation of the National Youth Suicide Prevention Strategy*. Melbourne: Australian Institute of Family Studies.

National Center for Health Statistics. (1996). Advance report of final mortality statistics, 1994. *NCHS Monthly Vital Statistics Report, 45*, 63.

Nordentoft, M. (2007). Prevention of suicide and attempted suicide in Denmark. Epidemiological studies of suicide and intervention studies in selected risk groups. *Danish Medical Bulletin, 54*(4), 306–369.

Oatis, P. J., Fenn Buderer, N. M., Cummings, P., & Fleitz, R. (1999). Pediatric practice based evaluation of the steps to prevent firearm injury program. *Injury Prevention, 5*(1), 48–52.

Orbach, I., & Bar-Joseph, H. (1993). The impact of a suicide prevention program for adolescents on suicidal tendencies, hopelessness, ego identity, and coping. *Suicide & Life-Threatening Behavior, 23*(2), 120–129.

Overholser, J. C., Hemstreet, A. H., Spirito, A., & Vyse, S. (1989). Suicide awareness programs in the schools: Effects of gender and personal experience. *Journal of the American Academy of Child and Adolescent Psychiatry, 28*(6), 925–930.

Pena, J. B., & Caine, E. D. (2006). Screening as an approach for adolescent suicide prevention. *Suicide & Life-Threatening Behavior, 36*(6), 614–637.

Peters, K. D., Kochanek, K. D., & Murphy, S. L. (1998). Deaths: Final data for 1996. *National Statistics Report, 47*(9), 1–100.

Pfeffer, C. R. (1997). Childhood suicidal behavior: A developmental perspective. *Psychiatric Clinics of North America, 20*(3), 551–562.

Pfeffer, C. R., Martins, P., Mann, J., Sunkenberg, M., Ice, A., Damore, J. P. Jr., et al. (1997). Child survivors of suicide: Psychosocial characteristics. *Journal of the American Academy of Child and Adolescent Psychiatry, 36*(1), 65–74.

Portzky, G., Audenaert, K., & van Heeringen, K. (2005a). Adjustment disorder and the course of the suicidal process in adolescents. *Journal of Affective Disorders, 87*(2–3), 265–270.

Portzky, G., Audenaert, K., & van Heeringen, K. (2005b). Suicide among adolescents. A psychological autopsy study of psychiatric, psychosocial and personality-related risk factors. *Social Psychiatry and Psychiatric Epidemiology, 40*(11), 922–930.

Ramsay, R. F., Cooke, M. A., & Lang, W. A. (1990). Alberta's suicide prevention training programs: A retrospective comparison with Rothman's developmental research model. *Suicide & Life-Threatening Behavior, 20*(4), 335–351.

Randell, B. P., Eggert, L. L., & Pike, K. C. (2001). Immediate post intervention effects of two brief youth suicide prevention interventions. *Suicide & Life-Threatening Behavior, 31*(1), 41–61.

Reynolds, W. M., & Mazza, J. J. (1992). *Suicidal behavior in nonreferred adolescents*. Paper presented at the International Conference for Suicidal Behavior, Western Psychiatric Institute and Clinic.

Rotheram-Borus, M. J., Walker, J. U., & Ferns, W. (1996). Suicidal behavior among middle-class adolescents who seek crisis services. *Journal of Clinical Psychology, 52*(2), 137–143.

Runeson, B. S., & Beskow, J. (1991). Borderline personality disorder in young Swedish suicides. *The Journal of Nervous and Mental Disease, 179*(3), 153–156.

Rutz, W., von Knorring, L., & Walinder, J. (1992). Long-term effects of an educational program for general practitioners given by the Swedish committee for the prevention and treatment of depression. *Acta Psychiatrica Scandinavica, 85*(1), 83–88.

Sankey, M., & Lawrence, R. (2005). Brief report: Classification of adolescent suicide and risk-taking deaths. *Journal of Adolescence, 28*(6), 781–785.

Scott, M. A., Wilcox, H. C., Schonfeld, I. S., Davies, M., Hicks, R. C., Turner, J. B., et al. (2009). School-based screening to identify at-risk students not already known to school professionals: The Columbia suicide screen. *American Journal of Public Health, 99*(2), 334–339.

Shaffer, D., Garland, A., Vieland, V., Underwood, M., & Busner, C. (1991). The impact of curriculum-based suicide prevention programs for teenagers. *Journal of the American Academy of Child and Adolescent Psychiatry, 30*(4), 588–596.

Shaffer, D., Gould, M. S., Fisher, P., Trautman, P., Moreau, D., Kleinman, M., et al. (1996). Psychiatric diagnosis in child and adolescent suicide. *Archives of General Psychiatry, 53*(4), 339–348.

Shaffer, D., & Pfeffer, C. R. (2001). Practice parameter for the assessment and treatment of children and adolescents with suicidal behavior. American academy of child and adolescent psychiatry. *Journal of the American Academy of Child and Adolescent Psychiatry, 40*(7 Suppl.), 24S–51S.

Shaffer, D., Scott, M., Wilcox, H., Maslow, C., Hicks, R., Lucas, C. P., et al. (2004). The Columbia Suicide Screen: Validity and reliability of a screen for youth suicide and depression. *Journal of the American Academy of Child and Adolescent Psychiatry, 43*(1), 71–79.

Shaffer, D., Vieland, V., Garland, A., Rojas, M., Underwood, M., & Busner, C. (1990). Adolescent suicide attempters. Response to suicide-prevention programs. *Journal of the American Medical Association, 264*(24), 3151–3155.

Shaffer, D., Wilcox, H., Lucas, C., Hicks, R., Busner, C., & Parides, M. S. (1996). *The development of a screening instrument for teens at risk for suicide.* Paper presented at the 1996 meeting of the American Academy of Child and Adolescent Psychiatry.

Shenassa, E. D., Catlin, S. N., & Buka, S. L. (2003). Lethality of firearms relative to other suicide methods: A population based study. *Journal of Epidemiology and Community Health, 57*(2), 120–124.

Silbert, K. L., & Berry, G. L. (1991). Psychological effects of a suicide prevention unit on adolescents' levels of stress, anxiety and hopelessness: Implications for counselling psychologists. *Counselling Psychology Quarterly, 4*(1), 45–58.

Steele, M. M., & Doey, T. (2007). Suicidal behaviour in children and adolescents. Part 2: Treatment and prevention. *Canadian Journal of Psychiatry, 52*(6 Suppl. 1), 35S–45S.

Stuart, C., Waalen, J. K., & Haelstromm, E. (2003). Many helping hearts: An evaluation of peer gatekeeper training in suicide risk assessment. *Death Studies, 27*(4), 321–333.

Suter, B. (1976). Suicide and women. In B. B. Wolman & K. H. Kraus (Eds.), *Between survival and suicide* (pp. 129–161). New York: Gardner.

Tarrier, N., Taylor, K., & Gooding, P. (2008). Cognitive-behavioral interventions to reduce suicide behavior: A systematic review and meta-analysis. *Behavior Modification, 32*(1), 77–108.

Thompson, E. A., & Eggert, L. L. (1999). Using the suicide risk screen to identify suicidal adolescents among potential high school dropouts. *Journal of the American Academy of Child and Adolescent Psychiatry, 38*(12), 1506–1514.

Thompson, E. A., Eggert, L. L., & Herting, J. R. (2000). Mediating effects of an indicated prevention program for reducing youth depression and suicide risk behaviors. *Suicide & Life-Threatening Behavior, 30*(3), 252–271.

Thompson, E. A., Eggert, L. L., Randell, B. P., & Pike, K. C. (2001). Evaluation of indicated suicide risk prevention approaches for potential high school dropouts. *American Journal of Public Health, 91*(5), 742–752.

United Nations Department for Policy Coordination and Sustainable Development. (1996). *Prevention of suicide: Guidelines for the formulation and implementation of national strategies*. New York: United Nations.

Vieland, V., Whittle, B., Garland, A., Hicks, R., & Shaffer, D. (1991). The impact of curriculum-based suicide prevention programs for teenagers: An 18-month follow-up. *Journal of the American Academy of Child and Adolescent Psychiatry, 30*(5), 811–815.

Webster, D. W., Wilson, M. E., Duggan, A. K., & Pakula, L. C. (1992). Parents' beliefs about preventing gun injuries to children. *Pediatrics, 89*(5 Pt 1), 908–914.

White, J., & Jodoin, N. (1998). *Before-the-fact interventions: A manual of Best practices in youth suicide prevention*. Vancouver: University of British Columbia.

Wilcox, H. C., Kellam, S. G., Brown, C. H., Poduska, J. M., Ialongo, N. S., Wang, W., et al. (2008). The impact of two universal randomized first- and second-grade classroom interventions on young adult suicide ideation and attempts. *Drug and Alcohol Dependence, 95*(Suppl. 1), S60–S73.

Windle, M., Miller-Tutzauer, C., & Domenico, D. (1992). Alcohol use, suicidal behavior, and risky activities among adolescents. *The Journal of Research on Adolescence, 2*, 317–330.

World Health Organization. (1982). *Changing patterns in suicide behaviour.* Copenhagen: Regional Office for Europe.

World Heath Organization. (2000). *Preventing suicide a resource for teachers and other school staff.* Geneva: Mental and Behavioural Disorders Department of Mental Health World Health Organization.

Wyman, P. A., Brown, C. H., Inman, J., Cross, W., Schmeelk-Cone, K., Guo, J., et al. (2008). Randomized trial of a gatekeeper program for suicide prevention: 1-year impact on secondary school staff. *Journal of Consulting and Clinical Psychology, 76*(1), 104–115.

Zenere, F. J. 3rd, & Lazarus, P. J. (1997). The decline of youth suicidal behavior in an urban, multicultural public school system following the introduction of a suicide prevention and intervention program. *Suicide & Life-Threatening Behavior, 27*(4), 387–402.

About the Authors

Maurizio Pompili, MD, PhD, is Professor of both Suicidology and Epidemiological Psychiatry at Sapienza University of Rome where he received his MD degree, training in psychiatry (both summa cum laude), and doctoral degree in neurosciences. He is also part of the Community at McLean Hospital – Harvard Medical School, USA. He is the recipient of the American Association of Suicidology's 2008 Shneidman Award for "Outstanding early career contribution to suicidology." He has published more than 200 papers on suicide including original research articles, book chapters, and editorials. He edited and co-edited several national and international books including the latest *Suicide in the Words of Suicidologists* and *Suicide: A Global Perspective*. He provided validation studies for psychometric instruments to assess suicide risk and he is the Italian National Representative to the International Association for Suicide Prevention (IASP).

Marco Innamorati, PhD, is a psychologist and psychotherapist. He is a member of the International Association for Suicide Prevention.

Paolo Girardi, MD, is Associate Professor of Psychiatry at Sapienza University of Rome. He is Vice-Director of the residency training in psychiatry at the II Medical School of Sapienza and in charge of the psychiatric ward at the Sant'Andrea Hospital in Rome. He supervises many research projects involving psychopharmacology and clinical trials. He contributed to the Italian validation of the Beck Hopelessness Scale and delivered educational programs in the field of psychiatry to general practitioners and doctors of the various medical disciplines. He has published more than 300 scientific papers and several books.

Roberto Tatarelli, MD, is Full Professor of Psychiatry, Chairman of the Department of Neurosciences, Mental Health, and Sensory Functions at Sant'Andrea Hospital, Sapienza University of Rome, Italy, and Director of the residency training in psychiatry at the II Medical School of Sapienza. During his long-lasting career he has carried out numerous research projects in the field of psychopathology, psychotic disorders, mood disorders, and suicide. He is full member of the International Academy for Suicide Research. He contributed to the Italian validation of the Beck Hopelessness Scale and has published more than 400 scientific publications and several books.

David Lester has doctoral degrees from Cambridge University (UK) in social and political science and Brandeis University (USA) in psychology. He is Distinguished Professor of Psychology at the Richard Stockton College of New Jersey. He has been President of the International Association for Suicide Prevention, and he has published extensively on suicide, murder, and other issues in thanatology. His recent books include *Katie's Diary: Unlocking the Mystery of a Suicide* (2004), *Suicide and the Holocaust* (2005), *Is there Life after Death?* (2005), *Preventing Suicide: Closing the Exits Revisited* (2009), and *Understanding Suicide: Why We Don't and How We Might* (2010).

Maurizio Pompili
Department of Psychiatry
Sant'Andrea Hospital
Via di Grottarossa
1035 – 00189 Rome
Italy
Tel.: +390633775675
E-mail: mpompili@mclean.harvard.edu

Suicide Prevention in Late Life

Is There Sound Evidence for Practice?

Marco Innamorati,[1] Maurizio Pompili,[1,2] Mario Amore,[3]
Cristina Di Vittorio,[3] Gianluca Serafini,[1] Roberto Tatarelli,[1]
and David Lester[4]

[1]Department of Neurosciences, Mental Health and Sensory Functions, Suicide Prevention Center, Sant'Andrea Hospital, Sapienza University of Rome, Italy
[2]McLean Hospital, Harvard Medical School, Boston, MA, USA
[3]Department of Neurosciences Division of Psychiatry, University of Parma, Italy
[4]Department of Psychology, The Richard Stockton College of New Jersey, Pomona, NJ, USA

Suicide in late life is a critical public health problem. In a recent cross-national study of 62 developing and developed countries, Shah reported an increase in the suicide rates with age in males and females in 25 and 27 countries, respectively (Shah, 2007). The suicide rate for the elderly in many countries is higher than that of any other age group, with the rates among people aged 75 years and older roughly three times that of adolescents (World Health Organization, 1999). The rates of completed suicide in elderly people may vary locally as well as between countries. For example, Oyama, Fujita, Goto, Shibuya, and Sakashita (2006), Oyama, Goto, Fujita, Shibuya, and Sakashita (2006) and Oyama, Ono, et al. (2006) reported suicide rates of 275–360 per 100,000 inhabitants per year in two small Japanese towns.

Pooled international data published by the World Health Organization (2002) show a rise in the rate of completed suicide with age. For men, the rate increases from 19.2 per 100,000 inhabitants in the 15–24-year-old age group to 55.7 in those over 75. For women, the respective rates are 5.6 and 18.8. The male-to-female ratio for completed suicide in the elderly ranges between 3:1 and 4:1, which is similar to that of other age groups. Moreover, suicidal behavior in the elderly is undertaken with greater intent and with greater lethality than in younger age groups.

The aim of this chapter is to review the international literature investigating whether there is sufficient evidence for sound-based practice in the prevention of suicidal behaviors in the elderly and to find recommendations and guidelines.

Conwell and Duberstein (1995), following Fried (1990), indicated four guidelines for the development of effective preventive strategies of late-life suicide. These are:

- Guideline 1 – The potential benefit of a preventive measure is proportional both to the prevalence of the disease and to the severity of the morbidity associated with it.
- Guideline 2 – The goals of disease prevention must be based on an analysis of what beneficial outcome is most meaningful for the individual and society.
- Guideline 3 – To be effective in older people, preventive care must take into account the multiple dimensions that impact on their health: biological, psychological, and social.
- Guideline 4 – The effectiveness of a prevention measure depends on: (a) the identification of the risk factors characteristic of the individual or group; (b) the strength of the causal relationship between the risk factors and the disease; and (c) the "alterability" of the causal factors.

The guidelines for preventive strategies indicate that the effectiveness of an intervention is related in part to the strength of the causal relationship between the risk factor and the outcome, and in part to the alterability of that causal factor. Many factors influence suicide risk among the elderly, the modification of which may help prevent suicide.

Grek (2007) conducted a systematic literature review to identify the risk factors for suicide in the elderly. The search for risk factors yielded two relevant cohort studies (Ross, Bernstein, Trent, Henderson, & Paganini-Hill, 1990; Turvey et al., 2002) and 17 relevant case-control studies (Beautrais, 2002; Chiu et al., 2004; Conwell et al., 2000; Duberstein, Conwell, Conner, Eberly, & Caine, 2004; Duberstein, Conwell, Conner, Eberly, Evinger, et al., 2004; Erlangsen, Zarit, Tu, & Conwell, 2006; Harwood, Hawton, Hope, & Jacoby, 2001; Harwood, Hawton, Hope, Harriss, & Jacoby, 2006; Juurlink, Herrmann, Szalai, Kopp, & Redelmeier, 2004; Juurlink, Mamdani, Kopp, & Redelmeier, 2006; Kolves, Varnik, Tooding, & Wasserman, 2006; Preville, Hebert, Boyer, Bravo, & Seguin, 2005; Quan, Arboleda-Florez, Fick, Stuart, & Love, 2002; Rubenowitz, Waern, Wilhelmson, & Allebeck, 2001; Waern, 2003; Waern, Rubenowitz, et al., 2002; Waern, Runeson, et al., 2002). Grek concluded that sound risk factors for suicide are: (1) male sex, (2) mental illness (particularly depression), (3) physical illness, and (4) interpersonal discord. Three of these four risk factors are modifiable.

Method

We performed careful MedLine and PsycINFO searches from 1980 to 2008. The following search terms were used: "elderly" or "older adults," suicid* (which comprises suicide, suicidal, suicidality, and other suicide-related terms), risk factors, and prevention. In addition, each category was cross-referenced with the others using the MeSH (Medical

Subjects Headings) method. Function limits were used to select meta-analyses, controlled trials, and other quantitative studies. The selection of papers suitable for this study allowed the inclusion of only those articles that were published in the English peer-reviewed journals. Included were those studies that added an original contribution to the literature.

When possible, we indicated the strength of the recommendations included in the published clinical guidelines (Shekelle, Woolf, Eccles, & Grimshaw, 1999). The strength of a recommendation is evaluated on a scale ranging from A to D, based on the available body of evidence. These levels are: (A) the recommendation is based on Category I of evidence; (B) the recommendation is directly based on Category II of evidence, or extrapolated from Category I of evidence; (C) the recommendation is directly based on Category III of evidence or extrapolated from Category I or II of evidence; and (D) the recommendation is directly based on Category IV of evidence, or extrapolated from Category I, II, or III of evidence. The categories of evidence for treatments are (Shekelle et al., 1999): (Ia) evidence from meta-analyses of randomized controlled trials; (Ib) evidence from at least one randomized controlled trial; (IIa) evidence from at least one study without randomization; (IIb) evidence from at least one other type of quasi-experimental study; (III) evidence from nonexperimental descriptive studies (comparative studies, correlation studies, and case-control studies); and (IV) evidence from expert committee reports or opinions and/or clinical experience of respected authorities.

Suicide Prevention Strategies in the Late Life

We found seven quantitative studies that evaluated programs directed toward reduction or prevention of suicidality in elders, or including data for interventions suitable for suicide risk reduction in the elderly (Bruce et al., 2004; De Leo, Carollo, & Dello Buono, 1995; De Leo, Dello Buono, & Dwyer, 2002; Eli Lilly and Company, 2005; Nelson, Delucchi, & Schneider, 2007; Szanto, Mulsant, Houck, Dew, & Reynolds, 2003; Unutzer et al., 2006). Another research study (Lapierre, Dube, Bouffard, & Alain, 2007), despite involving only adults aged 50–65 years, was included in the review because of its potential usefulness in the prevention of suicidality in late life. Moreover, we found a meta-analysis (Oyama et al., 2008) that included five previous quasi-experimental studies evaluating community-based interventions using depression screening (Oyama, Fujita, et al., 2006; Oyama, Goto, et al., 2006; Oyama, Koida, Sakashita, & Kudo, 2004; Oyama, Ono, et al., 2006; Takahashi et al., 1998). Finally, we found two clinical sets of guidelines with recommendations for suicide prevention (Blow, Bartels, Brockmann, & Van Citters, 2006; Canadian Coalition for Seniors' Mental Health, 2006), although only one set indicated the strengths of the recommendations (Canadian Coalition for Seniors' Mental Health, 2006).

Antidepressants for the Reduction of Suicidal Ideation

Szanto et al. (2003) performed a secondary analysis on the data from three federally funded treatment studies on late-life major depression and analyzed the occurrence and course of suicidality in the participants. The trials investigated the role of antidepressants and interpersonal psychotherapy in the reduction of suicidal ideation. The first study was an open study of maintenance therapies in patients with recurrent major depression. The participants were treated with nortriptyline (plasma level, 80–120 ng/mL) and weekly interpersonal psychotherapy. The second study was an open study of maintenance therapies in patients with major depression. The participants were treated with paroxetine (dosage, 10–40 mg/day) and weekly interpersonal psychotherapy. The third study was a double-blind randomized trial comparing nortriptyline (plasma level, 50–120 ng/mL) and paroxetine (dosage, 20–40 mg/day). All patients (n = 395; age range: 59–95 years) met the criteria for a major depressive episode. The participants were classified into three groups based on the highest level of suicidality reported in the week before the treatment and during treatment (as measured via Item 3 of the Hamilton rating scale for depression – HAM-D): a high-risk group (recent attempt or current suicidal ideation), a moderate-risk group (recurrent thoughts of death), and a low-risk group (neither suicidal ideation nor thoughts of death). The analysis was limited to the first 12 weeks of the trials (The third study investigated only acute antidepressant treatment of major depression).

The results indicated that the baseline levels of suicidal ideation or thoughts of death were similar in patients treated with nortriptyline (7.8%) or paroxetine (8.0%). Thoughts about death and suicidal ideation improved during the 12-week intervention in the whole group, regardless of treatment assignment (18.4% versus 77.5%; $p < .001$). At week 12, none of the patients who remained in treatment reported suicidal ideation, but 4.6% still reported thoughts of death. Of these, most of them were treatment responders or partial responders. Furthermore, one patient attempted suicide during maintenance treatment, and one more patient completed suicide after leaving the study and discontinuing treatment against medical advice. Both patients had suicidal ideation during the current episode. There were no statistical differences in the drop-out rates among the groups of patients ($p = .37$). At the end of the treatment, high-risk patients had significantly lower response rates and longer time to respond than low-risk patients. Finally, combined treatment with interpersonal psychotherapy added no additional impact, while nortriptyline and paroxetine were not significantly different in their efficacy.

Nelson et al. (2007) investigated the effects of sertraline on suicidal thinking and behavior in patients with late-life major depression. The investigators conducted an 8-week, multicenter placebo-controlled, double-blind randomized trial at 66 clinical sites. The inclusion criteria were outpatients aged 60 years and older with nonpsychotic major depression, a current depressive episode with a duration of at least 4 weeks, and a HAM-D score of 18 or above. Patients took sertraline (50–100 mg/day) or placebo for 8 weeks. Suicidal ideation and behavior were measured via Item 3 of the HAM-D. The authors reported an adjusted odds ratio of 0.70 for the sertraline group when compared with the placebo group on Item 3 of the HAM-D at the last observation, indicating lower suicidal ideation. The authors also investigated emergent suicidal ideation. Among all patients rating zero on Item 3 at the baseline, no patient on sertraline developed active suicidal ideation during treatment (Item 3 = 3) (versus only one patient in the placebo group). When investigating the change in Item 3 over time, using a mixed-effects model analysis, the estimates of the treatment effect were 0.65 ($z = 2.48$; $p < .05$) and 0.55 ($z = 2.41$; $p < .05$), respectively, for the patients who reported Item 3 scores higher than zero at the baseline and for the whole sample. However, the results of the study are limited because the patients judged to be at significant suicide risk were excluded from the final sample. In fact, over 35% of patients enrolled both in the sertraline group and in the placebo group scored zero on Item 3 of the HAM-D at baseline.

One trial of the Ely-Lilly Study (F1J-MC-HMBV) (Eli Lilly and Company, 2005), recently published by Raskin, Wiltse, et al. (2008), Raskin et al. (2007), and Raskin, Xu, and Kajdasz (2008), investigated the efficacy of acute therapy (9 weeks) with duloxetine 60 mg/day ($N = 167$) versus placebo ($N = 85$) in elderly patients (65+ years) who met the criteria for major depressive disorder and had a HAM-D score of 18 or higher and a Mini-Mental State Exam score of 20 or higher. The results indicate a least-square-mean change of −0.07 ($SE = 0.06$) in the placebo group and −0.35 ($SE = 0.04$) in the duloxetine group ($t_{242} = -3.93$; $p < .001$). However, the results of this trial are also limited because its summary failed to record whether the patients had a positive anamnesis for previous suicidal behavior and attempts.

Bruce et al. (2004) determined the effect of a primary care intervention on suicidal ideation and depression in older patients (PROSPECT – Prevention of Suicide in Primary Care Elderly: Collaborative Trial). PROSPECT hypothesized that, in a heterogeneous sample of older, depressed primary care patients, patients randomized to receive the intervention compared with usual care (usual care was enhanced by initially educating physicians about the treatment guidelines and notifying them when a patient met criteria for a diagnosis of depression) would demonstrate: (1) a greater reduction in suicidal ideation and (2) a greater reduction in depressive symptoms, increased response rates, and greater remission rates in depressive symptoms. Enrollment included patients with a major depression or a clinically significant minor depression as defined by the Diagnostic and Statistical Manual of Mental Disorders, Fourth Edition (DSM-IV), and a random sample of patients who screened negative ($N = 598$; 320 intervention; 278 usual-care). The study was conducted in 20 primary care practices from greater New York City, Philadelphia, and Pittsburgh. The sociodemographic characteristics of the intervention and the usual-care patients did not differ statistically. However, a larger proportion of intervention patients reported suicidal ideation than the usual-care patients (29.4% versus 20.1%; $p = .01$).

The results indicated that intervention patients were significantly more likely than usual-care patients to report depression treatment at each follow-up period (4, 8, and 12 months). Intervention patients had higher rates of medication-only ($p < .001$) and psychotherapy-only ($p < .001$) treatments. The small proportions of patients receiving combination treatment did not differ between the groups ($p = .23$). Despite the fact that patients in the intervention group were more likely to report suicidal ideation at baseline than patients in the usual-care group, by four months and at each subsequent follow-up period, the rates of suicidal ideation no longer differed between the groups reflecting a significantly greater decline in suicidal ideation in the intervention group after adjusting for the baseline difference. In the intervention group, raw rates of suicidal ideation declined 12.9% points

(29.4% to 16.5%) compared with 3.0% points (20.1% to 17.1%) in the usual-care group ($p = .01$). Adjusting for the baseline difference, the omnibus test for change over time was significant among all the depressed patients ($p = .01$) and among patients with major depression ($p = .006$). The differences were not significant among patients with minor depression ($p = .98$). The interaction between the intervention and depression diagnosis on reduced suicidal ideation was not statistically significant ($p = .64$).

Two sets of post hoc analyses examined the effect of the PROSPECT intervention stratified by both depression diagnosis and suicidality. Among patients who reported suicidal ideation at baseline, suicidal ideation had resolved by 4 months in 66.7% of intervention patients compared with 58.7% of patients receiving usual care ($p = .34$). The difference between the groups was more pronounced and statistically significant at 8 months (70.7% versus 43.9%; $p = .005$). By 12 months, more than two-thirds of both groups no longer expressed suicidal ideation (68.7% versus 65.8%; $p = .89$). Consistent with the group difference peaking at 8 months, the omnibus test for change across time was significant ($p = .03$). The pattern was similar within the major depression and the minor depression subgroups, although the omnibus test did not reach statistical significance in either group (major depression, $p = .09$ and minor depression, $p = .09$).

Intervention patients had significantly greater decreases in the HAM-D scores compared with patients receiving usual care whether or not at baseline they reported suicidal ideation (all depressed patients, $p < .001$ and patients with major depression, $p < .001$), or no suicidal ideation (all depressed patients, $p < .001$ and patients with major depression, $p < .001$). The majority (87%) of patients with minor depression did not report suicidal ideation, and the impact of the intervention on their depressive symptoms was not significant overall ($p = .72$). In contrast, patients with minor depression but also suicidal ideation in the PROSPECT intervention group had a significantly greater overall decrease in depression severity relative to usual-care patients ($p = .03$). However, the study design may have limited validity. For example, 36% of patients identified as receiving the "interpersonal therapy only" condition also used antidepressive medication (SAMHSA, 2007).

Unutzer et al. (2006) examined the long-term (2-year) effects on suicidal ideation of the Improving Mood: Promoting Access to Collaborative Treatment (IMPACT) for Late-Life Depression in Primary Care program, a collaborative-care program for late-life depression. It was hypothesized that individuals assigned to the IMPACT care model would report less suicidal ideation than usual-care patients during the 12-month intervention period and the 12-month follow-up period. The IMPACT trial was conducted in 18 primary care clinics affiliated with eight diverse healthcare organizations in five US states. Inclusion criteria were age 60+ years and current major depression, dysthymia, or both on the Structured Clinical Interview for the Diagnostic and Statistical Manual of Mental Disorders, Fourth Edition (SCID). Exclusion criteria included current alcohol abuse, severe cognitive dysfunction, a history of bipolar disorder or psychosis, and acute risk of suicide. Primary care patients were randomized to receive either collaborative care or usual care by their family doctors.

The intervention was a 1-year collaborative-care program that included a depression-care manager (DCM) working in the patient's primary care clinic to support the patient's regular primary care clinician. The DCMs were registered nurses with and without prior mental health experience and psychologists who worked in the clinics. DCMs completed an initial assessment visit to all patients and provided education about the treatment options, including antidepressant medications and psychotherapy. All patients were encouraged to engage in behavioral activity (physical activity or pleasant events scheduling) and were offered a choice of treatment with antidepressant medications, prescribed by the patient's regular primary care providers or Problem-Solving Treatment in Primary Care (PST-PC), a brief behavioral intervention lasting between four and eight sessions that nonmental health providers could provide in primary care. The DCMs were supervised every week by the primary care providers with geriatric expertise and a psychiatrist to monitor the progress of cases and to adjust the treatment plans according to a stepped-care treatment algorithm (Unutzer et al., 2001). This algorithm provided guidance for acute and continuation therapy and relapse-prevention recommendations over the 12-month intervention period.

The DCMs followed the patients in person or by telephone approximately every 2 weeks during the acute-phase treatment and approximately every month during the continuation-phase treatment. The DCMs were trained during a 2-day workshop that focused on the IMPACT care model, suggested treatment algorithms (Unutzer et al., 2002), and included didactic training and role-playing in key intervention skills such as behavioral activation and PST-PC. The primary outcome was the reporting of suicidal ideation according to a single item from a symptom checklist. Collaborative care consisted of closely supported antidepressant medication management or problem-solving treatment. After 1 year of treatment, the odds ratio for intervention when compared with usual care was 0.54 (95% confidence intervals, 0.40/0.73). This association, of small magnitude, persisted for 6 months after the treatment ended; after 1 year, it was somewhat smaller, but still present.

The "Managing Retirement" Program

This program, called *"Managing Your Retirement Goals,"* is not directed toward elders, but toward middle-aged individuals (50–65 years). However, it may be useful in the prevention of suicidality in the late life because it is directed toward retirement maladjustment. Lapierre et al. (2007) investigated individuals who had experienced problems adjusting to retirement and analyzed the subsample of individuals who had expressed suicidal ideation. The authors hypothesized that the goal-intervention program would be effective in increasing psychological well-being and decreasing levels of depression in the participants with suicidal ideation. The program was designed to help participants define their goals and pursue them effectively in order to achieve enhanced and lasting well-being. The program is composed of a series of meetings (usually 11 weekly meeting of 2 hours, but they may vary according to the group's needs) subdivided into several steps:

(1) preliminary meetings, (2) goal setting, (3) goal planning, (4) goal pursuit, (5) outcome evaluation, and (6) follow-up meetings.

The first step has the objective of making the acquaintance of the group participants and giving information on the program. In the second step, the group members exchange their experience with regard to retirement transition. In the goal setting step, participants list their personal aspirations, goals, intentions, aspirations, and projects. This step also identifies irrational beliefs about these goals. Goals with high priority are selected, and each goal is evaluated according to its characteristics (e.g., effort, stress, enjoyment, difficulty, resources, conflict, control, and probability of attainment). Lastly, the goals are operationalized in concrete and precise terms as a target-behavior, and one goal is selected.

The goal-planning step has the objective of planning goal-related actions (where, when, and how), anticipating obstacles and identifying strategies to deal with them, and identifying social resources. Planning is reevaluated regularly with the help of other participants. The next step, goal pursuit, has the objective of executing the plan and facing any difficulties with emotional support from the group. When necessary, a revision of goal-planning and questioning of the priority of goals may have to be made.

In this research, suicidal ideation was assessed through one item, "During the last week, did you think about ending your life?" Twenty-seven individual of 354 participants of the original sample answered "yes" at baseline. The subsample with suicidal ideation was significantly different on retirement decision variables from the participants in the original sample who answered "no" to the question on suicidal ideation. The individuals with suicidal ideation were more likely to feel that they had had insufficient time to make their decision to retire and that they were forced into retirement. From the original 27 participants who had suicidal ideation, only 21 completed the study. However, there was no significant difference in the sociodemographic and well-being indicators between these participants and those who dropped out. The study included three measurement points: pretest, posttest at the end of the intervention program, and follow-up 6 months later. Preliminary analyses indicated that there were no significant differences between the experimental and the control groups on all dependent variables at pretest.

The results indicated that the participants in the experimental group improved significantly more over time than those in the control group on goal realization, hope, retirement experience, serenity, flexibility, depression, and psychological distress. These gains were maintained 6 months later. More importantly, 80% of the experimental group and only 36% of the control group reported the absence of suicidal ideation in the previous week at the 6-month follow-up. Although the results of the study are interesting, their generalization is limited by shortcomings in the methodology, such as the lack of random assignment to intervention groups and the small number of subjects.

Selective Preventive Strategies

The TeleHelp/TeleCheck service, a broad public health intervention program providing twice-weekly telephone support and emergency response for up to 20,000 elders, was established in Veneto (Italy) in 1988. The TeleHelp/TeleCheck service uses a portable alarm system and offers active contacts to clients by trained staff who could provide information, support, and rapid intervention in medical and psychological emergencies. Elderly people were typically offered the service because of their disability or social isolation, their psychiatric problems, their poor compliance with hospital outpatient regimes, or because they were waiting for admission to public or private social and healthcare institutions.

De Leo et al. (1995) first investigated the impact of the service on suicidal behavior in terms of primary prevention and crisis management. The study participants were over 12,000 individuals 65+ years who were connected to the TeleHelp/TeleCheck. The authors reported that, during the 4-year evaluation, 2,135 deaths occurred, but reliable information was gathered only for 1,875 deaths of individuals 65+ years of age. In the 4-year study, only one suicide occurred, and the ratio between observed and expected suicides was 1:7.44 (standardized mortality ratio = 13.44% [95% confidence intervals, 0.3/74.8]; $p < .05$). This indicates a lower suicide rate than would be expected on the basis of the general population suicide rates. The standardized mortality ratio for the female elders was 39.53% (95% confidence interval, 0.3/220; p = n.s.), whereas the standardized mortality ratio for the male elders could not be calculated, because there were no suicides among older men.

Because the results of this study were limited by the small numbers of suicides involved, the authors published further results in a more recent paper (De Leo et al., 2002). The new study included 18,641 individuals, 65 years of age or older, connected to TeleHelp/TeleCheck between 1 January 1988 and 31 December 1998. In this second study, the authors reported that the number of observed suicides ($n = 6$) of TeleHelp/TeleCheck users was significantly lower than the number expected ($n_{expected} = 20.86$; $p < .001$). The standardized mortality ratio was 28.8% (95% confidence interval, 11.5/62.5). Examination of the data indicated that the observed suicide rate of female users of the TeleHelp/TeleCheck was 5.99 times lower than the expected suicide rate, with a standardized mortality ratio of 16.7% (95% confidence interval, 2.0/59.9; $p < .01$). In contrast, there was no significant difference between the observed and the expected suicide rates in male elders ($p = .20$).

Impact of Community-Based Depression Screening Programs on the Risk of Completed Suicide

Recently, Oyama et al. (2008) reported a meta-analysis of studies on the effect of community-based depression screening on the risk of completed suicide among older adults. The authors included studies if they: (1) evaluated intervention trials involving screening for mental health conditions in the community setting and were targeted toward a whole community or group of individuals therein; (2) had target populations involving individuals over 60 years of age; and (3) used completed suicide incidence as the outcome measure. Five studies (Oyama, Fujita, et al., 2006; Oyama, Goto, et al., 2006; Oyama et al., 2004; Oyama, Ono, et al., 2006; Takahashi et al., 1998) that were conducted in Japan satisfied the inclusion criteria and were included in the meta-analysis. (Four of the five studies were coauthored by one or more authors of the meta-analysis.) All these studies used a quasi-experimental design, that is, a pre- and postimplementation design with neighboring community controls, using the intervention community as a historical control.

All the studies, except for one (Takahashi et al., 1998), compared the change in suicide risk with the secular trend. All the five studies described universal prevention programs including screening for depression, follow-up, and health education in a community setting. The five studies offered educational health workshops to residents and, in addition, two of the five studies offered group activities providing social and recreational activities and exercise (Oyama, Ono, et al., 2006; Takahashi et al., 1998). All the five studies also provided a voluntary, two-step screening using a self-report questionnaire (Zung's Self-Rating Depression Scale) in the first step and an assessment by public health nurses and psychiatrists in the second step. Because the studies employed two different types of specialists who clinically followed those positive for the risk of suicide on initial screening, the participants were divided into the following two groups: (1) community-based depression screening with follow-up by a psychiatrist and (2) community-based depression screening with follow-up by a general practitioner.

In the first group of studies, two of the five studies implemented almost the same program, providing a two-step screening performed by public health nurses and psychiatrists and the follow-up conducted by psychiatrists during a 7- or 10-year period (Oyama et al., 2004; Takahashi et al., 1998). In these two studies, between 60% and 80% of the targeted elder residents participated in the program during the implementation. Overall, meta-analysis of the targeted population involved 21,170 person-years and 19 suicides in the implementation, compared to 16,110 person-years and 51 suicides at baseline. The combined incidence rate ratio (IRR) (95% confidence intervals) for the six populations of each gender from the two studies were 0.30 (0.13/0.68) and 0.33 (0.14/0.80) for men, respectively, using the Mantel-Haenszel method and the DerSimonian-Laird method, and 0.33 (0.19/0.58) and 0.33 (0.19/0.60) for women, respectively.

In the five studies with community-based depression screening with follow-up by a general practitioner, three studies implemented almost the same program, providing a two-step screening performed by public health nurses and psychiatrists, and the follow-up conducted by general practitioners during a 10-year period (Oyama, Fujita, et al., 2006; Oyama, Goto, et al., 2006) or by general practitioners and to a lesser extent psychiatrists during a 6-year period (Oyama, Ono, et al., 2006). In the three studies, more than 60% of the men and more than 80% of the women from the targeted elder residents participated in the program during implementation. Overall, meta-analysis of the target population involved 27,865 person-years and 44 suicides in the implementation, compared to 23,340 person-years and 71 suicides at baseline. The combined IRR (95% confidence intervals) for the nine populations of each gender from the three studies were 0.73 (0.45/1.18) and 0.74 (0.45/1.23) for men, respectively using the Mantel-Haenszel method and the DerSimonian-Laird method, and 0.36 (0.21/0.60) and 0.39 (0.22/0.66) for women, respectively, using the Mantel-Haenszel method and the DerSimonian-Laird method.

The results of the meta-analysis demonstrated that the implementation of universal prevention programs involving community-based depression screening and health education is associated with a reduced risk of completed suicide among older residents. However, there seems to be a clear difference as to whether psychiatrists or general practitioners conducted the follow-up for the participants. The community-based depression screening with the follow-up conducted by general practitioners is associated with a less reduced or unchanged risk for older men. However, the meta-analysis of Oyama et al. (2008) was based on quasi-experimental studies (nonrandomized, concurrent comparative, and before-and-after designs) that are open to bias and confounding.

Available Clinical Guidelines to Manage Suicidality in Late Life

There are few clinical guidelines for the prevention of suicide in late life. One was prepared in 2006 by the Canadian Coalition for Seniors' Mental Health (2006). The authors developed clinical practice guidelines for clinicians who encounter people 65 years of age and older who are at high risk for suicide, because they are thinking about it or planning it, or have recently tried to harm or kill themselves. The recommendations are listed in Table 1. All the recommendations included in these guidelines are rated from B to D on the scale of strength of evidence. The authors found no sound evidence to justify recommendation to include in the first category [A].

First of all, the authors have urged clinicians to assess suicidal risk factors in elders, especially suicidal ideation. Healthcare professionals must ask directly whether the patients present death wishes and suicidal ideation [C] (see Table 2) because older adults may not mention these thoughts spontaneously with clinicians. When evaluating the suicide risk, the healthcare professionals have to evaluate the weight of risk factors and protective factors, facilitating strategies to develop or regain a sense of meaning and purpose in life [D]. When possible, psychometric-validated instruments should be used in the assessment of suicide risk [D]. After evaluation, healthcare providers working with suicidal older adults should provide evidence-based assessment and treatment for depression [B].

Other clinical guidelines were drafted by the Older Americans Substance Abuse and Mental Health Technical Assistance Center (Blow et al., 2006). The authors concluded their review of evidence by indicating that current prevention programs could reduce the rate of suicide among older women, but have shown more limited effectiveness among older men. Although there are few data to support the prevention of suicide of older adults, the authors adapted some goals and objectives from the National Suicide Prevention Strategy to meet the needs of older adults like to:

- Promote awareness of the fact that suicide in older adults is a public health problem that is preventable.
- Develop broad-based support for the prevention of suicide among elders.
- Develop and implement strategies to reduce the stigma associated with aging and the stigma of being a senior consumer of mental health, substance abuse, and suicide prevention services.

Table 1. Recommendations from the Canadian Coalition for Seniors' Mental Health (2006)

Recommendation	Strength
Health care providers should always assess the presence of risk factors for suicide among older adults.	**D**
When risk factors are present, assess for death ideation and suicide ideation. In those with death ideation and suicide ideation, assess for suicidal intent, suicidal plan, and current or past suicidal behaviour.	**C**
Repeatedly assess for suicide ideation throughout treatment for depression.	**D**
Consider hospitalization for elders who express severe suicidal ideation and/or a suicide plan.	**D**
Assess mood disorders, and comorbid mental disorders.	**C**
Assess substance use disorders.	**C**
Assess personality disorders, dysfunctional personality traits, and non-adaptive coping strategies.	**C**
Assess for the presence of real or perceived physical illness.	**C**
Carefully assess for suicidal intent among those endorsing a wish to hasten death.	**D**
Assess for additional recent life events and stressors.	**C**
Assess for functional decline.	**C**
Facilitate the development or regaining of a sense of meaning and purpose in life.	**D**
Facilitate the enhancement of social support and interpersonal activities.	**D**
Facilitate strategies for/with clients to encourage better health practices.	**D**
Consider the use of standardized assessment instruments to assess for the presence and severity of psychological factors potentially associated with increased suicide risk.	**D**
Assess suicide risk in a respectful way, in the context of an empathic acceptance of the patient.	**D**
Validate clients' experiences in order to encourage the expression of their thoughts and feelings.	**D**
Consult previous health providers and family members and/or significant others, for the assessment of suicide risk.	**D**
Seek assistance and supervising if you do not have specialized training in mental health or in suicide prevention.	**D**
Use evidence-based practice to assess and treat depression.	**D**
Promote hope in clients who are suicidal.	**D**
Promote meaning and purpose in clients' lives.	**C**

(continued on next page)

Table 1. Continued.

Recommendation	Strength
Promote a therapeutic relationship and feeling of connectedness.	**D**
Use a team approach.	**D**
Focus on your own emotional well-being too.	**D**
Keep detailed notes of the intervention.	**D**
Involve emergency services when adherence is at risk.	**D**
Restrict access to lethal means.	**D**
Establish an interdisciplinary and collaborative care model of intervention.	**B**
Involve community resources.	**D**
Provide education to elders and their caregivers about suicide and treatments.	**D**

Table 2. Questions to ask to assess suicide risk in the elders

In the last year:	True	False
1. Did you think life was not worth living?	☐	☐
2. Did you think that for you, and for your own family and friend, it was better to be dead?	☐	☐
3. Did you think of injuring yourself without the intention to die?	☐	☐
4. Did you think of voluntarily ending your life?	☐	☐
5. Did you plan a way for ending your life?	☐	☐
6. Did you try to take your life?	☐	☐

- Develop and implement community-based suicide prevention programs for older adults.
- Promote efforts to reduce access to lethal means and methods of self-harm by older adults.
- Implement training for the recognition and assessment of at-risk behavior and delivery of effective treatment to older adults.
- Develop and promote effective clinical and professional practices.
- Improve access to and community linkages with mental health, substance abuse, and social services designed for the evaluation and treatment of older adults in primary and long-term care settings.
- Improve reporting and portrayals of suicidal behavior, mental illness, and substance abuse among older adults in the entertainment and news media.
- Promote and support research on late-life suicide and suicide prevention.

- Improve and expand surveillance systems.
- Carry out interventions which aim to strengthen elders' social network and ease their feelings of loneliness.
- Increase access to geriatric specialty healthcare.

Discussion of Preventive Strategies in the Elders at Risk of Suicide

Our review of the literature indicates that there is little sound evidence for planning and practicing suicide prevention among the elderly. Controlled trials evaluating strategies to manage and to prevent suicide in the elderly are rare, and sometimes their methodology is poor. There are few randomized controlled trials, and often the objectives of the original study were not to analyze the efficacy of treatments on suicide behavior and ideation *per se*. A bias associated with these studies is the exclusion of severely suicidal patients, and this in turn results in many of the research conclusions having a limited utility for clinical practice.

However, we can point out some evidence that is useful for the prevention of suicides in the elderly. First of all, the data indicate that community-based depression screening programs could show some efficacy in the reduction of completed suicides among older adults (Oyama et al., 2008). This approach is in line with the data indicating that elderly suicides have often visited their family physicians in the 6 months before their suicide (Pompili et al., 2008; Salib, Rahim, El-Nimr, & Habeeb, 2005; Tadros & Salib, 2007). However, mood disorders are often underdiagnosed in older adults. Suominen, Isometsa, and Lonnqvist (2004) identified all the consecutive suicide attempters who were treated in the hospital emergency rooms in Helsinki during the period from January 1997 to January 1998. They also found that, during the last 12 months before the attempt, most of the elderly suicide attempters had contact with primary health care, but only 4% had been diagnosed with a mood disorder, although the rate of diagnoses rose to 57% after the attempt. Consistent with the study by Suominen and colleagues, Salib and Green (2003) found that a high proportion of suicides (38% and 16%, respectively, for men and women) had psychiatric morbidity, but were not known to clinical services.

We may question whether general practitioners could be involved in the screening for suicides in the elderly. For example, Pfaff and Almeida (2005) pointed out that there was nothing specific in the presentations of older people to alert the general practitioners as to the presence of suicidal ideas. Stoppe et al. (1999) indicated that almost 20% of the physicians interviewed said they would not talk about suicide to depressed individuals because either the patients would communicate the suicidal intent themselves or because they feared provoking suicide by asking the patients directly. Uncapher and Arean (2000) conducted a between-subjects experimental study that was designed to determine the influence of patient age on primary care physicians' recognition of suicidal symptoms and willingness to treat the suicidal patient. Primary care providers were mailed one of the two case vignettes of a suicidal, depressed patient. The only difference between the two vignettes was the age of the patient (38 or 78 years) and the employment status (employed versus retired). A questionnaire was included to determine provider recognition of suicidal ideation, and a scale was designed to detect the willingness to treat the patient. A total of 595 general practitioners were randomly selected from the 1996 University of California, San Francisco physician roster. Three hundred forty-two physicians (a 63% response rate) responded to the mailings. The analyses were based on the responses of 215 primary care physicians. The randomly assigned experimental group received a vignette of a geriatric, retired patient who was depressed and suicidal (n = 100 participants). The control group received an identical but younger, employed patient (n = 115 participants). The vignette described a suicidal patient with medical problems and many depressive symptoms. The physicians were not told that this was a study about mental health, illness, or aging, and the instructions on the survey did not indicate that this was a depressed or suicidal patient.

The physicians in this study recognized depression and suicidal risk in both the adult and the geriatric vignettes, but they reported less willingness to treat the older suicidal patient compared with the younger suicidal patient ($p < .05$). In addition, physicians reported that a suicidal statement made by older patients was more normal, rational, and acceptable than the identical suicidal statement made by younger patients ($F = 31.21, p < .001$). They were statistically equal in their ambivalence about the effectiveness of the ability of mental health providers to treat depressed and suicidal patients of any age ($F = 2.98$, $p = .09$), although there was a trend toward believing that treatment would be more useful for younger patients than for older patients. Physicians' overall faith in treatment for any suicidal patient was lower than expected. For instance, on Items 3–8, "I think psychiatrists or psychologists can help patients like Sam," the average rating of disagreement with this statement was only 6.5 on a 1–10 scale.

Finally, the meta-analysis of Oyama indicated clear differences in the results when either psychiatrists or general practitioners conducted the main follow-up activity for participants at risk. In fact, the community-based depression screening with the follow-up conducted by general practitioners is associated with less reduced or unchanged risk for older men than when the follow-up is conducted by a psychiatrist. Iliffe and Manthorpe (2005) asked in an editorial if the prevention of suicide in later life was a task for general practitioners and concluded that "vigorous screening of older people" is not an "acceptable or realistic task" for the general practitioners.

A preventive strategy supported by some evidence is the treatment of depressive symptoms by a standardized algorithm-driven care that may include antidepressants and psychotherapy. This approach is in line with the results of the studies by Kalmar et al. (2008) and by Barak, Olmer, and a Aizenberg (2006) who reported an association between antidepressant prescriptions and a reduction in suicide rates in the elderly. For example, Kalmar et al. (2008) investigated whether the effect of antidepressant exposure on suicide rate was modified by age and gender in Hungary, between 1999 and 2005. The study indicated that the suicide rate was inversely related to the increased use of antidepressants in both genders and age bands in the elderly, with a strong effect especially for the oldest elderly (70–79 age band: −0.86 and −0.75, respectively, for men and women; 80+ age band: −0.75 and −0.96, respectively, for men and women).

Studies supporting the use of antidepressants to reduce suicidal ideation in the elderly include some research using randomized controlled design (Eli Lilly and Company, 2005; Nelson et al., 2007). However, the results of these studies are limited by the exclusion of the more seriously suicidal subjects from the samples and the use of single-item measures. (Most of the studies reviewed used Item 3 of the HAM-D to assess suicidal ideation, a measure with limited reliability and validity.)

One of the most complex studies of the latter kind reviewed is the PROSPECT study that approached suicide risk reduction from a public health perspective by targeting factors that are strongly related to suicide risk, common in primary care and modifiable. The PROSPECT intervention focused on two major components of care. First was physician knowledge, addressed by a clinical algorithm for treating geriatric depression in a primary care setting (Mulsant et al., 2001). Second was treatment management, operationalized by DCMs. The algorithm recommended the use of selective serotonin reuptake inhibitors in all patients who had not received any antidepressant or who have been inadequately treated. The protocol specified citalopram because it is equally efficacious as other antidepressants and has limited drug interactions, a low potential for central nervous system activation, and an insignificant withdrawal syndrome.

PROSPECT recommended dosages (or blood concentrations for tricyclic antidepressants when they are used) based on published trials, recommendations from drug manufacturers, and clinical experience in older adults. The acute treatment phase has to last 12 weeks or more. After patients have been treated for 6 weeks, the target dosage is maintained if the patients have a reduction of 50% or higher on the HAM-D, whereas, in cases of partial response, the dosage is increased and, in cases of insignificant response, the treatment is discontinued. In patients who report severe side effects with citalopram, even at 10 mg dosage, the medication is switched first to bupropion SR and then to nefazodone. Alternatively, the choice is directed toward interpersonal psychotherapy. In patients who have no response to an antidepressant, PROSPECT recommends taking progressive steps: (1) optimize treatment with the current medication and (2) switch to another antidepressant (citalopram, bupropion SR, venlafaxine, nortriptyline, and mirtazapine).

Practice-based, depression-care managers collaborated with physicians by helping them recognize depression, offering guideline-based treatment recommendations, monitoring the clinical status, and providing an appropriate follow-up. The depression-care managers included trained social workers, nurses, and psychologists. They had psychiatric backup, weekly supervision by psychiatrist investigators, and monthly interpersonal therapy cross-site supervision. Research associates introduced the depression-care manager to patients directly following the baseline interview. The depression-care manager interacted with patients in person or by telephone at scheduled intervals and, when clinically necessary, monitoring depressive symptoms, medication adverse effects, and treatment adherence.

The study of Szanto et al. (2003) indicated that patients who report suicidal ideation or thoughts of death are significantly less likely to be full responders to antidepressant acute treatments than patients without suicidal ideation, and those who respond require a longer time to do so. Thus, suicidal elderly require increased and longer therapy than their nonsuicidal peers. Furthermore, residual symptoms such as death thoughts should be evaluated even at follow-up because they may be a risk factor for suicide (Waern, Beskow, Runeson, & Skoog, 1999).

Conclusions

In recent decades, research has failed to focus on suicide prevention in the late life. Few studies have investigated the topic, and even fewer have used methodologically sound research designs (e.g., randomized controlled trials). Therefore, clinicians have to base their practice on very little sound evidence. Most of the recommendations are based solely on evidence from expert committee reports, opinions, and the clinical experience of respected authorities, or extrapolated from studies investigating suicide treatments in the younger age bands, which means weaker evidence for evidence-based practice. In conclusion, in the next few years, geriatric psychiatry research needs make a "great leap forward" in the investigation of suicide prevention programs in the elderly.

References

Barak, Y., Olmer, A., & Aizenberg, D. (2006). Antidepressants reduce the risk of suicide among elderly depressed patients. *Neuropsychopharmacology, 31*, 178–181.

Beautrais, A. L. (2002). A case control study of suicide and attempted suicide in older adults. *Suicide & Life-Threatening Behavior, 32*(1), 1–9.

Blow, F. C., Bartels, S. J., Brockmann, L. M., & Van Citters, A. D. (2006). *Evidence-based practices for preventing substance abuse and mental health problems in older adults.* Retrieved May, 24 2009, from http://www.samhsa.gov/OlderAdultsTAC/EBPLiteratureReviewFINAL.pdf.

Bruce, M. L., Ten Have, T. R., Reynolds, C. F. 3rd, Katz, I. I., Schulberg, H. C., Mulsant, B. H., et al. (2004). Reducing suicidal ideation and depressive symptoms in depressed older primary care patients: A randomized controlled trial. *Journal of the American Medical Association, 291*, 1081–1091.

Canadian Coalition for Seniors' Mental Health. (2006). *National guidelines for seniors' mental health. The assessment of suicide risk and prevention of suicide.* Toronto: Canadian Coalition for Seniors' Mental Health.

Chiu, H. F., Yip, P. S., Chi, I., Chan, S., Tsoh, J., Kwan, C. W., et al. (2004). Elderly suicide in Hong Kong – A case-controlled psychological autopsy study. *Acta Psychiatrica Scandinavica, 109*, 299–305.

Conwell, Y., & Duberstein, P. R. (1995). Prevention of late life suicide: When, where, why and how. *Psychiatry and Clinical Neurosciences, 49*(Suppl. 1), S79–S83.

Conwell, Y., Lyness, J. M., Duberstein, P., Cox, C., Seidlitz, L., DiGiorgio, A., et al. (2000). Completed suicide among older patients in primary care practices: A controlled study. *Journal of the American Geriatrics Society, 48*, 23–29.

De Leo, D., Carollo, G., & Dello Buono, M. (1995). Lower suicide rates associated with a Tele-Help/Tele-Check service for the elderly at home. *American Journal of Psychiatry, 152*, 632–634.

De Leo, D., Dello Buono, M., & Dwyer, J. (2002). Suicide among the elderly: The long-term impact of a telephone support and assessment intervention in northern Italy. *British Journal of Psychiatry, 181*, 226–229.

Duberstein, P. R., Conwell, Y., Conner, K. R., Eberly, S., & Caine, E. D. (2004). Suicide at 50 years of age and older: Perceived physical illness, family discord and financial strain. *Psychological Medicine, 34*(1), 137–146.

Duberstein, P. R., Conwell, Y., Conner, K. R., Eberly, S., Evinger, J. S., & Caine, E. D. (2004). Poor social integration and suicide: Fact or artifact? A case-control study. *Psychological Medicine, 34*(7), 1331–1337.

Eli Lilly and Company. (2005). Duloxetine versus placebo in the treatment of elderly patients with major depressive disorder. Clinical study summary: Study F1J-MC-HMBV. Retrieved May 21, 2008, from http://www.clinicalstudyresults.org/documents/company-study_2651_0.pdf.

Erlangsen, A., Zarit, S. H., Tu, X., & Conwell, Y. (2006). Suicide among older psychiatric inpatients: An evidence-based study of a high-risk group. *American Journal of Geriatric Psychiatry, 14*(9), 734–741.

Fried, L. P. (1990). Health promotion and disease prevention. In W. R. Hazzard, R. Andres, E. L. Bierman, & J. P. Blass (Eds.), Principles of geriatric medicine and gerontology (2nd ed., pp. 192–200). New York: McGraw Hill.

Grek, A. (2007). Clinical management of suicidality in the elderly: An opportunity for involvement in the lives of older patients. *Canadian Journal of Psychiatry, 52*(6 Suppl. 1), 47S–57S.

Harwood, D., Hawton, K., Hope, T., & Jacoby, R. (2001). Psychiatric disorder and personality factors associated with suicide in older people: A descriptive and case-control study. *International Journal of Geriatric Psychiatry, 16*(2), 155–165.

Harwood, D. M., Hawton, K., Hope, T., Harriss, L., & Jacoby, R. (2006). Life problems and physical illness as risk factors for suicide in older people: A descriptive and case-control study. *Psychological Medicine, 36*(9), 1265–1274.

Iliffe, S., & Manthorpe, J. (2005). The prevention of suicide in later life: A task for GPs? *British Journal of General Practice, 55*(513), 261–262.

Juurlink, D. N., Herrmann, N., Szalai, J. P., Kopp, A., & Redelmeier, D. A. (2004). Medical illness and the risk of suicide in the elderly. *Archives of Internal Medicine, 164*(11), 1179–1184.

Juurlink, D. N., Mamdani, M. M., Kopp, A., & Redelmeier, D. A. (2006). The risk of suicide with selective serotonin reuptake inhibitors in the elderly. *American Journal of Psychiatry, 163*(5), 813–821.

Kalmar, S., Szanto, K., Rihmer, Z., Mazumdar, S., Harrison, K., & Mann, J. J. (2008). Antidepressant prescription and suicide rates: Effect of age and gender. *Suicide & Life-Threatening Behavior, 38*(4), 363–374.

Kolves, K., Varnik, A., Tooding, L. M., & Wasserman, D. (2006). The role of alcohol in suicide: A case-control psychological autopsy study. *Psychological Medicine, 36*(7), 923–930.

Lapierre, S., Dube, M., Bouffard, L., & Alain, M. (2007). Addressing suicidal ideations through the realization of meaningful personal goals. *Crisis, 28*(1), 16–25.

Mulsant, B. H., Alexopoulos, G. S., Reynolds, C. F. 3rd, Katz, I. R., Abrams, R., Oslin, D., et al. (2001). Pharmacological treatment of depression in older primary care patients: The PROSPECT algorithm. *International Journal of Geriatric Psychiatry, 16*(6), 585–592.

Nelson, J. C., Delucchi, K., & Schneider, L. (2007). Suicidal thinking and behavior during treatment with sertraline in late-life depression. *American Journal of Geriatric Psychiatry, 15*(7), 573–580.

Oyama, H., Fujita, M., Goto, M., Shibuya, H., & Sakashita, T. (2006). Outcomes of community-based screening for depression and suicide prevention among Japanese elders. *The Gerontologist, 46*(6), 821–826.

Oyama, H., Goto, M., Fujita, M., Shibuya, H., & Sakashita, T. (2006). Preventing elderly suicide through primary care by community-based screening for depression in rural Japan. *Crisis, 27*(2), 58–65.

Oyama, H., Koida, J., Sakashita, T., & Kudo, K. (2004). Community-based prevention for suicide in elderly by depression screening and follow-up. *Community Mental Health Journal, 40*(3), 249–263.

Oyama, H., Ono, Y., Watanabe, N., Tanaka, E., Kudoh, S., Sakashita, T., et al. (2006). Local community intervention through depression screening and group activity for elderly suicide prevention. *Psychiatry and Clinical Neurosciences, 60*(1), 110–114.

Oyama, H., Sakashita, T., Ono, Y., Goto, M., Fujita, M., & Koida, J. (2008). Effect of community-based intervention using depression screening on elderly suicide risk: A meta-analysis of the evidence from Japan. *Community Mental Health Journal, 44*(5), 311–320.

Pfaff, J. J., & Almeida, O. P. (2005). Detecting suicidal ideation in older patients: Identifying risk factors within the general practice setting. *British Journal of General Practice, 55*(513), 269–273.

Pompili, M., Innamorati, M., Masotti, V., Personne, F., Lester, D., Di Vittorio, C., et al. (2008). Suicide in the elderly: A psychological autopsy study in a north Italy area (1994–2004). *American Journal of Geriatric Psychiatry, 16*, 727–735.

Preville, M., Hebert, R., Boyer, R., Bravo, G., & Seguin, M. (2005). Physical health and mental disorder in elderly suicide: A case-control study. *Aging & Mental Health, 9*(6), 576–584.

Quan, H., Arboleda-Florez, J., Fick, G. H., Stuart, H. L., & Love, E. J. (2002). Association between physical illness and suicide among the elderly. *Social Psychiatry and Psychiatric Epidemiology, 37*(4), 190–197.

Raskin, J., Wiltse, C. G., Dinkel, J. J., Walker, D. J., Desaiah, D., & Katona, C. (2008). Safety and tolerability of duloxetine at 60 mg once daily in elderly patients with major depressive disorder. *Journal of Clinical Psychopharmacology, 28*(1), 32–38.

Raskin, J., Wiltse, C. G., Siegal, A., Sheikh, J., Xu, J., Dinkel, J. J., et al. (2007). Efficacy of duloxetine on cognition, depression, and pain in elderly patients with major depressive disorder: An 8-week, double-blind, placebo-controlled trial. *American Journal of Psychiatry, 164*(6), 900–909.

Raskin, J., Xu, J. Y., & Kajdasz, D. K. (2008). Time to response for duloxetine 60 mg once daily versus placebo in elderly patients with major depressive disorder. *International Psychogeriatrics/IPA, 20*(2), 309–327.

Ross, R. K., Bernstein, L., Trent, L., Henderson, B. E., & Paganini-Hill, A. (1990). A prospective study of risk factors for traumatic deaths in a retirement community. *Preventive Medicine, 19*(3), 323–334.

Rubenowitz, E., Waern, M., Wilhelmson, K., & Allebeck, P. (2001). Life events and psychosocial factors in elderly suicides – A case-control study. *Psychological Medicine, 31*(7), 1193–1202.

Salib, E., & Green, L. (2003). Gender in elderly suicide: Analysis of coroners inquests of 200 cases of elderly suicide in Cheshire 1989–2001. *International Journal of Geriatric Psychiatry, 18*(12), 1082–1087.

Salib, E., Rahim, S., El-Nimr, G., & Habeeb, B. (2005). Elderly suicide: An analysis of coroner's inquests into two hundred cases in Cheshire 1989–2001. *Medicine, Science, and the Law, 45*(1), 71–80.

SAMHSA. (2007). PROSPECT (Prevention of suicide in primary care elderly: Collaborative trial). Retrieved May 24, 2009, from http://www.nrepp.samhsa.gov/programfulldetails.asp?PROGRAM_ID=113.

Shah, A. (2007). The relationship between suicide rates and age: An analysis of multinational data from the World Health Organization. *International Psychogeriatrics/IPA, 19*(6), 1141–1152.

Shekelle, P. G., Woolf, S. H., Eccles, M., & Grimshaw, J. (1999). Clinical guidelines: Developing guidelines. *British Medical Journal, 318*(7183), 593–596.

Stoppe, G., Sandholzer, H., Huppertz, C., Duwe, H., & Staedt, J. (1999). Family physicians and the risk of suicide in the depressed elderly. *Journal of Affective Disorders, 54*(1–2), 193–198.

Suominen, K., Isometsa, E., & Lonnqvist, J. (2004). Elderly suicide attempters with depression are often diagnosed only after the attempt. *International Journal of Geriatric Psychiatry, 19*(1), 35–40.

Szanto, K., Mulsant, B. H., Houck, P., Dew, M. A., & Reynolds, C. F. 3rd. (2003). Occurrence and course of suicidality during short-term treatment of late-life depression. *Archives of General Psychiatry, 60*(6), 610–617.

Tadros, G., & Salib, E. (2007). Elderly suicide in primary care. *International Journal of Geriatric Psychiatry, 22*(8), 750–756.

Takahashi, K., Naito, H., Morita, M., Suga, R., Oguma, T., & Koizumi, T. (1998). Suicide prevention for the elderly in Matsunoyama Town, Higashikubiki County, Niigata Prefecture: Psychiatric care for elderly depression in the community. *Seishin Shinkeigaku Zasshi, 100*(7), 469–485.

Turvey, C. L., Conwell, Y., Jones, M. P., Phillips, C., Simonsick, E., Pearson, J. L., et al. (2002). Risk factors for late-life suicide: A prospective, community-based study. *American Journal of Geriatric Psychiatry, 10*(4), 398–406.

Uncapher, H., & Arean, P. A. (2000). Physicians are less willing to treat suicidal ideation in older patients. *Journal of the American Geriatrics Society, 48*(2), 188–192.

Unutzer, J., Katon, W., Callahan, C. M., Williams, J. W. Jr., Hunkeler, E., Harpole, L., et al. (2002). Collaborative care management of late-life depression in the primary care setting: A randomized controlled trial. *Journal of the American Medical Association, 288*(22), 2836–2845.

Unutzer, J., Katon, W., Williams, J. W. Jr., Callahan, C. M., Harpole, L., Hunkeler, E. M., et al. (2001). Improving primary care for depression in late life: The design of a multicenter randomized trial. *Medical Care, 39*(8), 785–799.

Unutzer, J., Tang, L., Oishi, S., Katon, W., Williams, J. W. Jr., Hunkeler, E., et al. (2006). Reducing suicidal ideation in depressed older primary care patients. *Journal of the American Geriatrics Society, 54*(10), 1550–1556.

Waern, M. (2003). Alcohol dependence and misuse in elderly suicides. *Alcohol and alcoholism (Oxford, Oxfordshire), 38*(3), 249–254.

Waern, M., Beskow, J., Runeson, B., & Skoog, I. (1999). Suicidal feelings in the last year of life in elderly people who commit suicide. *Lancet, 354*(9182), 917–918.

Waern, M., Rubenowitz, E., Runeson, B., Skoog, I., Wilhelmson, K., & Allebeck, P. (2002). Burden of illness and suicide in elderly people: Case-control study. *British Medical Journal (Clinical Research ed.), 324*(7350), 1355.

Waern, M., Runeson, B. S., Allebeck, P., Beskow, J., Rubenowitz, E., Skoog, I., et al. (2002). Mental disorder in elderly suicides: A case-control study. *American Journal of Psychiatry, 159*(3), 450–455.

World Health Organization. (1999). *Figures and facts about suicide* (No. WHO/MNH/MBD/99.1). Geneve: WHO.

World Health Organization. (2002). Distribution of suicides rates (per 100,000) by gender and age, 2000. Retrieved March 20, 2008, from http://www.who.int/mental_health/prevention/ suicide/suicide_rates_chart/en/index.html.

About the Authors

Marco Innamorati, PhD, is a psychologist and psychotherapist. He is a member of the International Association for Suicide Prevention.

Maurizio Pompili, MD, PhD, is Professor of both Suicidology and Epidemiological Psychiatry at Sapienza University of Rome where he received his MD degree, training in psychiatry (both summa cum laude), and doctoral degree in neurosciences. He is also part of the Community at McLean Hospital – Harvard Medical School, USA. He is the recipient of the American Association of Suicidology's 2008 Shneidman Award for "Outstanding early career contribution to suicidology." He has published more than 200 papers on suicide including original research articles, book chapters, and editorials. He edited and co-edited several national and international books including the latest *Suicide in the Words of Suicidologists* and *Suicide: A Global Perspective.* He provided validation studies for psychometric instruments to assess suicide risk and he is the Italian National Representative to the International Association for Suicide Prevention (IASP).

Professor Mario Amore, MD, received his master's degree in medicine and his post-graduate degree in neurology and psychiatry at the University of Bologna. In 1989 he became assistant professor of psychiatry at the Institute of Psychiatry, University of Bologna, and in 1999 associate professor of psychiatry at the Institute of Psychiatry, University of Parma. He is Head of the Division of Psychiatry of the University of Parma. He is author or co-author of 210 articles published in Italian and international scientific journals. The research field of Professor Amore is focused on several psychiatric topics: psychopathology of catatonia, somatopsychosis, psychopathology of schizoid states, mood disorders, anxiety disorders, psychopharmacology (psychopharmacological treatment of depression and panic disorder, studies regarding the neuroleptic malignant syndrome), acute confusional conditions in psychiatry, psychiatric disorders of the pregnancy and post-partum period, depression and anxiety disorders of the elderly, sleep disorders in psychiatry, psycopathology of aggressive behavior, the perinatal risk factor of schizophrenia's etiology, mood disorders of the elderly, and suicidal behavior, particularly in old age.

Cristina Di Vittorio, MD, received her degree in medicine at the University of Parma in October 2007. She currently attends graduate school in psychiatry at the Division of Psychiatry of the Department of Neuroscience at Parma University, where she carries out both inpatient and outpatient psychiatric activity with particular interest in psychotic disorders in young adult population. Her scientific activity comprises several psychiatric topics: mood and anxiety disorders of the elderly, psychopathology and treatment of aggressive behavior, sleep disorders, pathogenesis of schizophrenia and its treatment, with particular regard to the spectrum of suicidal behavior in general, and particularly in the elderly population.

Gianluca Serafini, PhD, received his PhD degree in medicine from Sapienza University of Rome in 2003. He worked as psychiatrist from 2007 and started his PhD studies in November 2008 on "Early Interventions in Psychosis." He was a Professor of Psychiatry at Sapienza University of Rome. Between 2005 and 2010 he has published over 30 papers in refereed national and international journals and around 20 in conference proceedings and books. He is a reviewer of papers for around 5 international journals. He was an active member of the center for suicide prevention at Sant'Andrea Hospital in Rome. His academic research interests are particularly focused in the area of suicide, mood disorders, and neuroimaging techniques. Currently, he is engaged in research on various aspects of neuroscience, particularly in biological abnormalities underlying suicide and mood disorders.

Roberto Tatarelli, MD, is Full Professor of Psychiatry, Chairman of the Department of Neurosciences, Mental Health, and Sensory Functions at Sant'Andrea Hospital, Sapienza University of Rome, Italy, and Director of the residency training in psychiatry at the II Medical School of Sapienza. During his long-lasting career he has carried out numerous research projects in the field of psychopathology, psychotic disorders, mood disorders, and suicide. He is full member of the International Academy for Suicide Research. He contributed to the Italian validation of the Beck Hopelessness Scale and has published more than 400 scientific publications and several books.

David Lester has doctoral degrees from Cambridge University (UK) in social and political science and Brandeis University (USA) in psychology. He is Distinguished Professor of Psychology at the Richard Stockton College of New Jersey. He has been President of the International Association for Suicide Prevention, and he has published extensively on suicide, murder, and other issues in thanatology. His recent books include *Katie's Diary: Unlocking the Mystery of a Suicide* (2004), *Suicide and the Holocaust* (2005), *Is there Life after Death?* (2005), *Preventing Suicide: Closing the Exits Revisited* (2009), and *Understanding Suicide: Why We Don't and How We Might* (2010).

Marco Innamorati
Piazza filattiera 12
00139 Roma
Italy
Tel.: +39068105981
E-mail: innamorati.marco@libero.it; marco.innamorati@tin.it

Evidence-Based Suicide Prevention by Lethal Methods Restriction

David Lester

Department of Psychology, The Richard Stockton College of New Jersey, Pomona, NJ, USA

Preventing suicide by restricting access to lethal methods for committing suicide is one of the most well-researched strategies in suicide prevention. Despite this body of research, there are still some doubts as to whether this strategy is truly effective. This chapter briefly summarizes the research, highlights the issues, and draws some definitive conclusions. The present chapter is based on a thorough, updated review of the literature on this topic by Lester (2009). Lester did not conduct a meta-analysis of the studies, but he did endeavor to locate every relevant article based on literature searches, perusal of the suicide-focused journals, and checking the references of relevant articles located.

The issues surrounding this strategy involve the following:

1. Can the method for committing suicide be totally eliminated or merely restricted. There is a great deal of research on whether restricting access to guns has an impact on suicide rates using guns. The problem here is that guns are never eliminated from a society. The stricter gun control laws that are passed typically delay access to guns (for a week or so) and prohibit the sale of guns to felons and psychiatric patients.
2. Was the method a popular method for suicide? A small proportion of suicides jump from bridges to their death. Bridges can have fences installed to prevent jumpers, but such a measure, while useful, usually has no impact on the overall suicide rate in the region.
3. Was the method a lethal method? There have been many studies on the impact of restricting sales of paracetamol (acetominophen) in England, but the majority of those ingesting paracetamol survive the attempt, and so restricting access will have little impact on the completed suicide rate.
4. Will people simply switch to another method for suicide if access to their preferred method is restricted? This is an interesting question for which very little research has been conducted. Obviously, some suicidal individuals will switch methods while others will not, but the ways in which these two groups of individuals differ are far from clear.

Let us review the research on each of the methods of suicide for which means restriction may be effective.[1]

Domestic Gas

Domestic gas was, for many years, coal gas which has a high concentration of carbon monoxide, resulting in a reasonably certain and quick death. As reserves of natural gas were discovered, many nations switched to natural gas for domestic use. Natural gas is much less toxic, and the would-be suicide has to die from suffocation rather than carbon monoxide poisoning.

Stengel (1964) first noted the impact of the switch from coal gas to natural gas, and Kreitman (1976) first documented accurately the impact on suicide rates in England. Not only did the suicide rate using domestic gas drop almost to zero, but the overall English suicide rate was also cut by about one third. Clarke and Lester (1989) documented the impact of the switch in England, the Netherlands, and the United States.

Lester (1995) studied the question of whether the detoxification of domestic gas always led to a reduction in the overall suicide rate. Lester compared the changes in suicide rates by domestic gas, by all other methods, and overall in six nations: Japan, the Netherlands, Northern Ireland, Scotland, Switzerland, and the United States. In three nations (Northern Ireland, Scotland, and Switzerland), the suicide rate using domestic gas was high initially, and in all of them the overall suicide rate declined as domestic gas was detoxified. In three nations (Japan, the Netherlands, and the United States), the suicide rate using domestic gas was low initially, and in all of them the overall suicide rate increased as domestic gas was detoxified. Thus, the total suicide rate appears to have been reduced by making toxic domestic gas less available only in those nations where it was a common method for suicide.

A problem associated with the detoxification of domestic gas is that suicide using car exhaust is a similar method. Clarke and Lester (1989) showed that, during the period when domestic gas was detoxified in England and the suicide rate using domestic gas declined, the use of car exhaust for suicide rose. Apparently, rise in the use of car exhaust was not large enough to offset the decline in the use of domestic gas, but it does look as if switching methods (also known as substitution of methods) did occur to some extent.

Car Exhaust

The evidence for the impact of the introduction of emission controls for car exhaust (which reduce its toxicity by removing much of the carbon monoxide) is mixed. In the

[1] Some methods of suicide, of course, such as hanging and drowning, are not amenable to means restriction.

United States, the introduction of emission controls was accompanied by a reduction in the suicide rate using car exhaust (Clarke & Lester, 1989). However, no such effect was observed in Australia.

Routley and Ozanne-Smith (1998) suggested several reasons why car-exhaust suicides had not declined. (1) Carbon monoxide emissions while a car is idling had not been measured for the new cars and could be higher than the levels measured when driving. (2) Carbon monoxide emissions have not been measured inside the cars, whose cabins vary in volume, when the car exhaust enters through a hose connected to the exhaust pipe. (3) Carbon monoxide content may be higher before the engine warms up. (4) Catalytic converters deteriorate over time.

Despite this disparity in the results of research, simple inexpensive changes in car design could reduce the attractiveness of this method for committing suicide, such as changing the shape of the exhaust pipe from a circle to a flattened slit, so that a tube would no longer fit easily over the pipe, or installing automatic turn-off systems if the car engine idles for more than 1 minute. However, car exhaust is not a very common method for suicide in most countries, and so reducing the use of car exhaust for suicide might not have a significant impact on the overall suicide rate.

Fencing in Bridges

Fencing in bridges has been shown to prevent suicides from those bridges. However, it has been noted that, in some situations, people switch to other bridges in the city from which to jump. On the other hand, some bridges have a special attractiveness for suicides. For example, Seiden and Spence (1982, 1983–1984) showed that people drove over the Bay Bridge between Oakland and San Francisco in California to jump off the Golden Gate Bridge, but rarely, if ever, do people drive over the Golden Gate Bridge to jump off the Bay Bridge. No out-of-state suicides jumped from the Bay Bridge. Thus, fencing in popular suicide venues might prevent suicides by those who end their lives by jumping.

Suicide by jumping is not a common method except in nations that are heavily urbanized and dotted with many tall buildings such as Hong Kong and Singapore, where suicide by jumping from high buildings is common. Fencing in bridges, therefore, does not typically have a major impact on the overall suicide rate.

Medications

Many medications, including some of those used for treating the psychiatrically disturbed individuals who may be suicidal, could be used to commit suicide. Restricting access to a particular medication, such as barbiturates, typically results in a reduction in the use of that medication for suicide, but switching to alternative medications is easily accomplished by would-be suicides. However, simple practices, such as reducing the size in the number of prescribed pills or placing each pill in a plastic blister, do appear to have an impact on the use of that medication for suicide (Lester, 2009).

Barraclough, Nelson, Bunch, and Sainsbury (1971) suggested

1. reducing the number of prescriptions for such medications,
2. reducing the size of prescriptions,
3. wrapping tablets individually in tin foil or in plastic blisters,
4. using nonbarbiturates (and other lethal medications) when less lethal medications exist for the same problems,
5. having family physicians recall unused tablets when the treatment is changed or stopped,
6. writing prescriptions in a way that would prevent forgery,
7. having pharmacists monitor large and excessive prescriptions,
8. not prescribing medications or refilling prescriptions without seeing the patient.

Paracetamol[2]

In Europe, the use of paracetamol (acetominophen) for suicide results in a fair number of deaths and many attempted suicides who often suffer from kidney damage. A great deal of research has been conducted on restricting access to paracetamol, the results of which are not altogether consistent.

Bateman et al. (2006) examined the impact on deaths consequent upon restricting sales of paracetamol in Scotland in 1998 and found that the legislation did *not* have a preventive impact on deaths. In fact, the number of deaths each quarter from paracetamol products increased for both men and women. The number of discharges from hospitals due to paracetamol poisoning dropped. However, most of the deaths occurred due to ingestion of co-proxamol (a combination of paracetamol and dextropropoxyphene, an opioid), for which the prescription rate declined only from 1.42 million in 1995 to 1.26 million in 2003. The restrictions affected only over-the-counter sales, not the prescribed paracetamol products.

Sandilands and Bateman (2008) noted that, after co-proxamol was withdrawn from the market, beginning in 2005, the number of deaths in Scotland from the ingestion of co-proxamol dropped (from 41 in 2004 to only 10 in 2006). Interestingly, deaths from all poisons also declined (from 173 in 2004 to 128 in 2006). After the withdrawal of co-proxamol, prescriptions for other analgesics (such as co-codamol and paracetamol) increased, but this was not accompanied by an increase in deaths from these medications, which remained roughly the same as before. Thus, switching of medications for suicide does not appear to have occurred, but Sandilands and Bateman did not examine changes in other methods for suicide or the overall suicide rate.

Gunnell, Murray, and Hawton (2000) reviewed many suggestions for reducing the role of paracetamol in overdoses, with their advantages and disadvantages, including

[2] The common brand name in the United States is Tylenol.

1. adding methionine to the tablets to reduce the toxic effects (but which may lead to side effects for some people),
2. public education about its dangers (which may instead highlight its possibilities for suicide),
3. warning notices on packets (which may also highlight its possibilities for suicide),
4. using blister packs,
5. restricting sale to pharmacies,
6. making paracetamol available only by prescription,
7. restricting the quantity which may be purchased at one time.

Suggestions (4) to (7) all lead to inconvenience to those who wish to use paracetamol legitimately. If the frequency of attempted suicides with paracetamol could be reduced, and if the severity of the medical consequences of the suicide attempts with paracetamol could be reduced, then at least the harm to those individuals could be lessened.

Pesticides

The problem of pesticides as a method for suicide is of current concern since the method is very common in developing nations. Efforts are being made to encourage farmers to store their pesticides safely, but many fail to follow the guidelines for this and, furthermore, the farmers and their families know where they are stored and usually have access to them. Other solutions have focused on making pesticides less toxic.

Gunnell and Eddleston (2003) suggested several tactics for reducing the use of pesticides for suicide:

1. Restricting their availability, directly by restricting their import or use, or indirectly by storing them in secure facilities in communities:
   - (i) introducing a "minimum" pesticide list and restricting use to a few, less toxic pesticides,
   - (ii) prohibiting sales of the most toxic pesticides,
   - (iii) subsidizing the cost of less toxic pesticides,
   - (iv) keeping all pesticides locked up with the keys held by licensed users,
   - (v) reducing their use in farming by implementing other methods of pest control,
   - (vi) returning unused pesticides to the vendor.
2. Improving public education about the dangers of pesticide ingestion and better labeling of pesticides.
3. Reducing the toxicity of pesticides:
   - (i) adding emetics or antidotes to pesticides,
   - (ii) making pesticides unpleasant to smell and taste,
   - (iii) producing less toxic pesticides.
4. Improving the medical management of pesticide poisoning.

So far, only the impact of restrictions on the sale of one or more pesticides has been studied, and this seems to result in would-be suicides switching to alternative pesticides for their demise.

Trains

There is good evidence that simple safety procedures, especially in subway systems, can reduce the risk of death by jumping in front of trains. For example, the provision of a pit in the floor beneath the tracks results in some jumpers falling into the pit, thereby not being hit and killed by the train. Barriers on the platform and surveillance have also been shown to prevent a few suicides. However, the safest way to prevent suicide is to wall in the platforms completely.

Law et al. (2009) used a natural quasi-experiment in the subways in Hong Kong where one system (Mass Transit Railway, MTR) installed platform screen doors (to reduce air-conditioning costs, as in Singapore), while the other system (Kowloon-Canton Railway, KCR) did not. The doors were installed during the period 2002–2005. On the MTR system, there were 38 suicides in the 5-year period 1997–2001 but only 7 in the 5-year period 2003–2007. In contrast, the corresponding numbers for the KCR system were 13 and 15, respectively. The reduction in suicides on the MTR system seemed to be present both for those with a psychiatric history and those without such a history. Suicide on the railway did not constitute a large proportion of the suicides in Hong Kong, and so the installation of platform doors did not impact the total Hong Kong suicide rate. Preventing suicide on open railway tracks is much more difficult since it is not feasible to fence in thousands of miles of open track.

Gun Control

The major area of debate in the research on the effectiveness of restricting access to lethal methods for suicide concerns the impact of gun control. Gun owners have powerful lobbies that argue against the imposition of any restrictions on gun ownership. Researchers too differ on whether they support stricter or looser gun control laws, and their personal beliefs undoubtedly affect the way in which they conduct their research and how they report and interpret their results. The situation is compounded by the fact that stricter gun control laws typically do not reduce the number of guns in a region. Rather they simply make it a little more difficult to obtain a gun.[3] Most of the research has been conducted in the United States and in Canada where the available data are limited.

3 Some gun control laws restrict the type of weapons that can be sold, but this is more relevant to mass murderers than to suicides.

For example, Canada has passed four gun control laws in the past 40 years (in 1968, 1977, 1991, and 1995), and there is only one set of time-series data available for examination. Lester (2009) recently reviewed all of the studies on the Canadian data and drew the following conclusions.

All of the studies were, by necessity, correlational, and so cause-and-effect conclusions cannot be drawn. However, nations rarely, if ever, introduce changes in public policy in a way that permits an experimental design. This could be done, for example, by introducing a change in public policy in some regions but not in others. (Ideally, the two sets of regions should be chosen randomly.) Political reality prevents such experiments.

The Canadian situation is complicated by the passage of several gun control bills. During this time period, many social and economic changes also occurred, thereby complicating and possibly confounding the impact of any one variable. The results are also complicated by the technique of analysis used. In a meta-analysis of studies on the impact of executions on the homicide rate, Yang and Lester (2008) found that the conclusions were different for time-series, ecological, and panel data sets. The studies reviewed by Lester (2009) on gun control in Canada employed all three methodologies and, therefore, it would not be surprising if the results depended on the methodology used.

For studies of gun control, it is also important to explore the enforcement of the laws. In the study of the deterrent effect of the death penalty, in the 1970s, the focus switched from the study of the existence or passage of a death penalty law to the study of the impact of actual executions. Only one study was identified that explored whether Canadians obey the gun control laws, and no studies were identified on the enforcement of the gun control laws.

One conclusion from the research was that gun control appeared to reduce the use of firearms for suicide, although the impact differed for different subgroups of the population (men and women and those of different ages). The evidence as to whether individuals switch to other means for killing themselves or murdering others was contradictory. The conclusion depended on the time period studied, the methodology used, and the particular subgroup of the population that is the focus of the study. The different analyses were split almost 50:50 on whether switching to other methods for suicide occurred.

Public policy is rarely made on the basis of social science research. However, an examination of the situation in Canada suggests that both opponents and advocates of gun control could agree on provisions such as the safe storage of firearms and safety training for those who purchase and own guns. The provision of licenses for purchasing and registering a gun is more controversial, but the requirements that people obtain licenses to drive cars and that cars must be registered do not have any significant impact on people's ownership of cars. Objections to similar requirements for firearms seem to rest on fears of a "slippery slope," that is, that passing such requirements is just the first step to much more stringent requirements. Similarly, restrictions on the type of firearm permitted are reasonable. After all, it is unlikely that any government would permit citizens to own missile launchers and missiles. The difficulty is in negotiating what firearms are allowed and which are not and assuaging fears of a "slippery slope" in this area.

Conclusion

The research on the impact of restricting access to lethal methods for suicide is quite clear. When it is possible to remove access to a method for suicide, its use for suicide declines dramatically. This was true for fencing in subway platforms and detoxifying domestic gas. However, it is not always possible to totally remove access to a method for suicide. Medications are necessary for psychiatric and medical disorders, and medications are often toxic in high doses. Guns cannot be taken away from the population – we can only make it a little more difficult to buy guns in the future.

The critical question is whether would-be suicides switch to alternative methods for suicide if their preferred method is no longer available. The research evidence is mixed on this. If the method now no longer available was a popular method for suicide, then the overall suicide rate in the nation is reduced, at least for many years. Even if the population as a whole eventually turns to another method for suicide, many lives have been saved in the interim.

It is interesting to note that many of the changes in the environment which have had the effect of reducing the suicide rate using particular methods were not introduced to prevent suicide. Domestic gas switched to natural gas because of its price and availability. Car emissions were detoxified to reduce pollution. Subway stations were fenced in to reduce air-conditioning costs. Gun control is introduced primarily in an effort to reduce the rates of murder and armed robbery, not suicide. Only the fencing in of bridges and the restrictions on medications and pesticides were introduced to prevent suicide. The conclusion seems to be that, despite words from government officials to the contrary, preventing suicide is not a high priority.

References

Barraclough, B. M., Nelson, B., Bunch, J., & Sainsbury, P. (1971). Suicide and barbiturate prescribing. *Journal of the Royal College of General Practitioners, 21*, 645–653.

Bateman, D. N., Gorman, D. R., Bain, M., Inglis, J. H. C., House, F. R., & Murphy, D. (2006). Legislation restricting paracetamol sales and patterns of self-harm and death from paracetamol-containing preparations in Scotland. *British Journal of Clinical Pharmacology, 62*, 573–581.

Clarke, R. V., & Lester, D. (1989). *Suicide: Closing the exits*. New York: Springer-Verlag.

Gunnell, D., & Eddleston, M. (2003). Suicide by intentional ingestion of pesticides. *International Journal of Epidemiology, 32*, 902–909.

Gunnell, D., Murray, V., & Hawton, K. (2000). Use of paracetamol (acetaminophen) for suicide and nonfatal poisoning. *Suicide & Life-Threatening Behavior, 30*, 313–326.

Kreitman, N. (1976). The coal gas story. *British Journal of Preventive & Social Medicine, 30*, 86–93.

Law, C. K., Yip, P. S. F., Chan, W. S. C., Fu, K. W., Wong, P. W. C., & Law, Y. W. (2009). Evaluating the effectiveness of barrier installation for preventing railway suicides in Hong Kong. *Journal of Affective Disorders, 114*, 254–262.

Lester, D. (1995). Effects of the detoxification of domestic gas on suicide rates in six nations. *Psychological Reports, 77*, 294.

Lester, D. (2009). *Preventing suicide: Closing the exits revisited.* Hauppauge, NY: Nova Science.
Routley, V. H., & Ozanne-Smith, J. (1998). The impact of catalytic converters on motor vehicle exhaust gas suicides. *Medical Journal of Australia, 168*, 65–67.
Sandilands, E. A., & Bateman, D. N. (2008). Co-proxamol withdrawal has reduced suicide from drugs in Scotland. *British Journal of Clinical Pharmacology, 66*, 290–293.
Seiden, R. H., & Spence, M. (1982). A tale of two bridges. *Crisis, 3*(1), 32–40.
Seiden, R. H., & Spence, M. (1983–1984). A tale of two bridges. *Omega, 14*, 201–209.
Stengel, E. (1964). *Suicide and attempted suicide.* Baltimore: Penguin.
Yang, B., & Lester, D. (2008). The deterrent effect of executions. *Journal of Criminal Justice, 36*, 453–460.

About the Author

David Lester has doctoral degrees from Cambridge University (UK) in social and political science and Brandeis University (USA) in psychology. He is Distinguished Professor of Psychology at the Richard Stockton College of New Jersey. He has been President of the International Association for Suicide Prevention, and he has published extensively on suicide, murder, and other issues in thanatology. His recent books include *Katie's Diary: Unlocking the Mystery of a Suicide* (2004), *Suicide and the Holocaust* (2005), *Is there Life after Death?* (2005), *Preventing Suicide: Closing the Exits Revisited* (2009), and *Understanding Suicide: Why We Don't and How We Might* (2010).

David Lester
The Richard Stockton College of New Jersey
PO Box 195
Jimmie Leeds Road
Pomona, NJ 08240-0195
USA
Tel.: +1 609 652 4512
E-mail: lesterd@stockton.edu

Psychopharmacology for Suicide Prevention*

Ross J. Baldessarini[1] and Leonardo Tondo[2]

[1]Professor of Psychiatry and Neuroscience, Harvard Medical School; Director Psychopharmacology Program McLean Hospital; Founding Director, International Consortium for Bipolar Disorder Research, McLean Division of Massachusetts General Hospital, Belmont, MA, USA
[2]Founding Director, Lucio Bini Mood Disorder Research Center, Cagliari, Sardinia; Associate Professor of Clinical Psychology, University of Cagliari; Lecturer, Department of Psychiatry, Harvard Medical School, Boston, MA; Principal Collaborator, International Consortium for Bipolar Disorder Research, McLean Division of Massachusetts General Hospital, Belmont, MA, USA

> The medical treatment of the propensity to suicide, whether prophylactic or therapeutic, differs not from that which is applicable in cases of ordinary insanity.
>
> George M. Burrows, M.D. (1828)

The worldwide annual suicide rate currently averages approximately 13/100,000 (0.013%/year), with higher average rates for men than women in all but a few countries, very low rates in children, and relatively high rates in elderly men (APA, 2003; Goldsmith, Pellmar, Kleinman, & Bunney, 2002; Simon & Hales, 2006; WHO, 2007). Suicide rates vary markedly among world regions, countries, and locales, in part reflecting differences in case-identification and reporting procedures (APA, 2003; Diekstra, 1993). Notably, reported suicide rates are extraordinarily high in Eastern Europe and relatively low in Latin America and Southern Europe. In the US, annual suicide rates (per 100,000 population) are far higher in Alaska (24.6) as well as in New Mexico (20.2) and other areas in the Southwest and the Intermountain West than on the East or West Coasts, with the lowest rates reported in Massachusetts and New York (6.5), and in the District of Columbia (6.0; Tondo, Albert, & Baldessarini, 2006). Internationally, the overall average suicide rate has been rising gradually over the past half-century, with increases reported in about half of the reporting nations, mainly among men, but moderate decreases found in another half, including in Northern Europe and North America. These improvements may reflect improved diagnosis and treatment of mood disorders in the same era (Baldessarini, Tondo, et al., 2007; Gruncbaum, Ellis, Li, Oquendo, & Mann, 2004; Isacsson, 2000; Tondo et al.,

* Reprinted by permission from: Tatarelli R., Pompili M., & Girardi P., (Eds.). 2007. Suicide in psychiatric disorders (pp. 193–213). New York: Nova Science, with updating in 2009.

2006; WHO, 2007). Paradoxically, the observed increases may in part reflect improved case-finding and reporting associated with overall improvements in national healthcare systems.

Estimated rates of suicide *attempts* are much less reliable than for completed suicides. Attempts average 20–30-times higher than rates of completed suicide in the general population, but are probably under-reported, and range widely in seriousness of methods and intent (Kessler, Berglund, Borges, Nock, & Wang, 2005; Tondo, Isacsson, & Baldessarini, 2003). The ratio of attempts/suicides in clinical samples of mood-disorder patients is much lower, suggesting greater lethality of suicidal behaviors (Baldessarini, Tondo, et al., 2006). It is important to point out that most cases of suicide (81–95%) in the general population involve psychiatric illnesses, nearly half of which (48.5%) are mood disorders (Roy, 2000).

In a study of men and women who attempted suicide and were evaluated in a medical emergency service (suggesting relatively serious attempts), later risk of completed suicide within 5 years was twice-higher among men than women (8.3% versus 4.3%), as expected, and most likely to occur within a year of follow-up (Nordstrom, Samuelsson, & Åsberg, 1995). The ratio of attempts to later suicides (A/S) also was half as great in men as in women (12:1 versus 23:1), consistent with greater lethality of suicide attempts in men. The risk of later suicide was higher in men below versus above the median age of 35 years (9.7% versus 7.0%), but also in women older than this median (6.0% versus 2.5%); accordingly, the relative risk among younger men was four-times higher than in younger women (9.7%/2.5%), whereas risks in older men and women scarcely differed (7.0%/6.0%), indicating that the lethality of suicidal behavior in women over age 35 approaches that of men of similar age.

Over the past decade, unprecedented interest has emerged in considering the excess mortality associated with major mental illnesses as an important and plausible therapeutic target (Baldessarini & Jamison, 1999). Excessive mortality in mood, psychotic, and substance-use disorders includes risks (2–3-times above the general population) due to medical illnesses, particularly stress-sensitive disorders, sometimes worsened by the weight-gain and metabolic disorders associated with many modern psychotropic drug treatments, or with complications of comorbid substance-use disorders, or accidents (Ahrens et al., 1995; Black, Winokur, & Nasrallah, 1987; Dening, 2004; Evans et al., 2005; Goodwin & Jamison, 1990; Katon et al., 2005; Khalsa, Salvatore, Hennen, Tohen, & Baldessarini, 2007; Sharma & Markar, 1994; Tsuang & Woolson, 1977). Indeed, deaths associated with cardiovascular disorders probably account for the largest *number* of deaths among persons with mood disorders, as in the general population.

By far, however, the greatest source of a proportional excess of mortality is suicide, rates of which among patients with mood disorders can exceed those in the general population by 20-fold, particularly in bipolar disorders and in severe, recurrent major depression, with lesser rates in psychotic, anxiety, or primary substance-use disorders (Harris & Barraclough, 1998; Tondo et al., 2003). General risk factors for suicide include the presence of a major mood disorder with hopelessness, especially if complicated by comorbid abuse of alcohol or illicit drugs (APA, 2003; Roy, 2000; Tondo et al., 1999, 2003). Risk is especially high among young, impulsive-aggressive and older, unmarried men (APA, 2003; Simon & Hales, 2006). The risk of suicide in bipolar disorder patients continues to be high, despite the introduction of a growing number of treatments with putative mood-stabilizing effects, reflecting the great difficulty in treating bipolar depressive and mixed manic-depressive states effectively. Indeed, approximately three-quarters of the surprisingly high proportion of unresolved morbidity among bipolar disorder patients (40–50%) of weeks of long-term follow-up, even from illness onset are depressive (Baldessarini et al., in press; Joffe, MacQueen, Marriott, & Trevor Young, 2004; Judd et al., 2002; Post et al., 2003). This high level of residual depressive morbidity in treated bipolar disorder patients, no doubt, strongly encourages high rates of utilization of antidepressants in their treatment, even though such treatment is neither approved by regulatory bodies nor well supported by available clinical research as either effective or safe in bipolar disorder patients (Baldessarini, Leahy, et al., 2007; Baldessarini, Henk, Sklar, Chang, & Leahy, 2008; Ghaemi, Wingo, Filkowski, Goodwin, & Baldessarini, 2008; Ghaemi, Hsu, Soldani, & Goodwin, 2003). Moreover, antidepressant treatments are associated in some patients with dysphoric-mixed-agitated or psychotic states that can increase suicidal risk (Akiskal, Benazzi, Perugi, & Rihmer, 2005; Koukopoulos & Koukopoulos, 1999; Maj, Pirozzi, Magliano, Fiorillo, & Bartoli, 2006).

The unusually high risk of suicide among bipolar disorder patients was supported by our recent review of the medical records of nearly 3,000 outpatients with major mood disorders evaluated at the Lucio Bini Mood Disorders Research Center in Cagliari, Sardinia. We found substantially greater suicide risks among bipolar disorder patients than in those with recurrent major depression (Tondo, Lepri, & Baldessarini, 2007). The risk of *suicides* among 843 bipolar I and II disorder patients was 150/100,000/year, or more than 10-times higher than in the general population of Sardinia, and three-times greater than among 1,983 patients diagnosed with recurrent major depressive disorder. These rates suggest risk of dying by suicide among bipolar disorder patients of nearly 10%, considering potential risk exposures of 60 years or more. The rate of *suicide attempts* was 1.26%/year among bipolar disorder patients, and 25% of these acts were violent, versus 0.48%/year among the unipolar cases and a rate of violent acts of only 12.5%, compared to approximate general population rates of 0.2–0.3%/year (Kessler et al., 2005; Roy, 2000; Tondo et al., 2003). The ratio of attempts/suicides (A/S) as a proposed *index of lethality* of suicidal behavior (Baldessarini, Tondo, et al., 2006) was 8.6:1 in bipolar disorder patients, and similar, at 9.6:1, in unipolar, recurrent major depression patients, compared to an estimated value of about 25:1 in the general population, indicating higher lethality among mood-disorder patients. A particularly important observation was that more than one third of all suicidal acts occurred within the first year from illness onset, and more than half within the first 5 years of illness – indicating the need for early diagnosis and intervention in major mood disorders (Tondo et al., 2007).

Effects of treatments on suicidal risk have been a topic of growing research interest in recent years. Evidence that most modern psychiatric treatments reduce *long-term* suicide risks is very limited, including methods as diverse as psychotherapy, rapid hospitalization, and even electroconvulsive treatment, which can be lifesaving in acute emergencies (APA,

2003; Oquendo, Chaudhur, & Mann, 2005; Rose, Burt, & Clayton, 1985; Simon & Hales, 2006; Weinger, 2000). Suicide rates are surprisingly high among persons diagnosed with anxiety disorders (Harris & Barraclough, 1998; Khan, Leventhal, Khan, & Brown, 2002) and severe anxiety may accompany suicidal behavior (Fawcett, 2001), but evidence that antianxiety medications alter suicidal risk in anxiety disorder patients is very limited (Khan, Warner, & Brown, 2000). The following sections summarize recent findings pertaining to the effects of other psychotropic drug treatments on suicidal behavior and ideation, including antipsychotics, mood-stabilizers, and antidepressants, for which most evidence is available.

Antipsychotic Drugs

The first US FDA-approved treatment with an antisuicide indication was clozapine for schizophrenia patients. This regulatory approval in 2003 was based largely on a single, remarkable randomized trial (InterSePT) comparing clozapine with olanzapine among not necessarily treatment-resistant schizophrenia patients at high suicidal risk (Meltzer et al., 2003), as well as other supportive evidence (Hennen & Baldessarini, 2005; Modestin, Dal Plan, & Agarwalla, 2005). The InterSePT trial supported a prolongation of time to interventions and reduced rates of suicide attempts, but not reduction of mortality. Other antipsychotic drugs have not been tested adequately for their effects on suicidal behavior, but there is suggestive evidence that olanzapine may have beneficial effects on suicidal ideation when given in combination with a mood-stabilizing agent (Houston et al., 2006).

Mood-Stabilizers

Many studies support a suicide risk-reducing effect of long-term treatment of bipolar and other manic-depressive disorder patients with lithium (Ahrens & Müller-Oerlinghausen, 2001; Angst, Angst, Gerber-Werder, & Gamma, 2005; Cipriani, Pretty, Hawton, & Geddes, 2005; Kessing, Søndergård, Kvist, & Andersen, 2005; Müller-Oerlinghausen, Ahrens, & Felber, 2006; Tondo, Hennen, & Baldessarini, 2001). We recently meta-analyzed data from nearly three-dozen studies of long-term lithium treatment in bipolar disorder or a mix of major mood-disorder patients (Baldessarini & Tondo, 2008; Baldessarini, Tondo, et al., 2006). The findings not only support a marked reduction in the risk of suicide attempts, but also of completed suicides (both by fivefold or about 80%). We also found a more than twofold higher proportion of attempts/suicides during treatment with lithium, suggesting reduced lethality of suicidal behavior. These findings include several randomised controlled trials (RCTs) against either a placebo or alternative mood-stabilizing agents (Baldessarini & Tondo, 2008; Baldessarini, Tondo, et al., 2006, Cipriani et al., 2005). The strength of the evidence concerning antisuicidal effects of long-term treatment of lithium served as a basis for a recent citizen's petition to the US FDA seeking regulatory recognition of an antisuicide effect of all lithium products in bipolar I disorder patients (Baldessarini & Goodwin, 2005).

In addition, in the data compiled from eight studies by meta-analysis, we found a fourfold (76%) lower risk of suicide and attempts in patients diagnosed with recurrent major depressive disorder, treated with lithium compared to other alternatives (risk ratio [RR] = 4.2 [95% confidence interval; CI: 1.5–12.0]; Guzzetta, Tondo, Centorrino, & Baldessarini, 2007).

The evident beneficial effects of lithium in reducing mortality due to suicide are all the more remarkable for its potentially lethal toxicity in acute overdoses. Suicide attempts with lithium have been reported to be rare (Waddington & McKensie, 1994), and we found none among more than 700 patients with major mood disorders treated with lithium for several years at the Lucio Bini Mood Disorders Center in Sardinia (Tondo et al., 2007). Moreover, protection from lethal toxicity is afforded by vomiting often induced by acute overdoses of lithium as well as by the unique ability of dialysis methods to clear lithium from the circulation rapidly and efficiently (Baldessarini & Tarazi, 2005; Eyer et al., 2006). Recent national survey data from the US indicate that risk of fatalities following overdoses of lithium was similar to that of second-generation antipsychotic drugs and of antidepressants of the serotonin reuptake inhibitor (SRI) type (Watson et al., 2004).

There is little research that directly compares suicidal risks during treatment with other mood-stabilizers (Oquendo et al., 2005), but at least two studies found nearly threefold average lower risks with lithium than with carbamazepine or divalproex among bipolar or schizoaffective disorder patients (Goodwin et al., 2003; Thies-Flechtner, Müller-Oerlinghausen, Seibert, Walther, & Greil, 1996). Nevertheless, there are some indications that anticonvulsants, themselves, may have some beneficial effects on suicidal behavior (Baldessarini & Tondo, 2009; Yerevanian, Koek, & Mintz, 2003).

Antidepressants

A highly controversial question is whether antidepressant treatment alters the risks of various aspects of "suicidality" among patients with major depressive disorders (Baldessarini, Faedda, & Hennen, 2005; Baldessarini, Pompili, et al., 2005; Baldessarini, Pompili, & Tondo, 2006; Healy, 2006; Klein, 2006; Mann et al., 2006; Moller, 2006).

Ecological Studies

Evidence that antidepressant treatment yields expected reductions in risk of suicides or attempts is mixed. It includes data from correlative or "ecological," pharmacoepidemiological studies that compare suicide rates by regions or years with concurrent rates of prescriptions for antidepressant drugs (Baldessarini, Tondo, et al., 2007). In some Nordic countries and the US, modern, less-toxic antidepressants emerged in the 1990s to dominate current clinical practice and were associated with generally moderate decreases in overall suicide rates, varying in sex and age groups (Baldessarini, Tondo, et al., 2007; Gibbons, Hur, Bhaumik, & Mann, 2005, 2006; Grunebaum et al., 2004; Helgason, Tómasson, & Zoëga, 2004; Henriksson & Isacsson, 2006; Isacsson, 2000; Ludwig & Marcotte, 2005; Reseland, Bray, & Gunnell, 2006; Søndergård, Kvist, Lopez, Andersen, & Kessing, 2006c). However, in the US and some Nordic countries, at least, similar trends toward falling suicide rates were in evidence at least a decade before the introduction of the SRI fluoxetine, the first clinically successful modern antidepressant (Baldessarini, Tondo, et al., 2007; Reseland et al., 2006).

In our recent review of this body of research, only 9 of 29 ecological studies found significant inverse correlations of increased use of modern antidepressants with diminishing national, regional, or temporal trends in suicide rates; another six found no relationships, and 14 found correlations in some sex or age subgroups that were inconsistent across studies. Moreover, our analysis of data from 78 reporting countries indicated that only about half of them (54%) experienced decreases in annual suicide rates between the 1950s (when antidepressants were not available) and the early 2000s (a decade after introduction of modern antidepressants), and that a similar proportion (46%) reported increases; the international distribution of decreases and increases between 1990 and the early 2000s was similar (Tondo & Baldessarini, 2006; WHO, 2007). Moreover, both types of changes have been reported from similar world regions, including decreases and increases in Western and Eastern Europe, Latin America, and Asia. These outcomes suggest random, or at least highly complex phenomena that are likely to reflect the impact of many contributing factors.

As noted above, it is plausible to consider that improvements in public health, changes in legal, cultural, or social prohibitions against suicide, and improvements in identifying and reporting suicides might, paradoxically, associate higher suicide rates with increased access to modern psychopharmacologic agents in some countries. Additional socioeconomic factors may also contribute to the complex findings from the ecological studies in question. For example, in the US, we found strong correlations between state suicide rates and economic and demographic measures likely to be associated with access to clinical care in general, including population density, clinicians/100,000 population, per capita income, access to medical insurance, and public support of mental health services (Tondo et al., 2006). These findings underscore the point that many factors, including access to clinical services or social supports, and not merely antidepressant prescription rates, are likely to be associated with regional and temporal variations in suicide rates. It is also important to emphasize that all these correlative studies suffer from a fundamental inability to relate medication exposure or other specific factors to suicidal behavior at the level of individuals (Freedman, 2002). At best, they may suggest hypotheses for further testing with less ambiguous methods, but they cannot prove a direct, causal relationship between antidepressant treatment and reduced suicidal risk at the level of individual persons.

Cohort and Case-Control Studies

Other sources of data concerning antidepressants include large cohorts of depressed patients from general practice or health-maintenance organization data sources, and relatively large, case-control comparisons of subgroups varying in exposure to antidepressants. Such studies include over 1-million, mainly clinically depressed, subjects in 17 reports (Angst et al., 2005; Barak, Olmer, & Aizenberg, 2005; Bauer et al., 2006; Didham, McConnell, Blair, & Reith, 2005; Jick, Dean, & Jick, 1995; Jick, Kaye, & Jick, 2004; Juurlink, Mamdani, Kopp, & Redelmeier, 2006; Leon et al., 1999; Martinez et al., 2005; Olfson, Marcus, & Shaffer, 2006; Oquendo et al., 2002; Simon, Savarino, Operskalski, & Wang, 2006; Søndergård, Kvist, Andersen, & Kessing, 2006a, 2006b; Tiihonen et al., 2006; Warshaw & Keller, 1996; Yerevanian, Koek, Feusner, Hwang, & Mintz, 2004). These studies yield inconsistent findings; many of them (n = 11) were designed to test for greater suicidal risks with SRI antidepressants compared to other agents or to nontreatment. The great majority of such studies (9/11) did not find evidence of greater suicidal risk in association with antidepressant treatment, and a majority of others addressing other related questions (4/6) found decreased or no difference in suicidal risk with more antidepressant treatment. Several of these studies encountered *greater* suicidal risk with more antidepressant treatment in general, or specifically with greater use of SRIs and other modern antidepressants, at least in some age groups, including small increases among adolescents (Olfson et al., 2006; Søndergård et al., 2006b), larger increases in elderly patients (Juurlink et al., 2006), or inconsistently, fewer completed suicides but more attempts (Tiihonen et al., 2006).

Interpretation of findings from such studies is severely compromised by their risk of "confounding by morbidity or by indication." That is, medical treatments, in general, are more likely to be sought and given to more severely ill patients at higher risk of suicide, and medicines with low risks of toxic effects on acute overdosing (such as the SRIs) are more likely to be selected clinically than more toxic agents (e.g., tricyclic antidepressants, TCAs) to treat patients considered to be at increased risk for suicide. The nonrandomized, clinically selected treatment in such studies can severely distort observed associations between greater suicidal risk and use of particular treatments.

Randomized Controlled Trials (RCTs)

RCTs should be the best source of data on effects of antidepressant treatment on suicidal risks, and hundreds of such trials support the licensing and clinical applications of modern and older antidepressants in major depressive and anxiety disorder patients. Individual trials are unlikely to include enough patients with identified suicidal acts to allow testing for treatment effects, especially since being acutely suicidal is usually a criterion for exclusion from such trials. However, pooling of data across many RCTs, such as by use of meta-analytic methods, may yield substantial numbers of suicide attempts and even completed suicides. Indeed, rates of suicide attempts and even of completed suicides may be at least as high in controlled trials as in clinical samples of patients diagnosed with major depressive disorder. For example, suicide rates pooled across several recent large meta-analyses of modern and older antidepressants or placebo (given similar rates with all treatments) averaged 862/100,000/year (Acharya et al., 2006; Khan, Khan, Kolts, & Brown, 2003; Khan et al., 2000), or 66-times above average international general population rate of 13/100,000/year (WHO, 2007)! In clinical samples of even relatively severely ill major depression patients, usually hospitalized at some time, the standardized mortality ratio (SMR) for suicide compared to the general population rarely exceeds 20-fold (Harris & Barraclough, 1998), and among less severely ill, ambulatory, depressed patients this RR may be about three-times lower (Bostwick & Pankratz, 2000). To considerable extent, these high observed rates of suicidal behaviors in RCTs reflect exaggeration arising from annualizing rates based on relatively brief exposure times (typically 8–12 weeks) encountered in most trials in acute depression and early in the course of treatment.

There have been several recent reports based on pooling data on rates of suicides and attempts from large numbers of RCTs and subjects involving modern antidepressants, older standard agents, and placebo (Acharya et al., 2006; Baldessarini, Pompili, et al., 2006; FDA, 2005; Fergusson et al., 2005; Gunnell, Saperia, & Ashby, 2005; Hammad, Laughren, & Racoosin, 2006a, 2006b; Khan et al., 2000, 2003; Laughren, 2006; Storosum, van Zwieten, van den Brink, Gersons, & Broekmans, 2001; Tollefson, Rampey, Beasley, Enas, & Potvin, 1994). With the exception of one report finding a significant overall excess of suicide attempts during treatment with SRI antidepressants (Fergusson et al., 2005), other meta-analyses have found only minor differences in the rates of suicidal behaviors between depressed patients treated with an SRI, other antidepressants, or a placebo, overall tending toward apparently greater risks with antidepressants, assuming that the trials analyzed were well randomized and remained so, with well-balanced exposures in both drug and placebo arms throughout the duration of the trials. We have pooled the data reported from these previous meta-analyses to summarize the findings (Table 1; Figure 1).

One of the largest of these analyses was recently organized by the US FDA to review all available data from 386 controlled trials of modern antidepressant drugs involving 112,875 patient-subjects with major depressive or other disorders (Laughren, 2006). By far, most of the identified suicidal events involved *thinking* considered to be suicidal, but of uncertain clinical significance. Reported instances of suicides (0.013%) and attempts (0.198%) may be low due to relatively brief exposure times averaging 2 months. Among adult patients diagnosed with major depressive disorder, the *observed suicide rate*, based on estimated exposure times averaging 8 weeks, was 77/100,000/year (6/45,580/0.17 year), or only six-times above the general population rate of 13/100,000/year (WHO, 2007), compared to suicide rates of 862/100,000/year found in similar controlled trials of modern antidepressants, as already noted (Acharya et al., 2006; Khan et al., 2000, 2003). There was no overall difference in the risk of "suicidality" (mainly suicidal ideation), even when previous data from earlier analyses of data from RCTs of SRIs versus placebo used to treat juvenile depressed or anxious patients were included (FDA, 2005;

Table 1. Summary of meta-analyses of randomized controlled trials of antidepressants versus placebo in major depression

	Suicides		Attempts	
Study	Drugs	Placebo	Drugs	Placebo
Khan et al. (2000)	32/16,560	2/3,079	115/16,560	15/3,079
Khan et al. (2003)	72/43,382	5/4,895	–	–
Fergusson et al. (2005)	–	–	80/14,859	5/3,273
Gunnell et al. (2005)	9/23,804	7/17,022	111/30,814	61/21,689
Acharya et al. (2006)	1/1,812	1/1,184	15/1,812	5/1,184
Laughren (2006)	5/30,707	1/14,873	61/30,707	29/14,873
Totals	119/116,265	16/41,053	382/94,752	115/44,098
Crude pooled rates (%)	0.102	0.039	0.403	0.261

Note that the trials data analyzed probably overlap, and are uncorrected for exposure times, which may not be identical in drug and placebo arms of all trials, and that the analysis by Fergusson et al. (2005) involved suicide attempts and no suicides. Nevertheless, the pooled data suggest moderately higher rates of suicide (2.62-fold) and attempts (1.54-fold) with antidepressants versus placebos. Estimated "lethality" (ratio of rates of attempt/suicides) for patients diagnosed with major depression was 4.16 (0.358/0.086); this ratio is much lower than the ratios of 20–30 found in the general population, indicating greater lethality of suicidal acts among depressed patients, including in randomized treatment trials. The observed suicide rate was 135/157,318 with antidepressants and placebo, or 85.8/100,000 in approximately 0.17 year (8 weeks), which would annualize to approximately 508/100,000/year – a rate that is congruent with suicide risk in clinical samples of depression patients.

Hammad et al., 2006a). However, secondary analyses, based on stratifying by age groups, suggested increased risk of broadly defined "suicidality" (mainly ideation) with modern antidepressants versus placebo at younger ages and possible beneficial effects in older patients (Figure 2).

These provocative findings, pertaining almost entirely to increased observed risks of presumably new suicidal ideation with SRIs and other modern antidepressants over placebo, among children, adolescents, and young adults up to age 24 years, extend initial impressions of similar trends in meta-analyses carried out in RCTs involving children and adolescents by the UK drug regulatory agency (MHRA, 2004) as well as the FDA (2005; Hammad et al., 2006b). In the initial FDA review of SRI trials data involving some 4,400 depressed or anxious children and adolescents, there were no suicides, but there were a few self-injurious acts considered by independent experts to represent suicide attempts. For such acts, there was a suggestively greater meta-analytic relative risk during treatment with SRIs versus placebo (RR = 1.90; 95% CI: 1.00–3.63; FDA, 2005; Baldessarini, Pompili, et al., 2006).

RCT data fail to support an expected overall reduction of risk of suicidal acts during treatment with antidepressants of all types, and even suggest that risk of suicide *attempts* and perhaps *suicides* may be greater during treatment with antidepressants of various

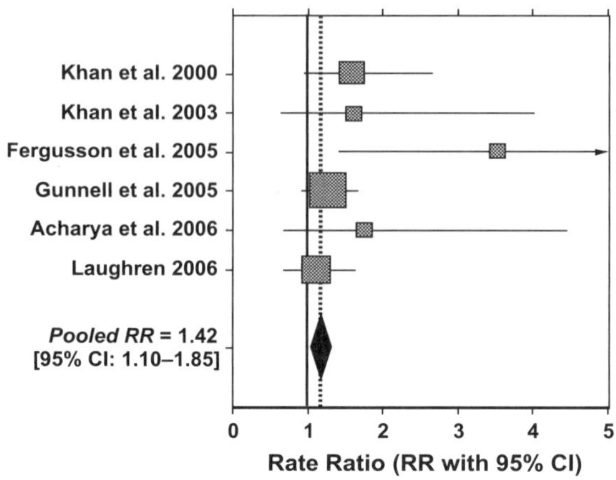

Figure 1. Forest plot of random-effect meta-analysis of reported summary findings from previous pooled analyses of data from randomized, placebo-controlled trials of antidepressants in adult major depression, based on the sum of *suicides and suicide attempts* (data in Table 1). The overall, pooled rate ratio (RR) and its 95% CI is 1.42 (CI: 1.10–1.85; z = 2.65, p = .008: black diamond and vertical dashed line; boxes are proportional to subject numbers and variance measures), compared to the null value of RR = 1.0 (vertical solid line). One study (Fergusson et al., 2005) had relatively large RR (3.52 [CI: 1.43–8.69]). In addition, the computed, overall, pooled risk difference (RD) was 0.0015 (CI: 0.00032–0.0027), or 0.15% (CI: 0.03–0.27%; z = 2.49, p = .013), indicating an estimated number-needed-to-harm (NNH) of 667 (CI: 373–3,135); without Fergusson et al. (2005): NNH = 1,307 (CI: 636–infinity, z = 1.86, p = .06). For completed *suicide*, RD = 0.022% (CI: 0.017–0.060%; z = 1.11, p = .27), with an estimated NNH of 4,651 (CI: 1,675–infinity); for suicide *attempts* RD = 0.163% (CI: 0.014–0.312%; z = 2.15, p = .03), with a correspondingly NNH = 613 (CI: 321–6,993). These results suggest that more than 600 depressed patients would have to be exposed to an antidepressant for approximately 2 months (or about 100 treated for a year), early in the course of an episode of acute major depressive disorder, when spontaneous suicidal risk is particularly high, to yield one excess suicide attempt, and over 4,500 to yield one excess suicide over the risk associated with untreated major depression itself.

types. However, many trials in adult depressive disorder patients have found substantially larger reductions in average ratings of suicidal *ideation* with antidepressants of various types than with placebo (Acharya et al., 2006; Beasley et al., 1991; Filteau, Lapierre, Bakish, & Blanchard, 1993; Pedersen, 2005; Tollefson et al., 1994). However, these findings are subjective, usually incidental or based on *post hoc* assessments of individual items on standard depression symptom-rating scales (Hamilton item 3 or Montgomery-Åsberg item 10), which may shift coincidentally with impressions of overall clinical improvement. Indeed, studies with antidepressants that explicitly consider suicidal ideation and behaviors as outcome measures remain to be carried out.

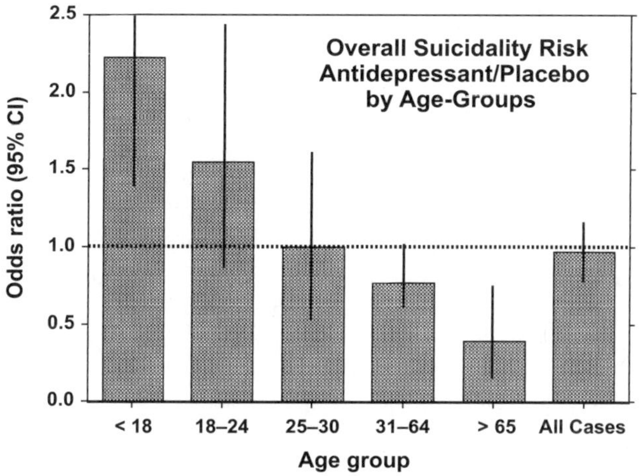

Figure 2. Overall suicidal risk in randomized, placebo-controlled trials of modern antidepressants, by age groups, as odds ratios (OR) for risk with drug versus placebo, with fixed-effect 95% CI (vertical lines) compared to the null value of 1.0 (horizontal dashed line). Note that there is a slightly but statistically nonsignificantly lower overall risk of new suicidal ideation and suicidal acts with antidepressants versus placebo (OR: 0.84; 95% CI: 0.69–1.02). Data are adapted from FDA analyses of spontaneous adverse-event reports from a total of 386 controlled trials involving 112,875 adult and juvenile patient-subjects with major depressive or other disorders (Laughren, 2006; Statistical section, p. 27). Most of the suicidal events pertain to ideation, whereas suicides and even attempts were rare. In addition, there was an age-associated decrease in risk of suicides and attempts (independent of treatment): < 18 years (0.55%), 18–24 (0.48%), 25–30 (0.19%), 31–64 (0.14%), > 65 (0.13%) (Laughren, 2006; Statistical Section, p. 37), whereas risk of emerging suicidality (acts plus ideation) was similar among men (OR for antidepressant versus placebo: 0.75; CI: 0.53–1.04) and women (OR: 0.89; CI: 0.70–1.13) (Laughren, 2006; Statistical section, p. 40).

It should be noted that even RCTs have limitations that can lead to artifacts and uncertainties. These include potential unreliability of essentially incidental, passive reporting of suicidal thoughts or behaviors in most RCTs based on currently typical "adverse-event reporting" systems, under conditions *not* designed explicitly to detect suicidal events. In addition, the relatively short duration of most trials of treatments for acute depression may not provide an adequate basis for evaluating the effects of treatment on rare suicidal behaviors, comparable to the long-term trials available for clozapine, lithium, and anticonvulsants already discussed. Moreover, much of what has been reported involves suicidal *ideation* of highly uncertain clinical significance and quantitatively very limited relationship to actual life-threatening behaviors. Another potential source of bias is that initial randomization in RCTs can break down during the conduct of trials. Premature, and potentially nonrandom, dropping out, owing usually to lack of perceived benefit, or emergence of intolerable adverse effects of treatment, is routinely encountered in most RCTs. More specifically, observed rates of "suicidal events" rarely are corrected for *actual* time of exposure of individual patient-subjects to specific treatments. This correction to reported adverse-event rates (events/persons/weeks) can be important if actual exposures are not closely matched across trial treatment arms, and particularly when rare events such as suicides and attempts are involved. For example, earlier dropping out of a trial arm involving ineffective placebo treatment can paradoxically limit observable suicidal risk with placebo, artifactually making active drug treatment *seem* "riskier" than placebo. The emergence of new suicidal behaviors among adults treated with antidepressants is very uncommon, involving perhaps 5/1000 patients within a year (Tondo, Lepri, & Baldessarini, 2008).

Recently, a meta-analytic review of large cohort and case-control studies of antidepressants found closely similar results as the FDA analyses. That is, younger patients experienced increased suicidal risks, whereas older adults had lower risks associated with antidepressant treatment (Barbui, Esposito, & Cipriani, 2009). These two *post hoc*, meta-analyses show remarkably similar risks versus age (Fawcett, Baldessarini, Coryell, Stein, & Silverman, 2009) that require prospective and controlled assessment.

Implications of Controlled Trials of Antidepressants

The preceding findings led to FDA requirements for revision of drug manufacturer information bulletins to include highlighted (black box) warnings of the findings just summarized, pertaining to possible increases in risk of suicidal thinking and perhaps behaviors during treatment of juvenile and young adult patients with SRIs and other modern antidepressants. The warnings also carry implications that special care is appropriate in the early treatment of young depressed or other patients being given an antidepressant (FDA, 2005). This recommendation is likely to further limit use of modern antidepressants in children, in addition to the fact that only fluoxetine is approved for juvenile major depression. The unique status of this agent is based on at least four controlled trials, some of which are large enough that their statistical power offsets the limited efficacy of SRIs and other antidepressants in children and adolescents (Tsapakis, Soldani, Tondo, & Baldessarini, 2007), particularly one very large federally funded trial with an unusually large separation of responses to the drug versus placebo (March et al., 2004). In 12 large trials of SRIs in juvenile major depression, the relative rate of responding to drug more than to placebo (RR) averaged 1.23 (95% CI: 1.14–1.33; $p < .0001$) and in 14 much smaller trials of TCAs, the pooled RR of 1.15 (CI: 0.98–1.34; $p = .098$) was of similarly modest magnitude but statistically nonsignificant (Tsapakis et al., 2007).

The findings pertaining to possible worsening of suicidal risks in young antidepressant-treated patients suggest potential scientifically and clinically very important developmental differences in affective and behavioral responses to antidepressants that require further study, especially with respect to risks of actual suicidal behavior. We presented evidence recently that SRIs may carry an unusually high risk of inducing switching from depression into agitated, dysphoric, irritable states in children, specifically below age

Table 2. Psychopharmacology and suicide: Summary of recent research findings

- Therapeutic research on suicide was virtually unknown a decade ago.
- Long-term treatment with lithium has strong evidence for up to fivefold reduced risks of suicide and attempts in bipolar and mixed samples of major affective disorders, and suggestive evidence of fourfold reduction of this risk in recurrent major depression.
- Long-term treatment with the anticonvulsant mood-stabilizers carbamazepine and divalproex appears to be less effective than lithium in reducing suicidal risk.
- Based on relatively limited data, clozapine has reduced risk of suicide attempts by nearly fivefold in schizophrenia patients and has unique FDA approval for this indication.
- A minority of ecological studies found minor decreases of suicide rates by region or time correlated with higher rates of prescribing modern antidepressants in the 1990s; these correlations are probably influenced by many factors associated with access to clinical care and may have begun earlier.
- Most large clinical studies suggest decreased suicidal risk with antidepressant treatment, but some find increases at various ages; these studies risk confounding by associating antidepressant treatment with more severe depression, and so with greater suicidal risk; this risk may decline in older adults.
- Data pooled from relatively brief, RCTs in acute major depression suggest increases in risk of suicide attempts, as well as increases in suicidal ideation in young patients, but decreases in older adults.
- Overall, antidepressants are not proved to have beneficial effects on risks of suicidal behaviors but may reduce suicidal ideation along with other symptoms of depression in adults.
- Differences between antidepressants and antipsychotic or mood-stabilizing agents may reflect differential benefits of the latter for irritability, anger, aggression, and impulsivity, which may worsen in some patients given antidepressants.
- Early depression requires particularly close clinical follow-up to identify emerging suicidal risks and treatable adverse behavioral reactions to treatment.

14 years (Baldessarini, Faedda, et al., 2005; Faedda, Baldessarini, Glovinsky, & Austin, 2004). These reactions are especially likely to arise among depressed juveniles previously not recognized as having bipolar disorders or other behavioral sensitivity to mood-elevating agents, but can arise also in adults (Pompili, Tondo, & Baldessarini, 2005; Tondo, Vázquez, & Baldessarini, 2009). Such responses might contribute to the reported excess of suicidal ideation in young patients treated with modern antidepressants (Hammad et al., 2006b).

Conclusions

Our main conclusions arising from this overview of current knowledge of the relevance of psychopharmacological treatments to suicidal risk in patients with major psychiatric disorders are summarized in Table 2. Since an initial case series reported soon after the introduction of fluoxetine (Teicher, Glod, & Cole, 1990), there have been repeated reports that a minority of depressed patients experience adverse behavioral and emotional responses to treatment with various types of mood-elevating medicines, and not only SRIs (Mann et al., 2006; Pompili et al., 2005). Typically, such responses arise early in treatment. Usually they can be identified clinically, and treatment appropriately modified, such as by removing antidepressant, adding sedating, antipsychotic, or mood-stabilizing treatments as well as providing additional individual support. The US FDA (2005) has encouraged a re-examination of what appears to have become somewhat casual routine practices in the use of relatively safe modern antidepressants to treat depressed patients and others at risk for suicide, calling for close early clinical follow-up of newly depressed persons not well known to a treating clinician.

Finally, a new hypothesis is suggested by the findings reviewed above. That antidepressant treatment appears to reduce suicidal ideation in depressed adults, whereas only clozapine and lithium have secure evidence of reducing risk of suicide attempts or suicides, suggests that "suicidality" is not usefully considered as a unitary clinical phenomenon or therapeutic target. Instead, there may be a differential pharmacology of particular aspects of suicidality. These probably include a need to limit rage, aggression, and impulsivity to reduce risks of attempts and suicides (Baldessarini, Tondo, et al., 2006). Such properties are more to be expected of antipsychotic or mood-stabilizing agents than of antidepressants.

Acknowledgments

This work was based in part on lectures at the McLean Division of Massachusetts General Hospital (RJB) on January 4, 2007, and the Upjohn Center for Depression Research, University of Michigan at Ann Arbor, on May 4, 2007 (RJB). This work was supported, in part, by USPHS-NIH NIMH Research Grant MH-073779 (to LT and RJB), a research grant from Janssen Pharmaceuticals, Titusville, New Jersey (to LT and RJB), a grant from the Bruce J. Anderson Foundation and the McLean Private Donors Research Fund for Mood Disorders and Psychopharmacology Research (to RJB), and by the Centro Bini Private Donors Mood Disorders Research Fund (to LT). Some of the research results summarized arose from a task force that analyzed research on antidepressants and suicide, chaired by Mauricio Tohen, MD, PhD for the Eli Lilly Research Center in Indianapolis, Indiana.

Disclosures: Dr. Baldessarini is a consultant to, or has collaborated in research with, the following corporations: Auritec, Biotrofix, IFI, Janssen, JDS, Eli Lilly, Merck, NeuroHealing, Novartis, and Solvay Corporations involved in the development and manufacture of a variety of psychotropic drugs. Dr. Tondo has received research support from Janssen Pharmaceuticals and Eli Lilly and Company. Neither author nor any family member holds equity positions in biomedical or pharmaceutical corporations.

References

Acharya, N., Rosen, A. S., Polzer, J. P., D'Souza, D. N., Perahia, D. G., Cavazzoni, P. A., et al. (2006). Duloxetine: Meta-analyses of suicidal behaviors and ideation in clinical trials for major depressive disorder. *Journal of Clinical Psychopharmacology, 26*, 587–594.

Ahrens, B., & Müller-Oerlinghausen, B. (2001). Does lithium exert an independent antisuicidal effect? *Pharmacopsychiatry, 34*, 132–136.

Ahrens, B., Müller-Oerlinghausen, B., Schou, M., Wolf, T., Alda, M., Grof, E., et al. (1995). Excess cardiovascular and suicide mortality of affective disorders may be reduced by lithium prophylaxis. *Journal of Affective Disorder, 33*, 67–75.

Akiskal, H. S., Benazzi, F., Perugi, G., & Rihmer, Z. (2005). Agitated "unipolar" depression re-conceptualized as a depressive mixed state: Implications for the antidepressant-suicide controversy. *Journal of Affective Disorder, 85*, 245–258.

American Psychiatric Association (APA). (2003). Practice guideline for the assessment and treatment of patients with suicidal behaviors. *American Journal of Psychiatry, 160*(11 Suppl.), 1–60.

Angst, J., Angst, F., Gerber-Werder, R., & Gamma, A. (2005). Suicide in 406 mood-disorder patients with and without long-term medication: A 40–44 years follow-up. *Archives of Suicide Research, 9*, 279–300.

Baldessarini, R. J., Faedda, G. L., & Hennen, J. (2005). Risk of mania with serotonin reuptake inhibitors vs. tricyclic antidepressants in children, adolescents and young adults. *Archives of Pediatrics & Adolescent Medicine, 159*, 298–299.

Baldessarini, R. J., & Goodwin, F. K. (2005). Antisuicidal efficacy of lithium products: Citizen's petition to the United States Food and Drug Administration, Washington, DC, September, 50 pp.– Available at www.fda.gov/ohrms/dockets/dockets/05p0402/05p-0402-cp00001-001- vol1.pdf – 10-17-2005 – Text Version. Accessed 20 May 2007.

Baldessarini, R. J., Henk, H. J., Sklar, A. R., Chang, J., & Leahy, L. F. (2008). Use of psychotropic medicines in bipolar disorder patients in the United States. *Psychiatric Services, 59*, 1175–1183.

Baldessarini, R. J., & Jamison, K. R. (1999). Effects of medical interventions on suicidal behavior: Summary and conclusions. *Journal of Clinical Psychiatry, 60*(Suppl. 2), 117–122.

Baldessarini, R. J., Leahy, L., Arcona, S., Gause, D., Zhang, W., & Hennen, J. (2007). Prescribing patterns of psychotropic medicines in the United States for patients diagnosed with bipolar disorders. *Psychiatric Services, 58*, 85–91.

Baldessarini, R. J., Pompili, M., & Tondo, L. (2006). Suicidal risk in antidepressant trials. *Archives of General Psychiatry, 63*, 246–248.

Baldessarini, R. J., Pompili, M., Tondo, L., Tsapakis, E., Soldani, F., Faedda, G. L., et al. (2005). Antidepressants and suicidal behavior: Are we hurting or helping? *Clinical Neuropsychiatry, 2*, 73–75.

Baldessarini, R. J., Salvatore, P., Khalsa, H.-M. K., Gebre-Medhin, P., Imaz, H., Gonzales-Pinto, A., et al. (in press). Morbidity in 303 first-episode bipolar I disorder patients. *Bipolar Disorders*.

Baldessarini, R. J., & Tarazi, F. I. (2005). Drug therapy of depression and anxiety disorders, psychosis and mania. In L. L. Brunton, J. S. Lazo, & K. L. Parker (Eds.), *Goodman and Gilman's The Pharmacological Basis of Therapeutics* (pp. 429–500). New York: McGraw-Hill.

Baldessarini, R. J., & Tondo, L. (2008). Lithium and suicidal risk. *Bipolar Disorders, 10*, 114–115.

Baldessarini, R. J., & Tondo, L. (2009). Meta-analytic comparison of antisuicidal effects of lithium versus anticonvulsants. *Pharmacopsychiatry, 42*, 72–75.

Baldessarini, R. J., Tondo, L., Davis, P., Pompili, M., Goodwin, F. K., & Hennen, J. (2006). Decreased suicidal risk during long-term lithium treatment: Meta-analysis. *Bipolar Disorder, 8*, 625–639.

Baldessarini, R. J., Tondo, L., Strombom, I., Dominguez, S., Fawcett, J., Oquendo, M., et al. (2007). Analysis of ecological studies of relationships between antidepressant utilization and suicidal risk. *Harvard Review of Psychiatry, 15*, 133–145.

Barak, Y., Olmer, A., & Aizenberg, D. (2005). Antidepressants reduce the risk of suicide among elderly depressed patients. *Neuropsychopharmacology, 31*, 178–181.

Barbui, C., Esposito, E., & Cipriani, A. (2009). Selective serotonin reuptake inhibitors and risk of suicide: A systematic review of observational studies. *Canadian Medical Association Journal, 180*, 291–297.

Bauer, M. S., Wisniewski, S. R., Marangell, L. B., Chessick, C. A., Allen, M. H., Dennehy, E. B., et al. (2006). Are antidepressants associated with new-onset suicidality in bipolar disorder? A prospective study of participants in the systematic treatment enhancement program for bipolar disorder (STEP-BP). *Journal of Clinical Psychiatry, 67*, 48–55.

Beasley, C. M. Jr., Dornseif, B. E., Bosomworth, J. C., Sayler, M. E., Rampey, A. H. Jr., Heilgenstein, J. H., et al. (1991). Fluoxetine and suicide: A meta-analysis of controlled trials of treatment for depression. *British Medical Journal, 303*, 685–692.

Black, D. W., Winokur, G., & Nasrallah, A. (1987). Is death from natural causes still excessive in psychiatric patients? A follow-up of 1593 patients with major affective disorder. *The journal of Nervous and Mental Disease, 175*, 674–680.

Bostwick, J. M., & Pankratz, V. S. (2000). Affective disorders and suicide risk: A reexamination. *American Journal of Psychiatry, 157*, 1925–1932.

Burrows, G. M. (1828). *Commentaries on the causes, forms, symptoms, treatment, moral and medical, of insanity.* London: Underwood.

Cipriani, A., Pretty, H., Hawton, K., & Geddes, J. R. (2005). Lithium in the prevention of suicidal behavior and all-cause mortality in patients with mood disorders: Systematic review of randomized trials. *The American Journal of Psychiatry, 162*, 1805–1819.

Dening, T. R. (2004). Lithium and motor vehicle crashes: Perhaps bipolar disorder is the risk, not its treatment. *British Medical Journal, 328*, 895–896.

Didham, R. C., McConnell, D. W., Blair, H. J., & Reith, D. M. (2005). Suicide and self-harm following prescription of SSRIs and other antidepressants: Confounding by indication. *British Journal of Clinical Pharmacology, 60*, 519–525.

Diekstra, R. F. W. (1993). Epidemiology of suicide and parasuicide. *Acta Psychiatrica Scandinavica, 371*(Suppl.), 9–20.

Evans, D. L., Charney, D. S., Lewis, L., Golden, R. N., Gorman, J. M., Krishnan, K. R., et al. (2005). Mood disorders in the medically ill: Scientific review and recommendations. *Biological Psychiatry, 58*, 175–189.

Eyer, F., Pfab, R., Felgenhauer, N., Lutz, J., Heemann, U., Steimer, W., et al. (2006). Lithium poisoning: Pharmacokinetics and clearance during different therapeutic measures. *Journal of Clinical Psychopharmacology, 26*, 325–330.

Fawcett, J. (2001). Treating impulsivity and anxiety in the suicidal patient. *Annals of the New York Academy of Sciences, 932*, 94–105.

Fawcett, J. A., Baldessarini, R. J., Coryell, W. H., Silverman, M. M., & Stein, D. J. (2009). Defining and managing suicidal risk in patients taking psychotropic medications. *Journal of Clinical Psychiatry, 70*, 782–789.

Faedda, G. L., Baldessarini, R. J., Glovinsky, I. P., & Austin, N. B. (2004). Treatment-emergent mania in pediatric bipolar disorder: A retrospective case review. *Journal of Affective Disorders, 82*, 149–158.

FDA (US Food and Drug Administration. (2005). Antidepressant use in children, adolescents, and adults. Available at: http://www.fda.gov/cder/drug/antidepressants Accessed 22 June 2006.

Fergusson, D., Doucette, S., Glass, K. C., Shapiro, S., Healy, D., Hebert, P., et al. (2005). Association between suicide attempts and selective serotonin reuptake inhibitors: Systematic review of randomized controlled trials. *British Medical Journal, 330*, 396–402.

Filteau, M. J., Lapierre, Y. D., Bakish, D., & Blanchard, A. (1993). Reduction in suicidal ideation with SSRIs: Review of 459 depressed patients. *Journal of Psychiatry & Neuroscience, 18*, 114–118.

Freedman, D. A. (2002). The ecological fallacy Accessible at http://www.stat.berkeley.edu/ ~census/ ecofall.txt. 2002. Accessed 10 January, 2007.

Ghaemi, S. N., Hsu, D. J., Soldani, F., & Goodwin, F. K. (2003). Antidepressants in bipolar disorder: The case for caution. *Bipolar Disorders, 5*, 421–433.

Ghaemi, S. N., Wingo, A. P., Filkowski, M. A., Goodwin, F. K, & Baldessarini, R. J. (2008). Effectiveness of long-term antidepressant treatment in bipolar disorder: A meta-analysis. *Acta Psychiatrica Scandinavica, 118*, 347–356.

Gibbons, R. D., Hur, K., Bhaumik, D. K., & Mann, J. J. (2005). The relationship between antidepressant medication use and rate of suicide. *Archives of General Psychiatry, 62*, 165–172.

Gibbons, R. D., Hur, K., Bhaumik, D. K., & Mann, J. J. (2006). The relationship between antidepressant prescription rates and rate of early adolescent suicide. *American Journal of Psychiatry, 163*, 1898–1904.

Goodwin, F. K., Fireman, B., Simon, G. E., Hunkeler, E. M., Lee, J., & Revicki, D. (2003). Suicide risk in bipolar disorder during treatment with lithium and divalproex. *JAMA, 290*, 1467–1473.

Goodwin, F. K., & Jamison, K. R. (1990). *Manic-depressive illness* (pp. 150–154). New York: Oxford University Press.

Goldsmith, S. K., Pellmar, T. C., Kleinman, A. M., & Bunney, W. E. (Eds.), *Reducing suicide*. Washington, DC: Institute of Medicine of the US National Academies of Science.

Grunebaum, M. F., Ellis, S. P., Li, S., Oquendo, M. A., & Mann, J. J. (2004). Antidepressants and suicide risk in the United States, 1985–1999. *Journal of Clinical Psychiatry, 65*, 1456–1462.

Gunnell, D., Saperia, J., & Ashby, D. (2005). Selective serotonin reuptake inhibitors (SRIs) and suicide in adults: Meta-analysis of drug company data from placebo controlled, randomized controlled trials submitted to the MHRA's safety review. *British Medical Journal, 330*, 385–388.

Guzzetta, F., Tondo, L., Centorrino, F., & Baldessarini, R. J. (2007). Lithium treatment reduces suicidal risk in recurrent major depressive disorder. *Journal of Clinical Psychiatry, 68*, 380–383.

Hammad, T. A., Laughren, T. P., & Racoosin, J. A. (2006a). Suicide rates in short-term randomized controlled trials of newer antidepressants. *Journal of Clinical Psychopharmacology, 26*, 203–207.

Hammad, T. A., Laughren, T., & Racoosin, J. A. (2006b). Suicidality in pediatric patients treated with antidepressant drugs. *Archives of General Psychiatry, 63*, 332–339.

Harris, E. C., & Barraclough, B. (1998). Excess mortality of mental disorder. *British Journal of Psychiatry, 173*, 11–53.

Healy, D. (2006). Did regulators fail over selective serotonin reuptake inhibitors? *British Medical Journal, 333*, 92–95.

Helgason, T., Tómasson, H., & Zoëga, T. (2004). Antidepressants and public health in Iceland: Time series analysis of national data. *British Journal of Psychiatry, 184*, 157–162.

Hennen, J., & Baldessarini, R. J. (2005). Suicidal risk during treatment with clozapine: A meta-analysis. *Schizophrenia Research, 73*, 139–145.

Henriksson, S., & Isacsson, G. (2006). Increased antidepressant use and fewer suicides in Jamtland county, Sweden, after a primary care educational programme on the treatment of depression. *Acta Psychiatrica Scandinavica, 114*, 159–167.

Houston, J. P., Ahl, J., Meyers, A. L., Kaiser, C. J., Tohen, M., & Baldessarini, R. J. (2006). Reduced suicidal ideation in bipolar I disorder mixed-episode patients in a placebo-controlled trial of olanzapine combined with lithium or divalproex. *Journal of Clinical Psychiatry, 67*, 1246–1252.

Isacsson, G. (2000). Suicide prevention – A medical breakthrough? *Acta Psychiatrica Scandinavica, 102*, 113–117.

Jick, S. S., Dean, A. D., & Jick, H. (1995). Antidepressants and suicide. *British Medical Journal, 310*, 215–218.

Jick, H., Kaye, J. A., & Jick, S. S. (2004). Antidepressants and the risk of suicidal behavior. *JAMA, 292*, 338–343.

Joffe, R. T., MacQueen, G. M., Marriott, M., & Trevor Young, L. (2004). A prospective, longitudinal study of percentage of time spent ill in patients with bipolar I or bipolar II disorders. *Bipolar Disorders, 6*, 62–66.

Judd, L. L., Akiskal, H. S., Schettler, P. J., Endicott, J., Maser, J., Solomon, D. A., et al. (2002). The long-term natural history of the weekly symptomatic status of bipolar I disorder. *Archives of General Psychiatry, 59*, 530–537.

Juurlink, D. N., Mamdani, M. M., Kopp, A., & Redelmeier, D. A. (2006). The risk of suicide with selective serotonin reuptake inhibitors in the elderly. *American Journal of Psychiatry, 163*, 813–821.

Katon, W. J., Rutter, C., Simon, G., Lin, E. H., Ludman, E., Ciechanowski, P., et al. (2005). Association of comorbid depression with mortality in patients with type-2 diabetes. *Diabetes Care, 28*, 2668–2672.

Kessing, L. V., Søndergård, L., Kvist, K., & Andersen, P. K. (2005). Suicide risk in patients treated with lithium. *Archives of General Psychiatry, 62*, 860–866.

Kessler, R. C., Berglund, P., Borges, G., Nock, M., & Wang, P. S. (2005). Trends in suicide ideation, plans, gestures, and attempts in the United States, 1990–1992 to 2001–2003. *JAMA, 293*, 2487–2495.

Khalsa, H.-M. K., Salvatore, P., Hennen, J., Tohen, M., & Baldessarini, R. J. (2008). Suicidal events and accidents in 216 first-episode bipolar-I disorder patients: Predictive factors. *Journal of Affective Disorders, 106*, 179–184.

Khan, A., Khan, S., Kolts, R., & Brown, W. A. (2003). Suicide rates in clinical trials with SRIs, other antidepressants, and placebo: Analysis of FDA reports. *American Journal of Psychiatry, 160*, 790–792.

Khan, A., Leventhal, R. M., Khan, S., & Brown, W. A. (2002). Suicide risk in patients with anxiety disorders: A meta-analysis of the FDA database. *Journal of Affective Disorders, 68*, 183–190.

Khan, A., Warner, H. A., & Brown, W. A. (2000). Symptom reduction and suicide risk in patients treated with placebo in antidepressant clinical trials: Analysis of the FDA database. *Archives of General Psychiatry, 57*, 311–317.

Klein, D. F. (2006). FDA post-marketing safety decisions. *Journal of Clinical Psychiatry, 67*, 1305–1306.

Koukopoulos, A., & Koukopoulos, A. (1999). Agitated depression as a mixed state and the problem of melancholia. *Psychiatric Clinocs of North America, 22*, 547–564.

Laughren, T. P. (2006). Overview of a meeting of the Psychopharmacology Drug Advisory Committee (PDAC). Concerning suicidal risk in trials of antidepressant drugs in juvenile and adult patients, pp. 27ff – Accessible at: http://www.fda.gov/ohrms/dockets/ac/06/briefing/2006-4272b1-index.htm. Accessed 26 December 2006.

Leon, A. C., Keller, M. B., Warshaw, M. G., Mueller, T. I., Solomon, D. A., Coryell, W., et al. (1999). A prospective study of fluoxetine treatment and suicidal behavior in affectively ill subjects. *American Journal of Psychiatry, 156*, 195–201.

Ludwig, J., & Marcotte, D. E. (2005). Antidepressants, suicide, and drug regulation. *Journal of Policy and Analysis Management, 24*, 249–272.

Maj, M., Pirozzi, R., Magliano, L., Fiorillo, A., & Bartoli, L. (2006). Agitated "unipolar" major depression: Prevalence, phenomenology, and outcome. *Journal of Clinical Psychiatry, 67*, 712–719.

Mann, J. J., Emslie, G., Baldessarini, R. J., Beardslee, W., Fawcett, J. A., Goodwin, F. K., et al. (2006). ACNP task force report on SRIs and suicidal behavior in youth. *Neuropsychopharmacology, 31*, 473–492.

March, J., Silva, S., Petrycki, S., Curry, J., Wells, K., Fairbank, J., et al. (2004). Treatment for adolescents with depression study (TADS) team. Fluoxetine, cognitive-behavioral therapy, and their combination for adolescents with depression: Treatment for adolescents with depression study (TADS) randomized controlled trial. *JAMA, 292*, 807–820.

Martinez, C., Rietbrock, S., Wise, L., Ashby, D., Chick, J., Moseley, J., et al. (2005). Antidepressant treatment and the risk of fatal and non-fatal self harm in first episode depression: Nested case-control study. *British Medical Journal, 330*, 389–392.

Meltzer, H. Y., Alphs, L., Green, A. I., Altamura, A. C., Anand, R., Bertoldi, A., et al. (2003). International suicide prevention trial study group. Clozapine treatment for suicidality in schizophrenia: International suicide prevention trial (InterSePT). *Archives of General Psychiatry, 60*, 82–91.

MHRA (UK Medicines and Health Regulatory Agency). (2004). Selective serotonin reuptake inhibitor (SSRI) antidepressants: Committee on Safety of Medicines (CSM) working group findings http://www.mhra.gov.uk/news/2004/2004.htm. Accessed 22 September 2005.

Modestin, J., Dal Plan, D., & Agarwalla, P. (2005). Clozapine diminished suicidal behavior: Retrospective evaluation of clinical records. *Journal of Clinical Psychiatry, 66*, 534–538.

Moller, H. J. (2006). Evidence for beneficial effects of antidepressants on suicidality in depressive patients: Systematic review. *European Archives of Psychiatry and Clinical Neuroscience, 256*, 329–343.

Müller-Oerlinghausen, B., Ahrens, B., & Felber, W. (2006). The suicide-preventive and mortality-reducing effect of lithium. In M. Bauer, P. Grof & B. Müller-Oerlinghausen (Eds.), *Lithium in Neuropsychiatry* (pp. 179–192). London: Informa Healthcare.

Nordstrom, P., Samuelsson, M., & Åsberg, M. (1995). Survival analysis of suicide risk after attempted suicide. *Acta Psychiatrica Scandinavica, 91*, 336–340.

Olfson, M., Marcus, S. C., & Shaffer, D. (2006). Antidepressant drug therapy and suicide in severely depressed children and adults: Case-control study. *Archives of General Psychiatry, 63*, 865–872.

Oquendo, M. A., Chaudhury, S. R., & Mann, J. J. (2005). Pharmacotherapy of suicidal behavior in bipolar disorder. *Archives of Suicide Research, 9*, 237–250.

Oquendo, M. A., Kamali, M., Ellis, S. P., Grunebaum, M. F., Malone, K. M., Brodsky, B. S., et al. (2002). Adequacy of antidepressant treatment after discharge and the occurrence of suicidal acts in major depression: A prospective study. *American Journal of Psychiatry, 159*, 1746–1751.

Pedersen, A. G. (2005). Escitalopram and suicidality in adult depression and anxiety. *International Clinical Psychopharmacology, 20*, 139–143.

Pompili, M., Tondo, L., & Baldessarini, R. J. (2005). Suicidal risk emerging during antidepressant treatment: Recognition and intervention. *Clinical Neuropsychiatry, 2*, 66–72.

Post, R. M., Denicoff, K. D., Leverich, G. S., Altshuler, L. L., Frye, M. A., Suppes, T. M., et al. (2003). Morbidity in 258 bipolar outpatients followed for 1 year with daily prospective ratings on the NIMH life chart method. *Journal of Clinical Psychiatry, 64*, 680–690.

Reseland, S., Bray, I., & Gunnell, D. (2006). Relationship between antidepressant sales and secular trends in suicide rates in the Nordic countries. *British Journal of Psychiatry, 188*, 354–358.

Rose, R. M., Burt, R. A., & Clayton, P. J. (1985). Consensus development conference statement: Electroconvulsive therapy. *JAMA, 254*, 2103–2108.

Roy, A. (2000). Suicide. In B. J. Sadock & V. A. Sadock (Eds.), *Kaplan and Sadock's comprehensive textbook of psychiatry* (7th ed., Vol. 2, pp. 2031–2040). Philadelphia: Lippincott Willians and Wilkins..

Sharma, R., & Markar, H. R. (1994). Mortality in affective disorder. *Journal of Affective Disorders, 31*, 91–96.

Simon, R. I., & Hales, R. E. (Eds.), 2006. Textbook of suicide assessment and management. Washington, DC: American Psychiatric Press.

Simon, G. E., Savarino, J., Operskalski, B., & Wang, P. S. (2006). Suicide risk during antidepressant treatment. *American Journal of Psychiatry, 163*, 41–47.

Søndergård, L., Kvist, K., Andersen, P. K., & Kessing, L. V. (2006a). Do antidepressants prevent suicide? *International Clinical Psychopharmacology, 21*, 211–218.

Søndergård, L., Kvist, K., Andersen, P. K., & Kessing, L. V. (2006b). Do antidepressants precipitate youth suicide? – A nationwide pharmacoepidemiological study. *European Child & Adolescent Psychiatry, 15*, 232–240.

Søndergård, L., Kvist, K., Lopez, A. G., Andersen, P. K., & Kessing, L. V. (2006c). Temporal changes in suicide rates for persons treated and not treated with antidepressants in Denmark during 1995–1999. *Acta Psychiatrica Scandinavica, 114*, 168–176.

Storosum, J. G., van Zwieten, B. J., van den Brink, W., Gersons, B. P., & Broekmans, A. W. (2001). Suicide risk in placebo-controlled studies of major depression. *American Journal of Psychiatry, 158*, 1271–1275.

Teicher, M. H., Glod, C., & Cole, J. O. (1990). Emergence of intense suicidal preoccupation during fluoxetine treatment. *American Journal of Psychiatry, 147*, 207–210.

Thies-Flechtner, K., Müller-Oerlinghausen, B., Seibert, W., Walther, A., & Greil, W. (1996). Effect of prophylactic treatment on suicide risk in patients with major affective disorders: Data from a randomized prospective trial. *Pharmacopsychiatry, 29*, 103–107.

Tiihonen, J., Lonnqvist, J., Wahlbeck, K., Klaukka, T., Tanskanen, A., & Haukka, J. (2006). Antidepressants and the risk of suicide, attempted suicide, and overall mortality in a nationwide cohort. *Archives of General Psychiatry, 63*, 1358–1367.

Tollefson, G. D., Rampey, A. H. Jr., Beasley, C. M. Jr., Enas, G. G., & Potvin, J. H. (1994). Absence of a relationship between adverse events and suicidality during pharmacotherapy for depression. *Journal of Clinical Psychopharmacology, 14*, 163–169.

Tondo, L., Albert, M., & Baldessarini, R. J. (2006). Suicide rates in relation to health-care access in the United States. *Journal of Clinical Psychiatry, 67*, 517–523.

Tondo, L., & Baldessarini, R. J. (2006). Trends in suicide rates: An international perspective (abstract). *Italian Journal of Psychopathology, 12*(Suppl. 2), 202–203.

Tondo, L., Lepri, B., & Baldessarini, R. J. (2007). Risks of suicidal ideation, attempts and suicides among 2826 men and women with types I and II bipolar, and recurrent major depressive disorders. *Acta Psychiatrica Scandinavica, 116*, 419–428.

Tondo, L., Baldessarini, R. J., Hennen, J., Minnai, G. P., Salis, P., Scamonatti, L., et al. (1999). Suicide attempts in major affective disorder patients with comorbid substance use disorders. *Journal of Clinical Psychiatry, 60*(Suppl. 2), 63–69.

Tondo, L., Hennen, J., & Baldessarini, R. J. (2001). Reduced suicide risk with long-term lithium treatment in major affective Illness: A meta-analysis. *Acta Psychiatrica Scandinavica, 104*, 163–172.

Tondo, L., Isacsson, G., & Baldessarini, R. J. (2003). Suicide in bipolar disorder: Risk and prevention. *CNS Drugs, 17*, 491–511.

Tondo, L., Lepri, B., & Baldessarini, R. J. (2008). Suicidal status during antidepressant treatment in 789 Sardinian patients with major affective disorder. *Acta Psychiatrica Scandinavica, 118*, 106–115.

Tondo, L., Vázquez, G., & Baldessarini, R. J. (2009). Mania associated with antidepressant-treatment: Comprehensive meta-analysis. *Acta Psychiatrica Scandinavica.* Advance online publication. doi: 10.1111/j.1600-0447.2009.01514.x.

Tsapakis, E., Soldani, F., Tondo, L., & Baldessarini, R. J. (2008). Efficacy of antidepressants in depressed children and adolescents: a meta-analysis. *British Journal of Psychiatry, 193*, pp. 10–17.

Tsuang, M. T., & Woolson, R. F. (1977). Mortality in patients with schizophrenia, mania, depression and surgical conditions. A comparison with general population mortality. *British Journal of Psychiatry, 130*, 162–166.

Waddington, D., & McKensie, I. P. (1994). Overdose rates in lithium-treated vs. antidepressant-treated outpatients. *Acta Psychiatrica Scandinavica, 90*, 50–52.

Warshaw, M. G., & Keller, M. B. (1996). The relationship between fluoxetine use and suicidal behavior in 654 subjects with anxiety disorders. *Journal of Clinical Psychiatry, 57*, 158–166.

Watson, W. A., Litovitz, T. L., Klein-Schwartz, W., Rodgers, G. C. Jr., Youniss, J., Reid, N., et al. (2004). 2003 Annual report of the American Association of Poison Control Centers Toxic Exposure Surveillance System. *American Journal of Emergency Medicine, 22*, 335–404.

Weinger, R. D. (Ed.), 2000. Practice of electroconvulsive therapy: Recommendations for treatment, training, and privileging. A task force report of the American Psychiatric Association (2nd ed.). Washington, DC: American Psychiatric Press..

World Health Organization (WHO) (2007). International suicide rates Accessible at www.who.int/mental_health/prevention/suicide/country_reports/en/index.html. Accessed 10 January 2007.

Yerevanian, B. I., Koek, R. J., & Mintz, J. (2003). Lithium, anticonvulsants and suicidal behavior in bipolar disorder. *Journal of Affective Disorders, 73*, 223–228.

Yerevanian, B. I., Koek, R. J., Feusner, J. D., Hwang, S., & Mintz, J. (2004). Antidepressants and suicidal behavior in unipolar depression. *Acta Psychiatrica Scandinavica, 110*, 452–458.

About the Authors

Dr. Ross J. Baldessarini was born in western Massachusetts (1937), graduated from Williams College (highest honors in chemistry, 1959), Johns Hopkins University (MD, 1963), and trained at Boston City Hospital (medical intern, 1963–64), NIH (neuroscience postdoctoral fellow, 1964–66), and Johns Hopkins Hospital (psychiatry, 1966–69). Since 1969, he has directed laboratory neuropharmacology and clinical psychopharmacology research programs at Massachusetts General and McLean Hospitals in Boston, is a tenured professor of psychiatry (neuroscience) at Harvard Medical School (1977–), and has contributed to basic understanding of central monoaminergic neurotransmission systems and their relationships to neuropsychiatric disorders. He has over 1,950 publications, including the chapters on psychopharmacology in the standard American textbook of pharmacology, and his own monograph on psychopharmacology. He has received several honorary degrees, research prizes, and the ISI listing of most-cited authors in pharmacology and psychiatry. He has trained 160 laboratory and clinical investigators and a generation of clinicians.

Dr. Leonardo Tondo is Director of Mood Disorder Lucio Bini Center in Cagliari (Italy), Lecturer in Psychiatry at the Harvard Medical School-McLean Hospital, founding member of the International Consortium for Research in Bipolar Disorder and formerly Associate Professor of Clinical Psychology at the University of Cagliari. He authored three books and more than 200 peer-reviewed articles and book chapters in mood disorders. He received the Nola-Maddox Falcone Prize (2003) for outstanding achievement in research of affective disorder and the Suicide Prevention Award (2004) for research on lithium treatment and prevention of suicide risk.

Ross J. Baldessarini
Harvard Medical School
Boston
Mailman Research Center 312
McLean Division of Massachusetts General Hospital
115 Mill Street
Belmont, MA 02478-9106
USA
Tel.: +1 617 855 3203
E-mail: rjb@mclean.org

Evidence-Based Approaches for Specific Disorders and Behaviors

Risk Is Not Static Over the Lifespan

Accurately Accounting for Suicide Prevalence in Major Mental Illness

John Michael Bostwick

Mayo Clinic, Rochester, MN, USA

For nearly 40 years, despite mounting evidence to the contrary, the accepted lifetime prevalence of suicide in affective disorders has been 15%, a number that major textbooks continue to cite indiscriminately, without consistently specifying type or severity of affective illness, treatment status of patients, or times of particular risk in illness course to which the statistic applies (Andreasen & Black, 2006, p. 371; Brendel, Lagomasino, Perlis, & Stern, 2008, p. 734; Dubovsky, Davies, & Dubovsky, 2004, p. 244; Melvin, Posner, Stanley, & Oquendo, 2008, p. 2480; Shear, 2008, p. 2519; Sudak, 2005, p. 2447). For schizophrenia, the textbooks persist in reporting that accepted lifetime prevalence is 10–13%, again without specific consideration of dynamic factors in illness course or treatment (Andreasen & Black, 2006, p. 371; Brendel et al., 2008, p. 734; Fenton, 2001, p. 1058; Ho, Black, & Andreasen, 2004, p. 207; Shear, 2008, p. 2519; Sudak, 2005, p. 2447).

Compounding the errors that resulted in these inflated suicide prevalence figures has been misapplications or misunderstandings of basic epidemiological concepts, either by the original investigators or by those who cited them in subsequent publications and reviews. The author of this chapter published two meta-analyses during the last 10 years that seek to debunk received wisdom that makes little sense on more than cursory consideration.

The 15% statistic appeared in a 1970 paper in the British Journal of Psychiatry by Guze and Robins (1970), Washington University professors who were prominent proponents of objective-descriptive or "medical psychiatry." They compared and contrasted 17 studies of patients with "primary affective disorders," by which they meant "affective disorders, depressive or manic episodes in patients who have been psychiatrically well previously, or who have episodes of mania or depression without other psychiatric illnesses." The studies were from Northern Europe and the United States, and had follow-up periods ranging from 1 to 20 years. They concluded that the relative risk of suicide was highest early in the course of the illness and was projected using a crude scatter plot that the suicide rate ultimately converged on 15% in these studies. They did not explicitly state that these studies almost exclusively involved inpatients. They could not have known that the definition of affective disorder in decades subsequent to 1970 would broaden to include less severe psychopathology such that the frequency of "depression" in the American population increased from 2–3% to 10–20%, simply by altering definitions (Klein & Thase, 1997). They certainly did not advocate the 15% figure being applied indiscriminately – as it frequently has been – to all forms of depressive illness.

The 15% figure gained even more legitimacy when Goodwin and Jamison (1990) updated and extended the original Guze and Robins meta-analysis in the first edition of their magisterial textbook, "Manic-Depressive Illness," the definitive text on bipolar disorder. Using a similar analytic approach, they added 13 studies to the original 17, concluding that 18.9% of depressed patients – nearly one in five – would eventually succumb to suicide. This and the Guze-Robins figure were the ones I was taught during psychiatry residency in the early 1990s. These were the answers I knew would be correct – and would likely still be correct – if I encountered a question about suicide in affective illness on a board examination (Perlis & Stern, 2004, p. 407).

In reality (as opposed to dogma), the figure – without serious qualification – seemed unbelievable, at least with my experience with the growing number of patients I was following and in the practices of my teachers and supervisors. No clinician I knew had lost one in six of their depressed patients to suicide. While nearly all of them had experienced at least one patient suicide during their careers and such an event was inevitably devastatingly memorable, it was hardly a commonplace occurrence. Guze and Robins had implied that they were not writing about *all* affectively ill patients. In a 1999 paper, Simpson and Jamison observed that the long-accepted 15% rate in major depression was probably too high because of sampling bias from early studies based on severely ill inpatients rather than the much larger numbers of depressed individuals treated as outpatients. Tondo, Isacsson, and Baldessarini (2003) pegged the suicide prevalence in never-hospitalized patients with moderately severe illness at less than 5%. Goodwin and Jamison themselves, in the second edition of their textbook, revised their earlier 18.9% estimate, declaring that "the rate today has dropped by about one half, except for patients early in the course of the illness" (2007, p. 248). Their revised figure has not yet gained widespread parlance, however. Enhanced by its propounders' statures, the earlier blanket generalizations that defy common sense have become gospel truth.

It was to see if we could redact the gospel that we embarked upon our first meta-analysis. Initial efforts consisted of accumulating as many studies as possible that contained information about the number of deaths and specifically the number of suicides that had occurred in an affectively ill cohort. Having amassed literally hundreds of papers, we needed to settle on a method to winnow this trove. Following the lead of Harris and Barraclough (1997), we adopted comparably stringent inclusion criteria for the meta-analysis. To be part of the pool, a patient cohort specifically identified as having affective illness had to be followed for at least 2 years with no more than 10% of the sample lost to follow-up. The 2-year requirement related to the period of highest risk for suicide after hospitalization, the entry point for most of the studies. The stipulation of at least 90% follow-up was premised on the common sense assumption that those unable to be accounted for were more likely to have killed themselves. We also took pains to establish treatment status – inpatient, outpatient, mixed – at the time of enrollment, and took notice of when studies stipulated that the observation period had begun with subjects in suicidal crisis, either with ideation or after an actual attempt.

A by-product of extracting vital status information – number of patients, number of those dead, number of dead to suicide – was the ability to determine how many were still alive. While trying to parse the reasoning behind the percentage of suicide deaths cited in the Guze and Robins, and Goodwin and Jamison publications, we observed that in many, a large proportion of the patients were still alive, and that in most of the studies, the percentage of suicides cited was based not on the number of suicides relative to the total sample of both living and dead subjects but rather on the proportion of the dead the suicides represented. These figures thus represented proportionate mortality (PM) rather than case fatality (CF) figures and were strongly biased toward overestimating suicide prevalence.

Neither PM nor CF is able to completely describe lifetime suicide risk, given that they each have to make assumptions about the status of those who have not died and who are still in active follow-up. PM assumes that the suicide rate among those who have not yet died will remain constant throughout the lifetime of those originally enrolled in the studies and CF assumes that all suicides in the study set will have already occurred. To demonstrate the difference between PM and CF, imagine a sample size of 100 individuals in which 10 have died, 5 by suicide. The PM for suicide is 5/10, or 50%. The CF is 5/100, or only 5%, an order of magnitude less than PM. Which number represents the true figure? If CF is used, it may underestimate risk because data are lacking about how the 90 still living will die. If PM is used, it will overestimate suicide risk unless suicide occurs at a constant rate over the lifespans of the 100 subjects. Only after all 100 subjects have died does PM equal CF.

I took up the issue with the statistician on both papers, Pankratz, and we hypothesized that the 15% figure, a PM statistic, likely overestimated suicide risk. Nonlinear regression methods that accounted for study-specific differences through the use of per-study random effects were constructed to model the intersection of PM and CF as a function of follow-up time. These models permitted the extrapolation of follow-up times to the point where CF and PM converged on a common figure. Thus, the already-observed patterns of PM and CF over the observed study-specific follow-up times provided information that enabled us to project a less biased estimate of lifetime suicide prevalence when the data were integrated in a single nonlinear regression model.

We had sufficient data to differentiate the studies into three categories: (1) inpatients enrolled after being admitted in suicidal crisis, (2) inpatients enrolled without specification of suicidality at admission, and (3) outpatients. Lifetime suicide prevalences calculated according to these methods were much less than 15% in all scenarios. A major finding of our study was that suicide risk layered out according to acuity, with a lifetime prevalence of 8.6% for category 1, 4.0% for category 2, and 2.2% for category 3 (Bostwick & Pankratz, 2000). Analyzed separately, both the Guze and Robins, and the Goodwin and Jamison samples had CF rates similar to our category of inpatients enrolled without specification of suicidality. This makes sense, since neither pair of authors distinguished between suicidal and nonsuicidal patients at enrollment. With this meta-analysis, we had shown not only that the lifetime suicide prevalence was not 15% but that prevalence varied based on treatment status at enrollment, a distinction the two pairs of authors we were refuting did not consider in their analyses.

While the prominence of depression in suicidal states remains a central tenet of suicide theory, contemporary thinkers emphasize that depression is neither necessary nor sufficient to explain why individuals are driven to self-harm. Mann's diathesis-stress model incorporates both predisposing characteristics – diatheses – and superimposed events – stresses – that interact to generate a suicidal crisis (Mann, 1998). Diatheses are chronic, including such genetic predispositions as family history of suicide, alcoholism, or affective illness; adverse early-life experience resulting in epigenetic changes in the ability to tolerate stress; a tendency toward impulsive action; chronic medical illness; and chronic substance abuse, particularly alcohol. Stresses are acute, including exacerbation of psychiatric illness; intoxication with alcohol or other drugs that result in disinhibition; medical illness causing pain, disfigurement, or alterations in brain function; and adverse life events.

What causes clinicians to hospitalize affectively ill patients? It is not primarily depression per se that gets their attention and elevates the situation to an emergency. Rather it is the suicidal ideation, the agitation, the impulsivity, and the hopelessness. These are the toxic, potentially life-threatening by-products that result when stress or trauma butts up against genetic or experiential predisposition.

While we did propose a revision that much diminished the 15% figure, the intent of our first meta-analysis was not to downplay suicide's significance in psychiatric populations. With the lifetime prevalence of suicide approximately 1% in the American general population, a 1969 study from Monroe County, New York illustrates how psychiatric patients disproportionately contribute to general population suicide prevalence (Babigian & Odoroff, 1969). Monroe County, population 625,000, home of Rochester, New York, had a psychiatric register that listed 39,475 individuals receiving some sort of mental health services in the county between 1960 and 1966. Over the 7 years of the study, the county had 408 suicides. Two thirds of these occurred in the 585,000 without a psychiatric history, one third in the 40,000 with a psychiatric history. Although twice as many suicides occurred in the nonpsychiatric sample, it was more than 14 times larger than the psychiatric sample, for a relative risk of suicide in the psychiatric sample seven times greater than in the nonpsychiatric one. In other words, the psychiatric patients comprised only one in 14 Monroe County residents, but accounted for one in three county suicides. From this finding, it can be deduced that a large number of American suicides – a number disproportionate to their representation in the general population – occurs in the mentally ill.

In the schizophrenic meta-analysis, for which Palmer was the first author, we explored not only the lifetime prevalence of suicide in this condition but also specific times of risk (Palmer, Pankratz, & Bostwick, 2005). Using in this second paper the same rigorous inclusion criteria as our affective disorders meta-analysis, we boiled 632 potential candidate studies down to 62 that met our standards and observed what appeared to be a bimodal suicide prevalence based on the point of subject entry to the study. Patient samples followed from illness onset or first admission appeared to have higher suicide rates than mixed patient samples – "all-comers" – containing both first-admission subjects and those enrolled at later points in this chronic illness.

When divided according to this specification, the first-admission group constituted 22,598 individuals abstracted from 29 papers, and the all-comers group 25,578 individuals from 32 papers. The first-admission group had a lifetime suicide prevalence of 5.6% (confidence interval, CI 3.7–8.5%), and the all-comers a lifetime suicide prevalence of 1.8% (CI 1.4–2.3%). Why the discrepancy? The dead cannot be counted, and the all-comers group misses suicides that have occurred in schizophrenics who killed themselves before they could be enrolled.

Given the tripling of rates between the all-comers and first-admission groups, one clear implication is that suicide is much more common in the early, actively psychotic years of the illness than in later decades than when psychotic symptoms have cooled and residual thought disorder assumes greater prominence. In this situation, PM illustrates how significant the contribution of suicide is to early death in schizophrenia. In the all-comers sample, the percentage of the deaths that were suicides was only 4.9%, while in the first-admission group, 30.6% – 3 in 10 of those who had died – had killed themselves.

Recognition that the relative importance of suicide declines over the illness course has important public health ramifications for resource allocation in schizophrenia. In a landmark 1978 study of 200 Iowa schizophrenics admitted to the University of Iowa Psychiatric Hospital between 1935 and 1944, Tsuang and Woolson (1978) showed that these individuals had an average life expectancy that was a decade shorter than the general population. Following them until 1974, when 53% had died, they found a higher than expected number of deaths due to suicide and accidents, and even though only 4% of the schizophrenics in their sample had died by suicide and a majority were not yet dead, they projected that 10% of the deaths would eventually be suicides, a projection that assumed a constant rate of suicide across the schizophrenic lifespan.

Forty years later, Capasso and colleagues replicated the Tsuang finding of reduced life expectancy, showing that mortality was even more significantly increased and lifespan even more reduced compared to Caucasian Americans of similar age, sex, and calendar year of birth (Capasso, Lineberry, Bostwick, Decker, & St. Sauver, 2008). They studied 319 schizophrenic or schizoaffective patients seen at the Mayo Clinic between 1950 and 1980, following them until 2005, when 44% of the sample had died. Their mortality plot is nearly identical to Tsuang and colleagues (Tsuang, Woolson, & Fleming, 1980), which was all the more startling because the average American's lifespan had increased by nearly 10 years during the second half of the 20th century. Capasso and colleagues shed light on other causes of death than accidents and suicide in explaining the attenuated average lifespan. Primary causes of death for 72% of the dead in their sample were medical, including cardiovascular (29%), neoplastic (19%, nearly half lung), and pulmonary disease (17%). The remainder succumbed to diabetes, stroke, and liver disease.

Known risk factors for most of these illnesses are rampant in the schizophrenic population. They point out that 70% of schizophrenics smoke cigarettes, 53% have elevated cholesterol, and 41% are physically inactive. Moreover, schizophrenics have reduced access to care. After a myocardial infarction, they are only 41% as likely to have cardiac catheterization, a procedure that is standard of care in the general population.

Only 3% of their sample had died by suicide, a number consistent with Tsuang and Woolson's 4%. Both statistics are in line with Palmer's lifetime suicide prevalence of 4.9%.

The methodologies of the two papers discussed in this chapter set the stage for what we hope will result in more accurate accounting of suicide prevalence and suicide risk in major mental illness. In neither affective disorders nor schizophrenia does suicide occur at a static rate across the lifespan. Early in the illness course, PM overestimates lifetime suicide prevalence while underscoring the outsized contribution suicide makes to early mortality. Unlike PM, which only considers the dead, CF factors in all subjects, promising greater accuracy, even as the fewer who have died, the more uncertain it is that CF approximates the true suicide rate. Whether PM or CF is used, therefore, an estimation of suicide prevalence should be taken with a grain of epidemiological salt until all subjects have died.

Even as our two papers do use sophisticated statistical techniques to arrive at more accurate projections of lifetime prevalence, the clinically useful pearl is not the figures we calculated but rather the evidence they provide for fluctuating risk depending on proximity to hospitalization and timing in the illness course. It appears that clinicians and public health specialists will be more likely to prevent suicide by investing resources in the early illness years for schizophrenics and in aftercare for both the affectively ill and the schizophrenic immediately after hospitalizations. Suicide risk conceptualized as a dynamic phenomenon offers the hope that high-risk periods can be anticipated and managed proactively, even as future research should seek to refine understanding of when these high-risk times are.

References

Andreasen, N. C., & Black, D. W. (2006). Psychiatric emergencies. In *Introductory textbook of psychiatry* (4th ed., pp. 365–378). Washington, DC: American Psychiatric Publishing.

Babigian, H. M., & Odoroff, C. L. (1969). The mortality experience of a population with psychiatric illness. *American Journal of Psychiatry, 126*, 470–480.

Bostwick, J. M., & Pankratz, V. S. (2000). Affective disorders and suicide risk: A reexamination. *American Journal of Psychiatry, 157*, 1925–1932.

Brendel, R. W., Lagomasino, I. T., Perlis, R. H., & Stern, T. A. (2008). The suicidal patient. In T. A. Stern, J. F. Rosenbaum, M. Fava, J. Biederman, & S. L. Rauch (Eds.), *Massachusetts General Hospital comprehensive clinical psychiatry* (pp. 733–745). Philadelphia: Mosby Elsevier.

Capasso, R. M., Lineberry, T. W., Bostwick, J. M., Decker, P. A., & St. Sauver, J. (2008). Mortality in schizophrenia and schizoaffective disorder: An Olmsted County, Minnesota cohort: 1950–2005. *Schizophrenia Research, 98*, 287–294.

Dubovsky, S. L., Davies, R., & Dubovsky, A. N. (2004). Mood disorders. In R. E. Hales & S. C. Yudofsky (Eds.), *Essentials of clinical psychiatry* (2nd ed., pp. 243–337). Washington, DC: American Psychiatric Press.

Fenton, W. S. (2001). Individual psychotherapies in schizophrenia. In G. O. Gabbard (Ed.), *Treatments of psychiatric disorders* (3rd ed., pp. 1045–1063). Washington, DC: American Psychiatric Press.
Goodwin, F. K., & Jamison, K. R. (1990). Suicide. In *Manic-depressive illness* (pp. 227–244). New York: Oxford University Press.
Goodwin, F. K., & Jamison, K. R. (2007). Suicide. In *Manic-depressive illness. Bipolar disorders and recurrent depression* (2nd ed., pp. 247–269). New York: Oxford University Press.
Guze, S. B., & Robins, E. (1970). Suicide and primary affective disorders. *British Journal of Psychiatry, 117*, 437–438.
Harris, E. C., & Barraclough, B. (1997). Suicide as an outcome for mental disorders: A meta-analysis. *British Journal of Psychiatry, 170*, 502–508.
Ho, B.-C., Black, D. W., & Andreasen, N. C. (2004). In R. E. Hales & S. C. Yudofsky (Eds.), *Essentials of clinical psychiatry* (2nd ed., pp. 189–241). Washington, DC: American Psychiatric Press.
Klein, D. F., & Thase, M. (1997). Medication versus psychotherapy for depression. *Progress Notes (American Society of Clinical Psychopharmacology), 8*, 41–47.
Mann, J. J. (1998). The neurobiology of suicide. *Nature Medicine, 4*, 25–30.
Melvin, G. A., Posner, K., Stanley, B. A., & Oquendo, M. A. (2008). Management of the suicidal patient. In A. Tasman, J. Kay, J. A. Lieberman, M. B. First, & M. Maj (Eds.), *Psychiatry* (3rd ed., pp. 2478–2490). West Sussex, England: Wiley-Blackwell.
Palmer, B. A., Pankratz, V. S., & Bostwick, J. M. (2005). The lifetime risk of suicide in schizophrenia: A reexamination. *Archives of General Psychiatry, 62*, 247–253.
Perlis, R. H., & Stern, T. A. (2004). Suicide. In T. A. Stern & J. B. Herman (Eds.), *Massachusetts General Hospital Psychiatry Update and Board Preparation* (2nd ed., pp. 405–410). New York: McGraw-Hill.
Shear, M. K. (2008). Death and bereavement. In A. Tasman, J. Kay, J. A. Lieberman, M. B. First, & M. Maj (Eds.), *Psychiatry* (3rd ed., pp. 2516–2525). West Sussex, England: Wiley-Blackwell.
Simpson, S. G., & Jamison, K. R. (1999). The risk of suicide in patients with bipolar disorders. *Journal of Clinical Psychiatry, 60*(Suppl. 2), 53–62.
Sudak, H. S (2005). Suicide. In B. J. Sadock & V A. Sadock (Eds.), *Kaplan & Sadock's comprehensive textbook of psychiatry* (pp. 2442–2453). Philadelphia: Lippincott Williams & Wilkins.
Tondo, L., Isacsson, G., & Baldessarini, R. J. (2003). Suicidal behavior in bipolar disorder: Risk and prevention. *CNS Drugs, 17*, 491–511.
Tsuang, M. T., & Woolson, R. F. (1978). Excess mortality in schizophrenia and affective disorders. *Archives of General Psychiatry, 35*, 1181–1185.
Tsuang, M. T., Woolson, R. F., & Fleming, J. F. (1980). Premature deaths in schizophrenia and affective disorders. *Archives of General Psychiatry, 37*, 979–983.

About the Author

Dr. John Michael Bostwick is consultant in psychiatry at the Mayo Clinic, Rochester, MN, and Professor of Psychiatry in Mayo Clinic College of Medicine. He is a member of the Aeschi Working Group, an international group of clinicians and researchers who strongly believe that new, patient-oriented models of understanding and treating suicidal patients must be developed. His foci in suicide research have included the epidemiology of suicide in affective disorders and schizophrenia, the nature of suicide in the general hospital environment, and the role of the dexamethasone suppression test in predicting eventual suicide.

J. Michael Bostwick
Mayo Clinic
200 First Street SW
Rochester, MN 55905
USA
Tel.: +1 507 284 3352
E-mail: Bostwick.John@mayo.edu

Evidence-Based Approaches for Reducing Suicide Risk in Major Affective Disorders

Isaac Sakinofsky

Department of Psychiatry and Dalla Lana School of Public Health, University of Toronto, Canada

> Suicide is never born out of exaltation or joy... The author of suicide is pain. This pain has various commonplace names: despair, loneliness, fear, anxiety, guilt, shame, depression, angst, and other more-or-less technical labels such as schizophrenia, affective disorders, depression, alcoholism, widowhood, mental illness (Shneidman, 1998).

Regardless of how momentary or drawn-out the interval from decision-making to suicide may be, no person *intentionally* takes his or her life without experiencing the cognitive equation ending in "therefore I must die." Even among those who have become resigned to their fate, dysphoria inevitably attends this equation, perhaps in the form of misery or anger mixed with despair. *Ecstatic suicide* (where the person is presumably impelled toward suicide by feelings opposite to depressed mood) is a rare curiosity in the suicide literature (Maltsberger, 1997). Shneidman labeled these painful feelings *psychache* to distinguish them from what he thought had become an overmedicalized term, *depression*, and to emphasize his belief that psychache was not necessarily a symptom of a nosologic psychiatric disorder (Pompili, Lester, Leenaars, Tatarelli, & Girardi, 2008; Shneidman, 1993, 1998). He postulated that severe mental pain arose in response to frustration of fundamental human needs, and suicide was an escape from this kind of pain. [This hypothesis goes only part of the way and does not explain the substantial group of those in mental pain who suffer from "endogenous depression," a term that is seldom employed in contemporary North American psychiatry, largely because we have moved away from dichotomizing endogenous versus nonendogenous mood disorders (Hagnell & Rorsman, 1978; Kendell, 1968) or endogenous versus exogenous (Lewis, 1979; Mayer-Gross, Slater, & Roth, 1960) or endogenous versus reactive (Carney, Roth, & Garside, 1965), it is still sometimes used even by those at the cutting edge (Mann et al., 1985), particularly in European psychiatry (Maruta, Yavdak, Denysenko, & Kharchenko, 2008). While "endogenous depression" seems unrelated to the effects of a desperate predicament impelling suicide (Sakinofsky, 2005) or negative life events, or the frustration of human needs, neurobiological mechanisms increasingly elucidate this real phenomenon. In any case a mix of endogenous and nonendogenous factors seems to account for most of the cases that we see in clinical practice and make the dichotomy pointless (Kendell, 1968).]

Orbach, Mikulincer, Sirota, and Gilboa-Schechtman (2003) developed an operational instrument (the OMMP) for measuring mental pain. Factor analysis yielded nine extracted factors; Factor 1, accounting for most of the variance (32%), expressed statements such as permanent loss, pain never going away, an unchangeable life situation, life having stopped, and pervading helplessness and hopelessness. The OMMP was tested on diagnostically comparable (major depression, bipolar depression, and psychotic depression) suicidal and nonsuicidal inpatients and on healthy community controls, and the suicidal inpatients scored significantly higher than the other two groups on "irreversibility," "loss of control," "emotional flooding," "freezing," "confusion," and "emptiness" (Orbach, Mikulincer, Gilboa-Schechtman, & Sirota, 2003).

To the psychiatrist, nonetheless, descriptors of psychache (hurt, anguish, soreness, aching, and psychological pain) *equate with depre*ssed *mood*, the term that is used professionally to indicate literally being pressed down by sadness. The Oxford English Dictionary (1992) defines depression as "a state of extreme dejection or morbidly excessive melancholy; a mood of hopelessness and feelings of inadequacy." These are emotions that are hardly distinguishable in practice from Shneidman's concept of psychache. For the purpose of organization of study and research, the psychiatrist groups all of them under the rubric of affective, mood, or depressive disorders. Hence, we are better able to strive for treatments that are evidence-based and may alleviate this kind of pain.

Cavanagh's comprehensive review of case-controlled psychological autopsy studies of suicide (Cavanagh, Carson, Sharpe, & Lawrie, 2003) showed that the median proportion of persons with affective disorder among the cases was 60% versus 10% of controls. Some form of diagnosable mental disorder was present in 90% of the cases and in 27% of controls. Harris and Barraclough (1997), in a systematic review of the follow-up studies, calculated the standardized mortality rate for the cases of major depression (DSM-III-R) as > 20 times that expected in the general public. For bipolar disorder, it was 15, dysthymia 12, mood disorders N0S 16, anxiety disorder 10, adjustment disorder NOS 15, and personality disorder (ICD-9) 7.

Early meta-analyses of observational follow-up studies of affective disorder estimated the ultimate suicide risk as 15–19% (Goodwin & Jamison, 1990; Guze & Robins, 1970; Miles, 1977), but these estimates have been periodically revised downward. Using contemporary data, the estimated lifetime risk of suicide in affective disorder reduced to 6% (Inskip, Harris, & Barraclough, 1998), but when outpatients were taken into account it was even lower, 3.5% (Blair-West, Mellsop, & Eyeson-Annan, 1997). This figure was almost identical to the estimations drawn up by Blair-West and colleagues who found the lifetime risk for suicide in an affective disorder in men to be 7% and in women to be 1%, respectively, with a combined risk of 3.4% (Blair-West, Cantor, Mellsop, & Eyeson-Annan, 1999). The male-to-female ratio for suicide risk in major depression in youths < 25 years was 10:1 and for adults this ratio was 5.6:1. Earlier studies had estimated *proportionate mortality* (the proportion of all deaths in the cohort attributable to suicide) and were criticized by Bostwick and Pankratz (2000) who applied *case fatality prevalences* (the proportion of the original cohort who ultimately succumbed to suicide) to the earlier studies and obtained lifetime risks of 8.6% in those affective disorder patients ever hospitalized for suicide risk, as compared with 4% for those hospitalized without specification of suicidality. For mixed inpatient/outpatient populations, it was 2.2% and for the nonaffectively ill population it was < 0.5% (Bostwick & Pankratz, 2000). Even though smaller than previously thought of, the suicide risk in patients with affective illness remains significant, and being hospitalized for suicide risk confers twice the risk of ultimately dying by suicide on affective disordered patients as compared with being hospitalized for the same illness without indications of suicidal thinking or behavior.

This chapter reviews the evidence that psychiatric treatment benefits suicidality (suicidal ideation, attempts, or completions) in affective disorders (i.e., ICD F30-F39) or mood disorders (DSM-IV-TR). Mood disorders encompass a wide variety of subtypes in DSM, including major depressive disorder (single episode and recurrent), dysthymia disorder, depressive disorder NOS, bipolar I disorder, bipolar II disorder, cyclothymic disorder, bipolar disorder NOS, schizoaffective disorder, and other mood disorders (due to medical conditions or substance induced). Then, there are such orphans of the DSM classification system as recurrent brief depressive episodes (ICD F 38.1) and depressive personality disorder (DSM-IV-TR, Appendix B). The latter was included among the proposals for new categories in DSM-IV that did not quite make adoption. These subtypes of mood disorders may not be mutually exclusive in practice, but have been separately delineated to facilitate interprofessional communication and research. Researchers are only lately performing prospective evaluation studies with suicide-related variables as their primary or even secondary outcomes of interest. Most of the evidence that we have for the effectiveness of treatments on suicidality in mood disorders has been obtained by the retrospective analysis of cohort studies or pharmaceutical trials that were primarily designed to test for the efficacy of compounds in treating such conditions as major depressive disorder (Oquendo & Mann, 2003). In these retrospective studies, a diligent collection of the data on nonfatal suicidality varies greatly between studies and may be unreliable. There are valid reasons for the paucity of trials that include ethical concerns and the low base rate for completed suicide that would necessitate impossibly large sample sizes (Gunnell & Frankel, 1994; Oquendo & Mann, 2003). This holds even for evaluating the suicide attempts, although these occur 28 times as frequently as suicide (Sakinofsky & Webster, 2010). For example, the international multicenter study for the evaluation of clozapine as an antisuicide agent in schizophrenia and schizoaffective disorders (InterSePT) utilized as endpoints completed suicide, suicide attempt, or requiring hospitalization to prevent an attempt. The sample size was 980, which would ordinarily be regarded as large. Although the study had sufficient power to enable it to demonstrate the significant effect for clozapine versus the comparator drug for nonfatal suicidality, the number of completed suicides in both study arms was too small to show a significant difference between the two drugs (Meltzer et al., 2003). Pooled data studies and meta-analyses of smaller studies are therefore often resorted to; but they too have their difficulties as regards heterogeneity of the underlying samples and research designs.

The most robust evidence for a specific effect of treatment on suicidality is with bipolar affective disorder and is reviewed in the next section. Even here, there is a dearth of evidence for or against antisuicidal properties of the commonly used drugs such as valproate, lamotrigine, SSRIs, and antipsychotics (Oquendo, Chaudhury, & Mann, 2005a). All the findings that are reported in this chapter about the treatment of suicidality across the mood disorders result from a systematic search of the literature that includes the Cochrane Library (which contains systematic reviews and a register of randomized controlled trials (RCTs) and meta-analyses culled from MEDLINE, EMBASE, CINAHL, PsycLIT, PSYNDEX, and LILACS). MEDLINE, EMBASE, and the author's personal database called SUICDATA were also individually searched. SUICDATA is the author's personal database on suicide-related topics in which are stored the citations and abstracts that were drawn weekly from MEDLINE and the ISI Web of Science for over 30 years. This database is further supplemented by other resources that have been gathered from the continuing self-directed medical education on suicide-related issues over the years, and currently totaling 50,602 entries.

The Web of Science search terms that contributed to the above-mentioned database were "suic*, attempted suic*, parasuicide, and self harm." For searching the Cochrane Library, the term "suicide" was used (797 studies of clinical trials where suicide cropped up in the title or abstract) and for MEDLINE search, the terms "suicide" or "attempted suicide" (38,152 hits), "affective" or "mood" (65,735), and "treatment" (608). Affective or mood combined with controlled trials yielded 40 studies. EMBASE, 1980–2009, yielded 7,850 references for affective or mood combined with suicidal behavior or suicidal attempt (30,618), and treatment and trial, 1,803. EMBASE, 1940–1979, ultimately yielded 57 studies. All the yields from the other databases were downloaded as text files and merged into SUICDATA, from which the relevant searches for this report were carried out and compiled, and finally the titles and abstracts were handsearched for those studies where suicidality was an outcome of interest, even though not necessarily the primary one.

In keeping with the hierarchy of evidence adopted throughout this book, the descending order of evidence will be systematic reviews and meta-analyses; RCTs with definitive results (i.e., confidence intervals that do not overlap the threshold, clinically significant effect); RCTs with nondefinitive results; cohort studies; case-control studies; cross-sectional surveys and, finally, case reports.

Bipolar Affective Disorder

As many as one fifth of the bipolar patients would eventually take their own lives (Goodwin & Jamison, 1990). The WHO Global Burden of Disease study ranked bipolar disorder sixth among all medical disorders in years of life lost to death or disability (Chavez-Leon, 2004). In the life of a patient suffering from bipolar disorder, considerably more time is spent depressed than manic (Post, 2005; Suppes, Kelly, & Perla, 2005; Thase, 2005) and the vast majority of suicides occur during depressive or mixed episodes; but there has been little evaluation of antisuicide properties in other drugs that are commonly used aside from lithium (Oquendo, Chaudhury, & Mann, 2005b).

Hawton, Sutton, Haw, Sinclair, and Harriss (2005) systematically reviewed studies reporting the risk factors for suicidality in bipolar affective disorder. Predictors for *completed suicide* included being male, having a family history of an affective disorder or suicide, a history of a previous suicide attempt, and hopelessness expressed at the admission to hospital. There was no association with rapid cycling or any sign of having suffered a psychotic disorder during their illness. The risk factors were somewhat different for *attempted suicide* or *deliberate self-harm*, and notably included being single, having a diagnosis of bipolar II disorder rather than bipolar I, being admitted to hospital as a result of depression, increasing severity of depressive or manic episodes, comorbid anxiety disorder, substance misuse, comorbid eating disorder, and having a mixed affective state at presentation (Hawton et al., 2005). A past history of a suicide attempt is probably the strongest predictor (Marangell et al., 2006; Valtonen et al., 2006), together with recurrent or refractory depressions (Oquendo, Currier, & Mann, 2006) and the percentage of days the person was depressed in the past year (Marangell et al., 2006).

It is salutary that 60% of bipolar suicide cases whose treatment was evaluated in an Australian study (Keks et al., 2009) "did not receive treatment at or above a benchmark standard, often due to illness and situational factors, but also possibly due to inadequate clinical interventions." The above-mentioned study identified 35 bipolar subjects from among the 3,752 suicides whose details were taken from coroners' records. The mean duration of illness was 12 years, and 86% had made at least one previous suicide attempt. The vast majority of patients (87%) were in the depressed phase at the time of death, 10% in mixed states, and only one patient (3%) suicided while manic (confirming the previous findings by Black, Winokur, & Nasrallah, 1987). The final episode was immediately preceded by hypomania in half of the cases. The duration of the preceding depressive episodes was quite short: < 1 month in half of the subjects and < 2 months in three-quarters of the subjects. Death occurred in 57% of the patients, while either still in hospital or within 6 weeks following discharge. Lithium had only been given to 11% at therapeutic levels and 31% had never been treated with it. Only 4 of 35 underwent a trial of electroconvulsive therapy (ECT) during the last episode. Psychosocial interventions in the year of death in 57% of cases did not meet the standards of adequacy set by the evaluative panel (meet with a designated clinician at least monthly). All in all, inadequacy both in pharmacotherapy and follow-up were the salient factors identified. However, problems with regard to treatment adherence were also noticed in half of the patients during the last 4 weeks, and an assertive outreach could have been, but was not, provided. Clearly, this study should put all the physicians on the alert with regard to regular follow-up and adequate treatment of their bipolar patients. It is significant that a manic illness preceded the depression in about half of the cases: With bipolar patients, it is likely that they would be admitted during the manic phase, but may go relatively unnoticed during the succeeding period of depression, which may supervene after discharge.

Pharmacotherapy

Lithium

Lithium continues to be the recommended first-line pharmacotherapy for bipolar disorder; despite being so its actual use still seems to be on the decline (Baldessarini & Tondo, 2009b; Blanco, Laje, Olfson, Marcus, & Pincus, 2002; Grandjean & Aubry, 2009a; Grof & Muller-Oerlinghausen, 2009). In an early multicenter study of mortality with lithium-treated patients, Muller-Oerlinghausen and colleagues retrospectively analyzed the risk among the affective patients who were treated in lithium clinics for an average of nearly 7 years and found the risk comparable to that in the general public (standardized mortality ratio, SMR = 0.89) (Muller-Oerlinghausen, Ahrens, et al., 1992). The overall mortality risk normalizes during the second year of lithium treatment (Grof & Muller-Oerlinghausen, 2009; Ahrens, Muller-Oerlinghausen, & Grof, 1993). A second study by these colleagues was focused on a subset of high-risk patients with a history of at least one suicide attempt prior to lithium treatment and compared the frequency of suicidal events on and off lithium treatment (Muller-Oerlinghausen, Muser-Causemann, & Volk, 1992). The frequency of suicide attempts dropped steeply during lithium treatment, particularly in the lithium responders but also in the nonresponders. Two patients completed suicide while on lithium, one a responder and the other a nonresponder, and four other patients suicided after discontinuation of lithium by their psychiatrists.

In 2005, Cipriani and colleagues in a Cochrane review systematically assessed 32 RCTs of the use of lithium in treating mood disorders (bipolar disorder and the broad spectrum of mood disorders) and identified seven of these studies that specifically reported suicide events, even though these events were not the primary outcome of interest (Cipriani, Pretty, Hawton, & Geddes, 2005). They concluded that patients who received lithium were less likely to die by suicide (2 suicides in the lithium arm and 11 among the comparators, odds ratio = 0.26; 95% CI = 0.09–0.77). A composite measure that included suicide and deliberate self-harm also favored lithium (odds ratio = 0.21; 95% CI = 0.08–0.50). However, only seven acts of deliberate self-harm were reported, probably indicative of underreporting, given the fact that acts of suicidality were not the primary outcome variable. There were also fewer deaths from all causes in patients who received lithium. But opposite conclusions were arrived at in a British NIHR evaluation study (Soares-Weiser et al., 2007) that had reviewed the clinical application and the cost-effectiveness of 45 controlled trials of relapse prevention in bipolar illness by pharmacological and psychosocial means. While the study concluded that lithium, lamotrigine, valproate, and olanzapine were significantly better for the prevention of all relapses than placebo (there were different findings for manic and depressive relapses specifically),

> there is insufficient information to permit any meaningful assessment of the relative tolerability of the treatments or their relative effects on suicide rate and mortality (Soares-Weiser et al., 2007).

Notwithstanding the overcautious conclusion of the above mentioned study, Baldessarini and Tondo published data on individual and pooled relative risks (RR) and risk differences (RD) for 34 relevant studies that their group had accumulated (Baldessarini & Tondo,

2009a). Their previous meta-analysis (Baldessarini et al., 2006) yielded 45 studies providing data on the rates of suicidal acts during lithium treatment; but only 34 of these also provided an arm without lithium therapy and only 31 of 34 were considered for inclusion in the meta-analysis after assessing their methodological quality. Three further studies were now able to be culled, in addition, from two published papers (Collins & McFarland, 2008; Yerevanian, Koek, & Mintz, 2007). For combined suicidal risks (suicide and attempted suicide), the revised, pooled RR value was 4.14 (95% CI = 3.02–5.67; $z = 8.82$, $p < .0001$) with and without lithium treatment. The recomputed value of RR for the effects of lithium on completed suicide only was 3.97 (95% CI = 2.65–5.93; 26 contrasts; $z = 6.71$, $p < .0001$) and on attempted suicide it was 4.74 (95% CI = 2.97–7.58; 19 contrasts; $z = 6.52$, $p < .0001$). Lower suicidal risks were demonstrated as well by meta-analytic derivations of RD (also called excess risk or attributable risk), the values which were positive in the 34 individual studies. The pooled RD for completed suicide and attempted suicide combined was 4.42% (95% CI = 4.06–4.77; 34 contrasts; $z = 24.5$, $p < .0001$), and the number needed to treat (NNT) was 23 (indicating that to avoid a suicidal act in one person, 23 patients would need to be treated with lithium). For completed suicide, the RD was 2.24% and the NNT 45, and for attempted suicide the RD was 5.16% and the NNT 19. [Note that an NNT $\leq$ 10 is usually considered as desirable.]

A recent Danish register linkage study provides an approximation of the degree of antisuicidal efficacy afforded by lithium in treating bipolar disorders in practice (Sondergard, Lopez, Andersen, & Kessing, 2008). All patients in Denmark who were discharged with the diagnosis of bipolar disorder from 1995 to 2000 were included in the investigation ($N = 5926$), yielding 51 suicides that took place during the study period. Although suicide rates were higher during periods when patients purchased anticonvulsants versus lithium (favoring lithium, 293 versus 136 per 100,000 person-years), the rates decreased similarly for both forms of pharmacotherapy in proportion to the number of prescriptions purchased. In patients initiated on anticonvulsants, switching to/augmenting with lithium was accompanied by a significantly reduced suicide rate (rate ratio = 0.28), but switching to/augmenting with anticonvulsant mood stabilizers by patients already on lithium had no effect, indicating lithium's antisuicidal superiority. Nonadherence to treatment was a problem in the Danish study: 27% of the bipolar patients and an identical proportion of the suicides did not purchase any mood stabilizers following discharge from inpatient or outpatient status of the hospital. Almost half of the suicided bipolar patients (43.1%) had lost touch with their psychiatric caregivers at the time of their suicide. A previous study by the same group also showed that discontinuation of lithium treatment is common: 25% stopped their treatment after about 6 weeks (Kessing, Sondergard, Kvist, & Andersen, 2007), underlining the major problem of lack of continuing adherence to treatment by bipolar patients and the need for continued psychosocial and psychoeducational input.

What may be the first prospective placebo-controlled trial of the efficacy of lithium in preventing suicidality in mood disorders ran into ethical constraints that may have led to a Type II error. Lauterbach et al. (2008) selected individuals from hospital emergency departments with a depressive spectrum diagnosis who had attempted suicide during the previous quarter and randomized them to treatment with lithium or placebo. Patients with borderline personality disorder with severe self-harm or substance disorders were excluded as were those with a clear indication for continued lithium treatment. Although 1,550 patients were assessed, only 167 (18%) could be randomized and this residual group was clearly without those patients classically treated with lithium, such as patients with bipolar disorder or recurrent affective illness. The small N so depleted the power of the study that only 14 suicide attempts (7 in each group) were counted over the follow-up year (Lauterbach et al., 2008). There was an excess of patients with personality disorders and with a previous history of multiple suicide attempts in the lithium compared to the placebo group, conceivably biasing the sample in favor of the placebo arm. The three cases of completed suicide, however, all occurred in the placebo arm, a narrowly significant difference ($p < .049$), leading the authors to arrive at the conclusion that this study supports lithium's antisuicidal effect. They argue that lithium exerts this effect by suppressing aggressivity and impulsivity.

Lithium has weathered controversies about its efficacy and has been shown to be helpful for mood stabilization, as an antimanic agent, or for augmenting antidepressants and preventing relapse in bipolar and recurrent depressive illnesses. It has now also been shown to be effective in preventing suicide in bipolar disorder, irrespective of whether the person is a "lithium-responder" or not (Grof & Muller-Oerlinghausen, 2009). Lithium is often referred to as "the cornerstone" or "keystone" of treatment in bipolar disorder. Why then is its popularity waning among physicians who prescribe medication for bipolar disorder?

The answer to this question must surely be complex and should include a marketing analysis of lithium versus alternative mood stabilizers (Goodwin et al., 2003). At the same time, we must recognize that the potential side effects and long-term complications of taking lithium may be daunting for both physician and patient. Grandjean extensively discussed the evidence pertaining to the safety of lithium (Grandjean & Aubry, 2009b). Typical complaints of patients on long-term therapy with lithium include gastrointestinal symptoms (discomfort, pain, and diarrhea), tremor, polyuria, nocturnal urination, psoriasis, and weight gain (30% of patients gain weight up to 10 kg). Nephrogenic diabetes insipidus may be a long-term sequela, and the glomerular filtration rate falls in 20% of patients. The risk increases with comorbid diseases and polypharmacy. Impairment in concentrating ability occasionally progresses to advanced chronic kidney disease from tubulointerstitial nephropathy. Biopsy and MRI findings in such cases include tubular atrophy and interstitial fibrosis interspersed with tubular cysts and dilatations (Grandjean & Aubry, 2009b; Kincaid-Smith et al., 1979; Markowitz et al., 2000). Cysts are in fact seen in 33–33% of patients undergoing long-term lithium therapy (Tuazon et al., 2008). The prevalence of overt and subclinical hypothyroidism may be increased, with circulating thyroid autoantibodies often found. Thyrotoxicosis also sometimes occurs, as well as hyperparathyroidism, hypercalcemia, or hypomagnesemia (Grandjean & Aubry, 2009b). Amiloride has been shown to improve the renal concentrating ability of lithium patients (Bedford et al., 2008).

These side effects and complications may be deterrents to prescribing practitioners and yet need to be balanced against the robust finding that lithium has been shown to normalize the overall mortality from all causes (not only suicide) among the long-term bipolar patients. It is important to balance the seriousness of nephrotoxicity against the fact that it is known to be relatively uncommon. One estimation of the frequency of drug-induced nephrogenic diabetes insipidus is that it may affect about 10% of patients treated long term (15 years or more). In this study (Bendz & Aurell, 1999), a search of the WHO adverse affect database also yielded only 159 reports – but these reports are not submitted systematically. Schou once declared that "systematically collected data indicates that even long-term treatment does not induce renal insufficiency" (Schou & Schou, 1997). The truth must lie somewhere in between these extremes of opinion. Gitlin commented that reviews of the effects of lithium on renal function have generally asserted the fact that no clinically significant effect on glomerular function is apparent even after many years; yet, a handful of studies persist to indicate the fact that a small minority of lithium-treated patients may develop rising levels of creatinine in the serum after a decade or more of treatment. His sample of 82 bipolar patients from a mood disorders clinic yielded 3 patients (3.7%) who developed creatinine levels in the serum above 2 mg per 100 ml and one of these patients progressed to hemodialysis (Gitlin, 1993). The risks and benefits must be clearly explained to the patients beforehand and a regular monitoring of the creatinine levels and the thyroid function at appropriate intervals needs to be maintained for as long as they are taking the drug.

Anticonvulsants

In the US, only lithium and lamotrigine have been licensed for the long-term maintenance treatment of bipolar disorder. While the prescriptions for lithium have been showing a decline in office-based psychiatric practice, those for divalproex (valproic acid and valproate) as a first-line maintenance therapy have been showing an increase (Baldessarini & Tondo, 2009b; Blanco et al., 2002). Greater educational promotion of valproate by pharmaceutical organizations targeting younger professionals may be a factor (Goodwin et al., 2003); but it is also possible, as stated above, that considerations of weight gain, cognitive dulling, or serious nephrotoxic effects in a minority of patients on lithium treatment (Alexander, Farliq, Mittal, Rennke, & Singh, 2008; Kincaid-Smith et al., 1979; Markowitz et al., 2000) could deter physicians and patients, even though lithium is considered to be safe and effective for the majority of patients when properly managed (Belmaker, 2004; Johnson, 1999; McCann, Daly, & Kelly, 2008). This being said, it is important to know whether anticonvulsants could provide the same protection against suicidal events as lithium.

There are relatively few evidence-based studies on the efficacy of maintenance therapy with anticonvulsants in suicide event reduction in bipolar disorder. Thies-Flechtner et al. undertook a prospective multicenter RCT in which patients with current episodes of bipolar disorder or schizoaffective disorder were randomized to prophylactic treatment with lithium or carbamazepine for 2.5 years (Thies-Flechtner, Muller-Oerlinghausen, Seibert,

Walther, & Greil, 1996). There were six suicides and one case of attempted suicide resulting in the bipolar group (N = 175) and two suicides and four attempts in the schizoaffective group (N = 110). None of the suicide events occurred in those who were taking lithium, but the suicides were evenly divided between those who were on carbamazepine or other medications (antidepressants, neuroleptics, or none at all). The suicide rate in participants taking carbamazepine was not different from what might have been expected in untreated bipolar patients.

Baldessarini and Tondo (2009b) carried out a meta-analysis of six controlled studies comparing lithium to anticonvulsants with nonzero risk of suicide or attempts as one of the outcomes. The anticonvulsants tested included carbamazepine, lamotrigine, and divalproex. Three of the studies (Bowden et al., 2003; Calabrese et al., 2003; Greil et al., 1997) were RCTs and three were chart reviews of nonrandomized, uncontrolled material (Collins & McFarland, 2008a; Goodwin et al., 2003; Yerevanian, Koek, & Mintz, 2003). Unfortunately, pooled rates were not calculated separately to distinguish the RCTs and chart studies, which clearly represent different levels of scientific evidence. A Forest plot of the risk ratios (RR) in the six studies favored lithium in every case. The problem in interpretation pertains to the fact that the suicide events were very infrequent in the RCTs (N = 0–2 in each arm), and the results must therefore be treated with caution. Greil et al. (1997) compared lithium versus carbamazepine in groups of 70 and 74 patients with bipolar affective disorder. At initiation, the lithium group reported 43% of participants with suicide events versus 34% in the carbamazepine group, but at study termination 2.5 years later there were zero events in the lithium arm and only one suicide and one attempt recorded in the carbamazepine group (computed RR 5.28). The other two RCTs shared the same research design, comparing relapse prevention with lithium or lamotrigine in bipolar patients with a recent manic (Bowden et al., 2003) or a recent depressed episode (Calabrese et al., 2003). In the first of these studies (patients recently diagnosed as manic), there was an imbalance for each study arm for a previous history of suicide attempts (percent of cases: lithium, 41%; placebo, 19%; and lamotrigine, data not supplied). This imbalance merits attention, given the fact that the strongest predictor of a future suicidal event is the previous history of same. No imbalance was reported in the Calabrese et al. study of the recently depressed bipolar patients, with 35% across study arms reporting previous suicide events. In the Bowden study, one patient in the lamotrigine group was reported to have attempted suicide (RR 2.35), and in the Calabrese study one death post-randomization in the lamotrigine group and one suicide attempt in the placebo arm (RR 2.14) were recorded. Small numbers such as these counsel caution while interpreting the results, in spite of the computed risk ratios on hand. These figures were arrived at based on the fact that suicidality was not included as an outcome at the outset of the study.

The other three studies were retrospective cohort chart reviews that were drawn up with the specific aim of comparing the risk of suicide attempt or suicide death in patients during treatment with lithium with that during treatment with anticonvulsants. Goodwin et al.'s (2003) investigation of two large managed care databases was by far the largest (N = 20,638), and consequently the suicidal outcome results were even greater (53 suicides and 980 attempts), giving the analysis a stronger statistical power. The risk of suicide death was 2.7 times greater during treatment with divalproex than with lithium after adjustment for possible confounders; for attempts with hospitalization, the hazard ratio was 1.7 and for attempts diagnosed in the ER but not admitted it was 1.8. The second study dealt with Medicaid bipolar patients ($N = 12{,}662$) and compared lithium, divalproex, gabapentin, and carbamazepine (Collins & McFarland, 2008). The recipients of lamotrigine and oxcarbazepine were too few (1.5%) to yield meaningful analysis. The RR for completed suicide was 2.6 for treatment with gabapentin versus lithium and 1.5 (NS) with divalproex. It was 2.74 for divalproex versus lithium in suicide attempts ($p < .001$). The third study culled bipolar patients from the private practice records of the senior investigator ($N = 140$) (Yerevanian et al., 2003). There was only one completed suicide (in a patient who had stopped taking his lithium). Suicide attempt rates/100 person-years for lithium did not vary significantly with those for carbamazepine or valproate in this study but rates of suicidal behavior were also compared with/without mood-stabilizing medications and were found to be significantly greater (a twofold increase) when not taking these medications. These investigators replicated their study using a larger sample ($N = 405$) (Yerevanian, Koek, & Mintz, 2007) and found the same results as in their earlier study. Taken as a whole, these retrospective studies favor the suicide-protective effect of lithium over other anticonvulsants and comprise much larger samples than would be possible with RCTs; but their conclusions are of course weakened by the investigations being nonrandomized and retrospective.

Geddes, Calabrese, and Goodwin (2009) undertook a systematic review and meta-analysis of the efficacy of lamotrigine versus placebo in bipolar depression based on five RCTs ($N = 1072$). Lamotrigine was modestly superior in relieving depression; this was more so in severe than in milder cases of bipolar depression (Geddes et al., 2009).

Oquendo recently reported the first prospective investigation comparing lithium and divalproex for suicidal behavior in high-risk bipolar attempters who were recruited in depressed or mixed phase and followed up for 2.5 years (Oquendo, 2007, 2009). Thirty-four percent of the sample recorded a suicidal event during follow-up, defined as suicide completion, attempts, or ideation with the plan requiring intervention. No overall differences were observed in the rates of suicidal events or attempts between the lithium and divalproex groups but, when the sample was split into those older and younger than 41, a greater protective effect of lithium was found for the older group. The age differences could not be explained by the inpatient status or by the presence of borderline personality disorder among younger patients. [This study has unfortunately so far only been available as an abstract.] The British systematic evaluation of relapse prevention in bipolar disorder found no difference in preventing new episodes between lithium and valproate or lamotrigine, but lithium was found to be superior to carbamazepine and imipramine. No placebo-controlled trials were available for testing the efficacy of carbamazepine and so its independent effectiveness over placebo could not be tested. The review could not arrive at a conclusion on the prevention of suicide or suicide attempts because the included trials did not provide the relevant data (Soares-Weiser et al., 2007).

Yet another observational cohort study of bipolar disorder patients employed register linkage of data on psychiatric diagnoses, pharmacoepidemiological data, and data on suicide (N = 5,926, 51 completed suicides) (Sondergard et al., 2008). Interestingly, 20% of these bipolar disorder patients did not purchase any mood-stabilizing drug after having been discharged from the hospital with the diagnosis of bipolar disorder; and even from among those who had purchased lithium or anticonvulsants, 5% and 7.5%, respectively, did so only once. Lithium monotherapy was present in 15% and in 36% monotherapy with anticonvulsants, highlighting the finding that use of lithium appears to be on the decline *vis-à-vis* other mood stabilizers. The suicide rates were higher when the patients purchased anticonvulsants than when purchasing lithium. Poisson regression analyses of suicide rates related to treatment showed that purchasing prescriptions twice or more times was associated with a decreased rate of suicide relative to single purchases. In both treatment groups, the suicide risk decreased with increasing number of prescriptions, that is, with presumed adherence. In patients initiated to treatment on anticonvulsants, a switch to or augmentation with lithium was associated with a significantly reduced suicide risk, but the reverse showed no additional effect on the suicide rate. The authors concluded that although both treatments are beneficial, there may be some advantage to lithium. Finally, one of the STEP-BD (Systematic Treatment Enhancement Program for Bipolar Disorder) studies (Goldberg et al., 2009) showed that bipolar patients on a combination regime of four or more agents (20% of the sample) were more likely to be struggling with bipolar depression and suicidality or to have been prescribed atypical antipsychotics. Use of traditional mood stabilizers (lithium, divalproex, or carbamazepine) was less likely to be associated with polypharmacy of four or more agents.

Antidepressants

A controversy exists over the use of *antidepressants in bipolar depression*. A considerable body of opinion holds the view that antidepressants worsen the outcome in bipolar disorder, thereby contributing to higher suicide risk, particularly in patients aged < 25 years, where bipolar disorder may masquerade as unipolar depression prior to being unmasked by a first attack of hypomania (O'Donovan, Garnham, Hajek, & Alda, 2008; Seemuller, Severus, Moller, & Riedel, 2009). The predominantly depressive polarity is associated with treatment with antidepressants during the long delay before diagnosis is made (Colom, Vieta, Daban, Pacchiarotti, & Sanchez-Moreno, 2006; Rosa et al., 2008). The mood state in bipolar I and II patients who are predominantly depressed and also have hypomanic features that are subsyndromal for mixed states may be worsened by antidepressant therapy, but respond to a combination of antipsychotics and mood stabilizers (Aizenberg et al., 2006; Keck, McIntyre, & Shelton, 2007). Yerevanian and colleagues, in a retrospective chart review (Yerevanian, Koek, Mintz, & Akiskal, 2007), found that rates of suicidal behavior were increased in patients taking antidepressants, and the only completed suicide in their sample was in a patient taking lithium combined with an antidepressant. However, these findings are tempered by the absence of randomization to different treatments in this study and may have been confounded by indication (patients with preexisting suicidality having been selected to receive antidepressant treatment).

Antidepressants also risk *switching* an episode of depression to mania (Post, 2005; Suppes et al., 2005), paradoxically incurring the risk of emergent suicidality, intensifying existing suicidality, or inducing rapid cycling (Yerevanian, Koek, Mintz, & Akiskal, 2007). Switching was found to be more likely (probability of 10%) with patients taking tricyclic antidepressants (Prien, Klett, & Caffey, 1973) and in the last two decades TCAs have therefore seldom been used in bipolar patients. The 2002 APA guidelines for treatment of bipolar depression advised that either lithium or lamotrigine be the first-line monotherapy (Hirschfeld et al., 2002). A Cochrane review and meta-analysis (Gijsman, Geddes, Rendell, Nolen, & Goodwin, 2004) analyzed 12 RCTs: five of these RCTs compared antidepressants with placebo, four of these RCTs compared an antidepressant with another antidepressant, and the remainder compared antidepressants with other medications. The trials were all relatively short term. The rate of switching to mania for TCAs was 10% and for all other antidepressants 3.2%. Antidepressants proved effective in the short-term treatment of bipolar depression. Ensuing correspondence defended the 2002 APA recommendations against using antidepressants, particularly given the fact that the RCTs reviewed by Gijsman and colleagues were short term and had not considered the emerging positive trials for lamotrigine (Ghaemi & Goodwin, 2005; Gijsman, Geddes, Rendell, Goodwin, & Nolen, 2005; Hirschfeld, Fochtmann, & McIntyre, 2005; Maharaj & Parasram, 1989).

Canadian guidelines (updated for 2009) recommend lithium, lamotrigine, or quetiapine as monotherapy, or olanzapine plus an SSRI, and lithium or divalproex plus an SSRI or bupropion as first-line options for bipolar depression (Yatham et al., 2009). The UK National Institute for Health and Clinical Excellence (NICE) guidelines (2006) recommend lithium, olanzapine, or valproate as monotherapy or if necessary in combination for the long-term management of bipolar disorder. In cases of bipolar depression that are moderate or severe, an SSRI (not paroxetine in pregnant women) or quetiapine (the latter if taking an antimanic drug that is not antipsychotic). Antidepressants should be avoided in rapid-cycling bipolar disorder, recent hypomanic episode, or recent functionally impairing rapid mood fluctuations. When antidepressants are used, the patient should be told about the possibility of manic or hypomanic switching. In such cases where antidepressants are to be avoided, the dose of the antimanic drug should be raised and a second one possibly added (including lamotrigine). Contrary to the American Psychiatric Association (APA) and Canadian Network for Mood and Anxiety Treatments (CANMAT) guidelines, lamotrigine is expressly not recommended in the NICE guidelines as monotherapy for routine maintenance in bipolar I disorder.

Of the first 425 participants (out of 2000) in the STEP-BD who developed fresh depressive episodes during an 18-month follow-up, only 6% had emergent suicidality (including two attempts and no fatalities) and there was no association with antidepressant treatment (Bauer et al., 2006). Grunze (2008) reviewed the evidence for antidepressants inducing switching, rapid cycling, and the probability of suicidality with antidepressants in bipolar patients and concluded that it had been overinterpreted; but, on the other hand, there was no strong evidence either to prove that antidepressants were effective as monotherapy for bipolar depression (Grunze, 2008). He also concluded that the risk of antidepressants causing switching or inducing rapid cycling and new-onset suicidality may have been overstated. The STEP-BD trial of adjunctive antidepressant therapy combined with a mood stabilizer versus a mood stabilizer combined with placebo gave further support to Grunze's view that antidepressants were relatively innocuous, but also ineffective (Sachs et al., 2007). Either paroxetine or bupropion was selected as the antidepressant for the trial because of its reputation for being associated with low rates of switching to mania or hypomania. The main outcome criterion to be met was 8 consecutive weeks of euthymia. Only 24% in the mood stabilizer plus antidepressant arm and 27% in the mood stabilizer plus placebo arm met this criterion by the end of the 26-week study, not significantly different. The rate of hospitalization for suicidal ideation was identical in both groups (2.5%). A better outlook for antidepressant treatment was reported comparing monotherapy with an antidepressant (fluoxetine or venlafaxine) in a series of studies of bipolar type II versus unipolar patients, the bipolar II patients faring at least as well as the unipolar patients (Amsterdam & Brunswick, 2003). Suicidality was not alluded to in this report. Depressed patients with bipolar II disorder seem less vulnerable to switch into hypomania or mania than bipolar I patients. In a 10-week trial of antidepressants (bupropion, sertraline, or venlafaxine) as an adjunct to mood stabilizers (lithium, valproate, or carbamazepine) in outpatients with bipolar depression, the switch rate was 12% for bipolar I and 2% for bipolar II patients (Altshuler et al., 2006).

McElroy, Kotwal, Kaneria, and Keck (2006) pointed out that there were no published prospective RCTs of antidepressants in bipolar disorders that evaluated *suicidality* as a primary outcome measure and that suicidality was usually an exclusion criterion for treatment studies of bipolar disorder. Suicidality as a secondary outcome was also neglected in treatment investigations (McElroy et al., 2006). The review found that five of the eight studies reported a positive relationship between antidepressant treatment and increased suicidality in patients with probable or definite bipolarity; but the association could also be explained by confounding by indication (the higher rate of suicidality in these patients may have led to their higher rate of antidepressant exposure). These studies also suggested some protection against emergent suicidality when antidepressants were combined with mood stabilizers, particularly lithium.

Prevailing guidelines suggest only cautious use of antidepressants in bipolar depression and never without combining with an anticonvulsant/mood stabilizer or antipsychotic (Fountoulakis, Grunze, Panagiotidis, & Kaprinis, 2008). In surely one of the longest naturalistic follow-up investigations of mood disorders (40–44 years), suicides occurred in 11% (SMR = 17.5). This study found antidepressants to be protective against suicide (the SMR for treated versus untreated depressed patients was 13.8 versus 33.3, $p < .05$). However in 68% of cases, the antidepressants were combined with neuroleptics, of which two thirds were atypical (clozapine or thioridazine). There were significantly fewer suicides among the medicated group, irrespective of whether they were treated with lithium, neuroleptics, or antidepressants. Even though the untreated group was shown to have been less seriously ill at the beginning of the prospective observation period, relatively more suicide cases were seen (Angst, Angst, Gerber-Werder, & Gamma, 2005). In another naturalistic follow-up of bipolar I and II patients (from Rome) (Tundo, Marchetti, & Lega, 2006), antidepressants did not contribute negatively to the outcome in suicidality during treatment. In EMBLEM, a European prospective, observational study on the outcomes of patients with a mixed or manic episode, one third of the mixed state patients were treated with antidepressants at baseline and throughout a 2-year follow-up period (Azorin et al., 2009). In any case, whatever available evidence might suggest that antidepressants should be used less frequently in patients with bipolar disorder, there is a large gap between the existence of this evidence and clinical practice in the real world (Schaffer, Cairney, & Veldhuizen, 2006).

Electroconvulsive Therapy

There are no studies that have specifically examined suicidality in cases of bipolar depression treated with ECT. Since the majority of suicides among bipolar patients occur during the depressive phase, it is arguable that any treatment that is effective in bipolar depression will reduce suicidality. Thase (2005) recommended venlafaxine, tranylcypramine, or ECT as options for refractory depressive episodes (Thase, 2005). Daly et al. (2001) compared ECT in unipolar and bipolar depression, and found no difference (after controlling for covariates) in the rates of response or remission; but the bipolar patients responded more quickly and required less treatments, a finding repeated by Sackeim (2005) and Sackeim and Prudic (2005). A short-term RCT without follow-up compared ECT and transcranial magnetic stimulation (rTMS) in the treatment of major depressive patients (unipolar or bipolar), and found that their scores on the Hamilton Depression Rating Scale improved to the same degree (59%) by the end of the study (Janicak et al., 2002). ECT seems to be efficacious in patients with mixed mania. Consecutively enrolled patients with mixed mania (41) and bipolar I (23) were assigned to ECT in a naturalistic study. Between-group comparisons showed that the patients with mixed mania showed significantly greater decreases in depression and suicidality in their Montgomery-Asberg Depression Rating scores (MADRS) (Ciapparelli et al., 2001). In a similar observational study, 96 bipolar I patients with either major depressive episode or a mixed state were given bilateral ECT with no difference between them in their global and depression remission rates (Medda et al., 2009).

ECT also has a place as maintenance therapy for refractory bipolar depression, but the evidence of its effectiveness rests on small observational studies (Vaidya, Mahableshwarkar, & Shahid, 2003). When ECT is resorted to for depression that is nonresponsive to a trial of two antidepressants in succession, it is better to switch the patient to a different antidepressant after the course of ECT. A retrospective chart review from Japan showed that these patients required readmission less frequently over a year of follow-up than those who were maintained on the same antidepressant to which they had not responded (Nakajima et al., 2009). It may not be necessary to stop an anticonvulsant during a course of ECT. In a small case series, nine patients were treated simultaneously with lamotrigine and ECT, and the concurrent use did not interfere with seizure adequacy (Penland & Ostroff, 2006). It is unfortunate that none of these investigations, except for one (Ciapparelli et al., 2001), had the foresight to include the measurement of suicidality as a secondary outcome and clearly this oversight needs to be remedied in the future investigations of the treatment of bipolar depression.

Antipsychotics

As with other drugs used in bipolar disorder (aside from lithium), there are almost no studies evaluating the impact of antipsychotics on suicidality in bipolar patients (Oquendo et al., 2005b). On the basis of RCTs, the FDA has licensed olanzapine and fluoxetine in combination and quetiapine as first- or second-line drugs in bipolar disorder. One recent RCT found the combination of olanzapine/fluoxetine to be superior to lamotrigine in ameliorating scores on the Clinical Global Impressions-Severity of Illness (CGI-S), MADRS, and the Young Mania Rating (YMRS) scales over 25 weeks. No difference was observed in the rates of relapse or treatment-emergent mania, but the olanzapine/fluoxetine group experienced more treatment-emergent adverse events and a greater incidence of weight gain and hypercholesterolemia (Brown et al., 2009). Two short-term RCTs tested olanzapine/fluoxetine versus olanzapine or fluoxetine alone in outpatients with treatment-resistant depression (Thase et al., 2007). In the first study, there was no significant difference in the MADRS scores, but in the second study the combination showed a significantly greater MADRS improvement. Pooling the results confirmed a significant difference in the MADRS scores and the pooled remission rates were 27% for olanzapine/fluoxetine, 17% for fluoxetine, and 15% for olanzapine alone, favoring the combination drug. The adverse effects (increased cholesterol and weight gain) were worse for the combination as previously found. Similar findings were reported elsewhere (Trivedi et al., 2009).

Shelton and Papakostas (2008) and Perlis (2007) reviewed the literature for olanzapine and other atypical antipsychotics augmenting antidepressants for treatment-resistant depressive disorder and found only observational studies. These reviews suggested there might be beneficial effects in combining them with antidepressants, but they also posed significant metabolic risks that needed to be weighed. One advantage with olanzapine/fluoxetine over olanzapine alone or placebo could be a greater percentage of early (within a week) persistent responders (32% versus 18% versus 13% in this study) (Dube et al., 2007). Augmentation of lithium or divalproex in bipolar I disorder mixed-episode patients has been shown to reduce suicidal ideation that was associated with somatic discomfort, agitated depression, and psychosis (Sturner, 1986).

The most recent CANMAT guidelines (issued collaboratively with the International Society for Bipolar Disorders) support quetiapine monotherapy as a first-line option for the management of bipolar depression along with lithium or lamotrigine monotherapy, olanzapine plus an SSRI, and lithium or divalproex plus an SSRI/bupropion (Yatham et al., 2009). The primary studies of quetiapine in bipolar disorder comprised the series known as the BOLDER (for bipolar depression) studies. Bipolar I and II patients were randomized to quetiapine or placebo, and a significant reduction in the MADRS total score was evidenced in both arms over placebo as well as in remission rates. MADRS items showed a lowering in suicidal thoughts as well as in core depressive items (Kemp, Muzina, McIntyre, & Calabrese, 2008; Thase et al., 2006) and quality-of-life (Endicott et al., 2007). There was no difference in efficacy between quetiapine at 300 mg or 600 mg/day. A post hoc analysis confirmed the findings on efficacy (Weisler et al., 2008).

Psychosocial

Rucci, Frank, and Kostelnik (2002) established lifetime rates of suicide attempts among patients with acute bipolar I disorder before entering a trial of lithium pharmacotherapy combined with adjunctive psychotherapy specific to bipolar disorder, or nonspecific, intensive clinical management involving regular visits with empathic clinicians. The rate of suicide attempts experienced a threefold reduction during the acute and maintenance treatment phases, and no patient with one or more previous suicide attempts repeated during the protocol. The study showed that a treatment program in a maximally supportive clinical environment could significantly reduce suicidal behavior in high-risk patients with bipolar I disorder (Rucci et al., 2002). In the STEP-BD, intensive psychotherapy lasting for up to 30 sessions over 9 months or brief psychoeducation was given in conjunction with protocol pharmacotherapy for bipolar I or II or bipolar depressed patients. The psychotherapy plus pharmacotherapy patients registered significantly higher recovery rates (64% versus 52%) and took a shorter time for recovery, but the effect on suicidal ideation or attempts (Miklowitz et al., 2007) is hardly mentioned. A pilot RCT for Mindfulness-based Cognitive Therapy (MBCT) in suicidal bipolar disorder patients in remission focused on between-episode anxiety and depressive symptoms. The results suggested that MBCT improved current anxiety and both bipolar and unipolar participants allocated to MBCT showed reductions in residual depressive symptoms compared with waitlist controls (Williams, Alatiq, et al., 2008). Sajatovic et al. (2004) reviewed 11 studies that showed interpersonal group therapy, cognitive behavioral therapy, group sessions for partners of persons with bipolar disorder, and patient and family psychoeducation as enhancing adherence to treatment (one third of bipolar patients take less than 30% of their medication and non-adherence is associated with rehospitalization and suicide). Negative conclusions about the value of psychotherapy in the treatment of bipolar disorder were drawn in another review (Colom et al., 1998), but concluded that none of these treatments had established the efficacy in controlled clinical trials with regard to hospitalization, recurrences, or suicidal behavior. The authors argued for a more systematic clinical research on psychotherapy applied to bipolar disorder.

Depressive Disorders

DSM-IV-TR recognizes a sequence of variants of mood disorders where depressed mood is a dominant feature: *major depressive disorder* (at least 2 weeks of depressed mood or anhedonia with at least four additional symptoms of depression), *dysthymic disorder* (at least 2 years of depressed mood with additional depressive symptoms that do not qualify for major depressive episode), and *depressive disorder NOS* (with depressive features that do not meet criteria for the above order for adjustment disorder with depressed mood or adjustment disorder with mixed anxiety and depressed mood) (2000). Depressive illness is prevalent in 45–70% of suicides (Barraclough, Bunch, Nelson, & Sainsbury, 1974; Cavanagh et al., 2003; Chynoweth, 1980; Rich, Young, & Fowler, 1986; Robins, 1959).

Harris and Barraclough (1998) carried out meta-analysis of the studies of mortality rates in the various types of mental disorders and found that the SMR for suicide in DSM-III-R major depression for both genders was 21, affective disorders NOS (including psychoses, manic depression, and depressive neuroses) 17, dysthymia 12, and bipolar disorder 12, similar to the rank order previously found by Newman and Bland (1991). Earlier consensus posited that 15% of patients with depressive illness would ultimately take their lives (Guze & Robins, 1970; Miles, 1977), but Bostwick and Pankratz (2000) revised this estimate downward, 8.6% for those depressed patients ever hospitalized for suicidality and 4% for those hospitalized without specifications of suicidality. Although we may debate its exact magnitude, the risk of suicide in depressive disorders is significant. It is unclear whether mood disorders increase the risk of suicide by creating a predisposition (diathesis) or act as a trigger or both (Sher, Oquendo, & Mann, 2001). The risk is greatest during the first attack: among depressed suicide completers, 75% were in the throes of their first major depressive episode, with declining frequencies occurring during subsequent depressive episodes (McGirr, Renaud, Seguin, Alda, & Turecki, 2008). A small study found the suicide SMR in recurrent major depressive episodes 47 for female depressed patients (Schneider, Muller, & Philipp, 2001). This high risk for suicide in women depressives accords with the findings from the Stirling County 40-year follow-up (Murphy et al., 2008), which showed that although in 1952 depression was somewhat more common among women than men (6% compared to 4%), it carried a significant overall mortality risk only among men (HR 2.7, 95% CI 1.6–4.7). However, at the follow-up in 1992, depression was associated with mortality risk equally for both genders (HR 2.2 for men and 2.1 for women). Unfortunately, although implicit as a major factor, suicide data were not specifically mentioned. Mechanisms that are usually proposed to account for excessive mortality among patients with depressive disorders include increased suicide rates, hazardous health behavior (smoking, alcohol use, and unhealthy eating), psychological reactions to developing a medical illness, biological dysregulation, and noncompliance with medical treatment (Cuijpers & Schoevers, 2004). An investigation of suicides that occurred over 1 year in the Canadian province of New Brunswick showed that efforts at suicide prevention among patients with mood disorders that ignore comorbid substance-related disorders and concomitant personality disorders would be less than successful (Seguin et al., 2006). Objective severity of the mood disorder does not necessarily identify those patients at high risk for suicidality (Sher et al., 2001). Given the fact that depressive spectrum disorders universally carry a high suicide risk, it should follow that treatment that ameliorates depressive illness should reduce suicide rates as well.

Antidepressants

For five decades, antidepressants have been the cornerstone of the management of depressive illness, but in the last decade important questions have been raised about their safety and efficacy (Brent, 2007; Sakinofsky, 2007a, 2007b; Thase, 2008). With regard to the question of efficacy, current evidence suggests that it is considerably more modest than what was previously thought of (e.g., remission rates in drug trials typically hover between 35% and 45%, Thase, 2008), whereas they were previously believed to have been about 70%. The effect sizes of antidepressants versus placebo in recent important meta-analyses (Cohen's *d*) were 0.31 and 0.32 (Turner & Rosenthal, 2008; Kirsch et al., 2008), which being < 0.4 is considered to be only a small effect in Cohen's categorization, which delineates 0.4–0.65 as medium and ≥ 0.7 as large (Cohen, 1977; Thase, 2008). An important reason for this small effect size appears to be the growing power of placebo response, which is possibly based on increased expectations by patients of improvement and also better clinical psychosocial support in the placebo arm than was previously the case. Paradoxically, the effect size differentiating the active drug and placebo is greater when the clinical sample is more severely ill; severity may in fact reduce both the placebo response and the positive effect of psychosocial support (Kirsch et al., 2008). The UK NICE has chosen a medium level of effect size of 0.5 as a minimum criterion for efficacy, which antidepressants clearly do not meet. However, Turner and Rosenthal argue that this is a misuse of Cohen's concepts and that, although relatively small, the effect size reached in antidepressant trials is measurable and significant, and that when considering the potential benefits of treatment with antidepressants one should be circumspect but not dismissive (Turner & Rosenthal, 2008). Efficacy measured in clinical trials is not so synonymous with effectiveness in clinical practice and clinical trials of efficacy do not usually also measure improved quality-of-life. It is an example of what Cohen called "confusion of the degree of relationship with its statistical significance" (Cohen, 1986).

We have also become more aware in the real world of clinical practice of widespread undertreatment of depression associated with suicide, in part because of poor compliance and adherence by patients, possibly culturally determined (Hirschfeld et al., 1997; Sakinofsky, 2007a). The impact of placebo response is growing not only in drug trials, but also in trials of the evidence-based psychotherapies, reducing their measured efficacy also (Nelson et al., 2008). The most robust evidence of the effectiveness of antidepressants is in relapse prevention of depression where a meta-analysis found them to reduce the risk of relapse by 70% (Geddes et al., 2003).

Primary studies that investigate the effectiveness of antidepressants in reducing suicidality (ideation, suicidal acts, attempts, or completions) are few and far between. Almost all of the drug trials in Phase III and Phase IV are industry-sponsored and carried out for the purpose of obtaining "labels" from authorities such as the FDA (Thase, 2008). Further, Phase III trials for depression enroll participants according to stringent inclusion and exclusion criteria, a history of previous suicide attempts usually being one of the reasons for exclusion (Wisniewski et al., 2009). In the STAR*D project (Sequenced Treatment Alternatives to Relieve Depression), only minimal exclusion criteria were employed and therefore only 22% of almost 3,000 participants would have met typical entry criteria (including a previous suicide attempt) for Phase III antidepressant drug trials. The 78% of participants who would not have met these criteria are what the psychiatrist deals with in the real world; the efficacy reported in most antidepressant trials may not be generalizable or indeed reflect the effectiveness in clinical practice of the antidepressants concerned (Wisniewski et al., 2009).

A wave of secondary analyses of the frequency of emergent suicidality were retrospectively undertaken following urgent questions about the possibility that antidepressant drugs may induce suicidality and even suicide in some patients (Healy & Aldred, 2005; Teicher, Glod, & Cole, 1993). These questions were initially prompted by anecdotal reports (Teicher, Glod, & Cole, 1990) (see also, Sakinofsky, 2007b) and were followed by a large number of meta-analyses of suicidal events reported during drug trials (Sakinofsky, 2007b). An FDA-sponsored meta-analysis of 372 double-blind randomized placebo-controlled trials ($N = 99{,}231$) demonstrated that the risk for emergent suicidality with antidepressants is age-related and dissipates with increasing age (Stone et al., 2009). For participants with nonpsychiatric indications, suicidal behavior and ideation were extremely rare (which must surely question the theory that emergent suicidality is specifically related to the antidepressant drug), but for those with psychiatric indications risk was associated with age. For suicidal behavior, the OR was 2.30 (95% CI, 1.04–5.09) for those aged < 25 and 0.87 (0.58–1.29) for those aged 25–64 and 0.06 (0.01–0.58) for those aged ≥ 65. When age was modeled as a continuous variable, the OR for suicidal behavior declined at a rate of 4.6% per year of age. These studies succeeded in raising the Black Box warning put out by the FDA against antidepressants except for fluoxetine to 25 years because the increased risk for suicidality and suicidal behavior among adults < 25 was found to approach that seen in children and adolescents. It is noteworthy that the net effect was concluded to be neutral on suicidal behavior, possibly protective for suicidal ideation in adults 25–64, and to reduce the risk of both suicidality and suicidal behavior in those aged ≥ 65. Bridge and colleagues, based on a meta-analysis of pediatric drug trials for major depression and obsessive-compulsive disorder, reported that the overall benefits of antidepressants in youth far outweighed the risks (Bridge, Birmaher, & Brent, 2007; Bridge, Iyengar, et al., 2007). Simon and Savarino (2007) reviewed claims from a prepaid health plan for prescriptions and probable suicide attempts, and found that the overall incidence of suicide attempts was highest for outpatients receiving prescriptions from psychiatrists (1,124 per hundred thousand), lower for those starting psychotherapy (778), and lowest for those receiving antidepressants in primary care (301). However, the pattern of attempts over time was the same in all three groups: Highest in the month before starting treatment, followed by the month after starting treatment and declining thereafter. The results were unchanged after eliminating patients who received overlapping treatment with medication and psychotherapy. The overall incidence of suicide attempts was higher in adolescents and young adults, but the time pattern was the same across all three treatments. The authors concluded that the results reflected referral patterns, with psychiatrists receiving the more severe cases, and that the differences over time showed the risk of suicide attempts to be highest before treatment and declining with improvement as a result of treatment (Simon & Savarino, 2007). Below we review specific evidence for reduction of suicidality in depressive illness categorized by time of life. Because of the statistical problems created by the low base rate of suicide, impossibly large numbers of participants would have to be included in the RCTs (Gunnell & Frankel, 1994). Therefore, surrogates of suicide such as suicidal ideation, suicide attempts, or preparations for a suicide attempt or "suicide events" are generally measured in these investigations, but we need to always keep in mind that these approximations probably do not accurately estimate the relative proportions of suicide completions.

General Adult Studies

McGrath et al. (2008) investigated whether *melancholic features* were predictive of response to the SSRI citalopram. The participants of the above mentioned study had received the drug in the first-step treatment of the STAR*D study and 24% at enrollment had melancholic features, greater rates of previous suicide attempts, and current suicide risk. Compared with nonmelancholic depressed patients, their chances of remission were significantly reduced by 24% (McGrath et al., 2008). Clearly, SSRIs may not be sufficient for this subset of depressed patients. Another neglected group in antidepressant trials concerns the *suicidal substance-abusing* disordered patients and as recently as 2001 only one RCT could be reported by Cornelius in 2001 (Cornelius, Salloum, Lynch, Clark, & Mann, 2001). This was a small 12-week study of 51 patients with comorbid depressive disorder and alcohol dependence. Depression and alcohol consumption in this group with suicidal ideation both improved significantly with fluoxetine, but changes in suicidal ideation were not documented (Cornelius et al., 1997). Unfortunately, this was also the case in 2004 (Pirkola, Suominen, & Isometsa, 2004) and continues to be the only RCT I could find in the literature on suicidal depressed substance-abusing patients, no doubt because of a large noncompliance factor.

A small pilot study (RCT) was designed by Reeves et al. (2008) for investigating the efficacy of risperidone augmentation to antidepressants in the acute management of suicidality and other core symptoms in major depressive disorder with suicidality. Subjects were randomly assigned to receive risperidone 0.25–2 mg/day or a placebo, while continuing on their antidepressant therapy. Risperidone significantly reduced suicidal ideation, and its overall effect appears to be superior to placebo. Treatment-resistant unipolar depressed patients who had responded to augmentation therapy with lithium were randomized into continuation with lithium augmentation versus placebo over a 4-month period. There were no relapses in the treatment group and one suicide occurred in the placebo group only (Bauer et al., 2006). As part of the STAR*D project, investigators randomized patients who had completed a trial of citalopram to either sustained-release bupropion (150–400 mg/day) or sertraline (50–200 mg/day) or venlafaxine XR (titrated to 375 mg/day). Remission was more likely among those who had no prior suicide attempts as well as a partial response to citalopram and remission was less likely in those who had concurrent generalized anxiety, obsessive-compulsive symptoms, panic, or other indications of anxiety. Similar findings were reported by Claassen et al. (2007).

Acharya and colleagues evaluated all completed duloxetine trials for major depressive disorder with data lock by February 2004 for suicide-related events with duloxetine versus placebo. In 12 placebo-controlled trials, there were no significant differences in the incidence of suicide-related events and changes in the HAMD suicidality score (item-3) showed more improvement with duloxetine and less worsening of suicidal ideation (Acharya et al., 2007). Another new drug, the SSRI escitalopram, was also evaluated in a number of RCTs and no suicide occurred among escitalopram-treated patients, and there were no significant differences with placebo in suicidal ideation and events (Baldwin, Reines, Guiton, & Weiller, 2007). A further metareview was carried out by a Cochrane group to evaluate short-term effectiveness and safety of antidepressants for depression (Cipriani, Geddes, Furukawa, & Barbui, 2007). Antidepressants were found to be efficacious in primary care settings, and there was slight but important evidence for differences in efficacy between them. However, there was no good evidence that combining with antipsychotic was superior to antidepressant monotherapy in cases of psychotic depression. There was evidence to suggest that SSRIs may increase suicidal thoughts, but not actual suicide in early phase therapy, leaving some uncertainty for the investigators. They recommended that clinicians assess the balance between risks and benefits for individual patients.

Elderly

In many countries, seniors ≥ 65 years of age have the highest suicide rates, although they are less likely to have a history of recurrent suicide attempts (Schaffer et al., 2008). The PROSPECT study (Prevention of Suicide in Primary Care Elderly-Collaborative Trial), carried out between 1999 and 2001, was a randomized, double-blind, placebo-controlled trial to determine whether placing a specially trained "health specialist" in collaboration with physicians in a primary care practice (Care Management) would benefit suicidal elderly patients, given that the majority of such patients who suicide have seen a primary care physician in preceding months (Bruce et al., 2004). The design was two-stage, involving age stratified patients with a diagnosis of depression (N = 598) with TAU (Treatment As Usual) controls. A treatment algorithm for antidepressant use was devised and guidelines given for changing antidepressants or for treatment with interpersonal psychotherapy (Mulsant et al., 2001). Rates of suicidal ideation declined faster in the intervention patients, peaking at 8 months, lagging behind improvement in depressed mood, which peaked at 4 months, regardless of the severity of the depression. Recently (Alexopoulos et al., 2009), the 24-month outcomes became available. Compared with patients receiving TAU, those receiving Care Management were much more likely to receive antidepressants and/or psychotherapy (85–89% versus 49–62%) and reported a 2.2 times greater decline in suicidal ideation over 24 months. The treatment response in the intervention group increased rather than attenuated from months 18 to 24 without the same response in the comparison group. More patients with major depression achieved remission of their dysphoria (45% versus 32%). Limitations in physical and emotional functions and significant anxiety predicted a poor remission rate in this study (Alexopoulos et al., 2005), and residual symptoms of anxiety and sleep disturbance independently predicted early recurrence (Dombrovski et al., 2007, 2008).

When elderly patients who had been treated in a 12-week trial with paroxetine or nortriptyline were classified as either nonsuicidal for having emergent, persistent, or resolved suicidality, the rates were 7.8%, 12.6%, and 15.6%, respectively. The patients with persistent suicidal ideation were more likely to have recurrent depression. Patients with emergent or persistent suicidality were more likely to maintain higher depression scores as well as levels of anxiety and agitation, leading to the conclusion that although emergence of suicidality is uncommon in treatment of late-life depression, it may signal treatment resistance. Emergent suicidality was not associated with akathisia (Szanto et al., 2007).

Elderly patients treated with ECT respond relatively well, although not as frequently as we used to believe, but are likely to relapse without continuation treatment. In an RCT of elderly patients who completed an ECT treatment phase, 159 of 290 (55%) met criteria for remission and of these 84 participated in a continuation study where they were randomly assigned to receive 24 weeks of placebo, nortriptyline, or combination nortriptyline and lithium. Thirty-nine percentage of patients taking the nortriptyline-lithium combination relapsed in 24 weeks, compared with 60% on nortriptyline and 84% of those in the placebo arm (Sackeim et al., 2007). Although this study did not specifically look at suicidality as an outcome, it clearly has relevance for preventing suicide during relapses of major depression.

Overall, the elderly depressed and suicidal patients are encouraging to treat. Szanto et al. (2001) reported on treatment outcomes in elderly suicidal and nonsuicidal patients with recurrent major depression who received combined treatment with pharmacotherapy and psychotherapy. Patients with suicidal ideation had identical remission rates (77–78%) to those without suicidal ideation, but they relapsed more frequently and suggested a brittle treatment response requiring continued use of adjunctive medication. Suicidal elderly patients with depression require special attention because of a lower and slower response rate. Although suicidal ideation was found to resolve fairly speedily in all treated patients, suicidal patients continued to have thoughts of dying (passive ideation) for quite a long time (Szanto, Mulsant, Houck, Dew, & Reynolds, 2003).

Youth

A smaller number of industry-sponsored antidepressant trials were carried out in youth relative to adults prior to the concern for the risk of emergent suicidality raised by researchers and by regulatory agencies, fluoxetine alone surviving the meta-analyses in the US (Sakinofsky, 2007b). In the midst of this furor researchers analyzing the treatment for adolescents with depression study (TADS) published findings of a multicenter 12-week trial in adolescents 12–17 years with major depressive disorder. The patients were randomized to receive fluoxetine alone, CBT alone, CBT with fluoxetine, or a placebo drug. The CBT was administered unblinded. Clinically significant suicidal ideation, present in 29% of the sample at baseline, improved significantly in all four treatment groups but fluoxetine with CBT showed the greatest reduction and fluoxetine alone was superior to CBT alone for ameliorating depression (March et al., 2004). The 36-week results were reported in the same order: 86% for combination therapy, 81% for fluoxetine alone, and 81% for CBT alone. Suicidal ideation decreased with treatment, but less so with fluoxetine than with the combination or CBT alone, so that the authors concluded that adding CBT to the SSRI enhances the safety of medication (March et al., 2007). A British study did not find CBT to be protective against suicidality. Goodyer et al. (2008) carried out a 28-week RCT of an SSRI or an SSRI with CBT, but found no significant differences in the effectiveness of treatment for the primary or secondary outcome measures. On average, there was a decrease across groups in suicidal thoughts and self-harm. Along the same lines, a smaller trial compared CBT, sertraline and their combination for adolescent depression but came up with different findings. Combined CBT-sertraline treatment was not superior to either treatment alone and CBT was found to be superior to the antidepressant over for the acute treatment of mild to moderate depression among youth (Melvin et al., 2006). March and colleagues meta-analyzed pooled trials of sertraline versus placebo in pediatric major depressive disorder and obsessive-compulsive disorder (March et al., 2006). The authors calculated the NNT for response and remission and the number needed to harm (NNH) for suicidality and their ratio for each clinical trial. The NNTs ranged from 2 to 10, indicating clinically meaningful benefits and the NNH for suicidality in major depressive disorder was 64. There were no suicidal events recorded in the OCD trials at all. Treatment emergent suicidality was more common in children (NNH = 28.7) than in adolescents (NNH = 706.3), indicating a positive benefit-to-risk ratio for sertraline in adolescents with major depressive disorder and in patients of all ages with OCD. A very large meta-analysis of antidepressant trials in youth was performed by Bridge and colleagues (Bridge, Iyengar, et al., 2007). There was an increased risk of suicidal ideation or attempt across all trials and indications for the active drug versus placebo; the pooled RD within each indication were not statistically significant and there were no completed suicides. In children younger than 12 years with major depressive disorder, only fluoxetine showed benefit over placebo. The investigators concluded that the benefits of antidepressants appear to be much greater than the risks from nonfatal suicidality. Recently, investigators analyzed the TADS database to determine whether suicidal events could have been predicted by severity of depression or other clinical characteristics. The suicidal events were defined according to the Columbia classification algorithm (Fernandez, Grataloup, & Posner, 2008; Posner, Oquendo, Gould, Stanley, & Davies, 2007). Most suicidal events occurred within in the context of persistent depression and inadequate improvements, and without evidence for medication-induced suicidal activation. The risk for suicidal events did not decrease after the first month of treatment, which suggested the need for careful clinical monitoring for several months after starting treatment. Severity of suicidal ideation and depressive symptoms predicted the emergence of suicidality during treatment (Vitiello et al., 2009). Emslie, Ventura, Korotzer, and Tourkodimitris (2009) found the incidence of suicidality in a trial of escitalopram versus placebo for adolescent depression to be similar for both groups.

Electroconvulsive Therapy

Carney et al. (2003) undertook a Cochrane meta-analysis of data of short-term efficacy from RCTs and found that real ECT was significantly more effective than simulated ECT and that treatment with ECT was significantly more effective than pharmacotherapy. Bilateral ECT was more effective than unipolar ECT (Carney et al., 2003). Geddes et al. (2003) reviewed RCTs of continuing treatment with antidepressant in patients with depressive disorders who responded to ECT and found that continuing treatment with antidepressants reduces the odds of relapse by 70% compared with treatment discontinuation. Kellner et al. (2005) reported the results of the first phase of a multicenter study to compare continuation ECT with pharmacotherapy for the prevention of relapse after a successful course of ECT. Expressed suicidal intent was scored at baseline and before each ECT session in 444 patients with unipolar depression. Twenty-nine percent of the patients reported suicidal thoughts and acts at baseline. Scores decreased to 0 after 1 week in 38%, after 2 weeks in 61%, and by the end of the course of treatment in 81%. The authors advised that ECT should be considered earlier and not as a last resort (Kellner et al., 2005).

Psychological Treatment

While there is a reasonable literature with regard to controlled trials on psychological treatment of depression, there is almost no literature pertaining to controlled trials of psychotherapy for suicidal people. MBCT proponents have, however, given the idea that this area of study merits considerable attention. Williams, Barnhofer, Crane, and Beck (2005) compared depressed patients with and without previous suicidality, and those having no history of depression on a problem-solving test (MEPS). Only the depressed patients with a history of suicidality produced significantly less effective problem solutions following mood challenge, consistent with their vulnerability for the recurrence of suicidal ideation and behavior (Williams et al., 2005). Once suicidal thoughts have emerged as a feature of depression then they are likely to be reactivated whenever sad mood reappears. The authors prospectively examined 69 individuals with a history of major depression over 12 months. Severity ratings of the symptom of major depression during a previous episode and at recurrence showed significant associations for suicidality, guilt, worthlessness, and thinking difficulties (Williams, Crane, Barnhofer, Van der Does, & Segal, 2006; Williams, Duggan, Crane, & Fennell, 2006). Individuals who reported suicidal ideation when depressed in the past had higher scores on the hopelessness/suicidality subscale of a measure of assessing cognitive reactivity and low mood (Williams, Van der Does, Barnhofer, Crane, & Segal, 2008). MBCT may reduce thought suppression in previously suicidal participants; thought suppression, a strategy aimed at mental control, may paradoxically increase the frequency of suicidal ideation (Hepburn et al., 2009). Recently, a preliminary study of the treatment of patients with chronic depression and a history of suicidal ideation with MBCT appeared (Barnhofer et al., 2009). MBCT was compared with treatment as usual and self-reported symptoms of depression decreased from severe to mild levels in the MBCT group, while there was no change for the TAU group. The sample of this study was small and it requires replication.

Emergent Suicidality

The furor over the risk that antidepressant treatment may paradoxically activate suicidal ideation or activity seems to have died down although reports of emergent suicidality continue to appear in the literature (Gaudiano, Andover, & Miller, 2008; Olfson & Marcus,

2008). There have been several previous reviews of the evidence with varying conclusions (Brent, 2007; Mann, 2008; Mann et al., 2006; Mann, Goodwin, O'Brien, & Robinson, 1993; Sakinofsky, 2007b; Healy et al., 2005). It is important to recognize that there has been no excess of suicide deaths reported in the meta-analyses of drug trials, only of suicidal ideation and events. Two case-control studies do report an excess of suicidal deaths but there is controversy over methodological questions and caution is counseled in their interpretation (Juurlink, Mamdani, Kopp, & Redelmeier, 2006; Juurlink, 2006; Olfson, Marcus, & Shaffer, 2006).

The FDA and other national safety agencies have ruled that antidepressants be withheld (with the exception of fluoxetine in the US but without exceptions in the UK), at first from children and adolescents <18, and then the bar was raised to age 25. Notwithstanding, expert and public consensus developed strategic clinical algorithms that allow the use of off-label SSRIs in the treatment of major depression in youth (Hughes et al., 2007). The algorithm emphasizes consultation with close family regarding their treatment preferences, thorough assessment and monitoring, as well as consideration of the role of alternative treatments such as CBT and interpersonal psychotherapy. [Three SSRIs (fluoxetine, sertraline, and citalopram) were previously shown in RCTs to be efficacious in major depression in adolescents and recently escitalopram has also been shown in RCTs to be safe and effective in adolescents, but not children (Wagner, Jonas, Findling, Ventura, & Saikali, 2006; Emslie et al., 2009).]

The recently published (but previously available on the Web) meta-analysis of 372 studies by the FDA (Stone et al., 2009) showed the risk to be very much related to younger age, with the OR for suicidal behavior declining at the rate of 4.6% of age. The risk was neutral from age 25 to 65 and antidepressants were protective thereafter. The FDA Black Box warnings had their intended effect and antidepressant prescribing to youth (presumably by pediatricians and primary care physicians) fell sharply, with the resultant fear that suicide rates in youth would rise, but this has not proved to be the case and they have resumed falling in the US, and continued to decline in the UK although the use of antidepressants fell sharply in 2003 and 2004 (Simon, 2008; Wheeler et al, 2008). Simon points out that treatment is probably too sporadic to affect overall suicide rates; only half of adults and a quarter of adolescents in the US with a major episode of depression in any given year take an antidepressant.

There is now an FDA requirement for all new drug trials to incorporate in their safety planning the prospective collection of suicidality adverse effects (AE) using a Columbia-developed standardized instrument for evaluating suicidal ideation and events during treatments (Posner et al., 2007; Posner, Oquendo, Stanley, & Gould, 2004; Fernandez et al., 2008). This should go some way to resolving the issue, and at the same time will henceforth in all US drug trials incorporate suicidality as an outcome measure and provide useful research data.

New pharmacogenetic studies are opening up the possibility of identifying patients who are more likely to develop emergent suicidality. Collaborating centers in the US and Sweden collected DNA samples from a representative cohort of 1,938 outpatients with major depressive disorder treated with citalopram under a standard protocol.

The DNA was genotyped for participants who developed treatment-emergent suicidal ideation and those who did not (Laje et al., 2006; Laje et al., 2007). Two markers were significantly associated with emergent suicidal ideation, both of them within genes involved in glutamate signaling (sensitivity = 57% and specificity = 99.8%). In concert, colleagues associated with the STAR*D project analyzed DNA from citalopram-treated outpatients for cyclic adenosine monophosphate response element binding (CREB) protein, based on previous knowledge that CREB1 is associated with the expression of anger in men with major depressive disorder. Polymorphisms spanning CREB1 were associated with treatment-emergent suicidality among men with depression but not women (Perlis et al., 2007). The corollary to the pharmacogenetic studies of treatment-emergent suicidality is the finding, in an offshoot of the same study, associations between genetic variations in the HTR2A and GRIK4 genes, with markers pinpointing those patients 23% more likely to experience response to treatment (Paddock et al., 2007). If these studies are replicated, eventually clinicians will be able to target treatment with antidepressants with greater confidence in anticipated safety and outcomes. The DNA studies may even become cost-effective for clinical use (Perlis, Patrick, Smoller, & Wang, 2009).

Summary

The pain of depression is associated with suicide less often than previously estimated but still problematic. Intolerable mental pain may precede suicide in the context of frustrated needs, unbearable predicament, and developmental and neurobiological vulnerability. Researchers have been slow to evaluate treatments for impact on suicidality with the exception of lithium. RCTs of antidepressants developed for satisfying regulatory agencies have neglected testing for antisuicidal potency until the possibility of drug-induced emergent suicidality led to a crisis in this state of affairs. Data from trials have since been retrospectively analyzed and meta-analyzed, and more recently the FDA has instructed that safety assessment be prospectively built into future pharmaceutical trials using the Columbia Suicide Severity Rating Scale.

Bipolar disorder:
Evidence for lithium's antisuicide efficacy is robust. Lithium offers protection to patients who persist with it for at least two years, whether or not they are lithium responders (in relapse prevention). Notwithstanding, prescriptions for a variety of anticonvulsants and antipsychotics appear to be overtaking lithium in clinical practice, possibly because of aggressive marketing or the fear of worrisome sequelae found in a minority of cases, especially nephrogenic. Lithium's antisuicide effect appears to exceed that of anticonvulsants or antipsychotics but this advantage was seen to diminish in a register-linkage study when patients adhered to any treatments. Manic episodes are more attention-grabbing but the clinician should remain focused on bipolar depression, since most bipolar patients who attempt or complete suicide do so during depressed or mixed phases and rarely during

manic episodes. In half the cases of suicide during bipolar depression, the episode was immediately preceded by hypomania or mania. Careful monitoring and psychosocial support should be maintained after patients are discharged from hospital. Antidepressant use for bipolar depression is controversial; tricyclics are contraindicated but SSRIs or bupropion may be cautiously used in combination with mood stabilizers or antipsychotics. ECT effectively improves bipolar I and mixed manic depression but only observational evidence confirms that it reduces suicidal ideation in bipolar patients. Quetiapine alone or olanzapine as augmentation may reduce suicidal ideation in bipolar patients. Psychotherapy has been inadequately evaluated.

Depression:
Depressive illness occurs in 45–70% of suicides and may operate as a diathesis, trigger, or both. Magnitude of severity does not necessarily identify high risk patients but certainly the highest risk is during the first attack. Comorbid substance abuse and concomitant personality disorders are important determinants of outcome. Antidepressants have been the cornerstone for 50 years but efficacy is clearly demonstrated only for suicidal ideation, an inexact surrogate for estimating completed suicide outcomes. Suicide rates are lower for those who continue purchasing (and presumably ingesting) antidepressants, than for those purchasing single prescriptions. This may signal antidepressant efficacy in suicide prevention or be due to confounding by indication. Antidepressant use among depressed lower educated men is less frequent than desirable and remains to be elucidated. Undertreatment of depression with antidepressants is general, with low proportions of suicides having evidence in their blood at autopsy. Yet there is good meta-analytic evidence that continued treatment with efficacious antidepressants greatly reduces risk of relapse of depressive illness.

Augmentation of antidepressant therapy with lithium or risperidone has been shown to reduce suicidal ideation. However, in the STAR*D those depressed patients with a history of suicide attempts or anxiety disorders were less likely to remit. RCTs have not shown escitalopram and duloxetine (novel antidepressants) to have emergent suicidality in adults. In the elderly, having a trained health assistant in collaboration with primary care physicians assures better care management for suicidal elders and relieves depression and suicidal ideation. Elderly patients show a brittle (relapse-prone) recovery from depression, including with ECT, and continuation treatment with nortriptyline and lithium has been helpful. With treatment, suicidal ideation in the elderly resolves speedily but thoughts of dying may persist for a long time.

The TADS showed better results from combination SSRI-CBT treatment for suicidal ideation than from either alone but other studies found that suicidal ideation fell across all treatments. Several studies show that antidepressant treatment benefits greatly outweigh the risks (e.g., an NNT<=10 vs. NNH = 64). Most youngsters will choose combination treatment with both CBT (a structured, quasi-educational therapy) and an antidepressant, as in the NIMH-sponsored TASA trial.

ECT is effective in depressive illness, bilateral more than unilateral, but the response does not last and continuing treatment with pharmacotherapy (or ECT) is advised. ECT has been shown to effectively reduce suicidal intent. Psychological therapies have not been adequately tested specifically for suicidality. A pilot study of MBCT in patients with chronic depression and a history of suicidal ideation relieved depression but is too small to be conclusive.

Emergent Suicidality:
The initial furor appears to have subsided. A large FDA meta-analysis of drug trials has shown it to be age-dependent, risky among youth, risk-neutral in those 25–65, and protective thereafter. The Black Box warnings resulted in a fall in prescribing to children and adolescents but did not raise suicide rates as was feared. A Texas algorithm for careful management of depression in youth with comprehensive treatment (including antidepressants where indicated) has been developed. The FDA has arranged for future drug trials to have prospectively built-in suicidality monitoring using a standardized instrument from Columbia University. This will provide important research data, not only about treatment emergence but also efficacy. Finally, there is promising pharmacogenetic research that may help identify both those at risk for suicidality emergence as well as those likely to respond to a specific antidepressant.

References

Acharya, N., Rosen, A. S., Polzer, J. P., D'Souza, D. N., Perahia, D. G., Cavazzoni, P., et al. (2007). Meta-analyses of suicidal behaviors and ideation in clinical trials for major depressive disorder. *Journal of Clinical Psychopharmacology, 26*, 587–594.

Ahrens, B., Muller-Oerlinghausen, B., & Grof, P. (1993). Length of lithium treatment needed to eliminate the high mortality of affective disorders. *British Journal of Psychiatry, 163*, 27–29.

Aizenberg, D., Olmer, A., Barak, Y., Aizenberg, D., Olmer, A., & Barak, Y. (2006) Suicide attempts amongst elderly bipolar patients. *Journal of Affective Disorders, 91*, 91–94.

Alexander, M. P., Farliq, Y. M., Mittal, B. V., Rennke, H. G., & Singh, A. K. (2008). Lithium toxicity: A double-edged sword. *Kidney International, 73*, 233–237.

Alexopoulos, G. S., Katz, I. R., Bruce, M. L., Heo, M., Ten Have, T., Raue, P., et al. (2005). Remission in depressed geriatric primary care patients: A report from the PROSPECT study. *American Journal of Psychiatry, 162*, 718–724.

Alexopoulos, G. S., Reynolds, C. F., Bruce, M. L., Katz, I. R., Raue, P. J., Mulsant, B. H., et al. (2009). Reducing suicidal ideation and depression in older primary care patients: 24-month outcomes of the PROSPECT study. *American Journal of Psychiatry, 166*, 882–890.

Altshuler, L. L., Suppes, T., Black, D. O., Nolen, W. A., Leverich, G. S., Keck, P. E., et al. (2006). Lower switch rate in depressed patients with bipolar II than bipolar I disorder treated adjunctively with second-generation antidepressants. *American Journal of Psychiatry, 163*, 313–315.

Amsterdam, J. D., & Brunswick, D. J. (2003). Antidepressant monotherapy for bipolar type II major depression. [Review] [62 refs]. *Bipolar Disorders, 5*, 388–395.

Angst, J., Angst, F., Gerber-Werder, R., & Gamma, A. (2005). Suicide in 406 mood-disorder patients with and without long-term medication: A 40 to 44 years' follow-up. *Archives of Suicide Research, 9*, 279–300.

Azorın, J. M., Aubrun, E., Bertsch, J., Reed, C., Gerard, S., & Lukasiewicz, M. (2009). Mixed states vs. pure mania in the french sample of the EMBLEM study: Results at baseline and 24 months – European mania in bipolar longitudinal evaluation of medication. *BMC Psychiatry, 9*.

Baldessarini, R. J., & Tondo, L. (2009a). Lithium and suicidal risk. *Bipolar Disorders, 10*, 114–115.

Baldessarini, R. J., & Tondo, L. (2009b). Suicidal risks during treatment of bipolar disorder patients with lithium versus anticonvulsants. *Pharmacopsychiatry, 42*, 72–75.

Baldessarini, R. J., Tondo, L., Davis, P., Pompili, M., Goodwin, F. K., & Hennen, J. (2006). Decreased risk of suicides and attempts during long-term lithium treatment: A meta-analytic review. *Bipolar Disorders, 8*, 625–639.

Baldwin, D. S., Reines, E. H., Guiton, C., & Weiller, E. (2007). Escitalopram therapy for major depression and anxiety disorders. *Annals of Pharmacotherapy, 41*, 1583–1592.

Barnhofer, T., Crane, C., Hargus, E., Amarasinghe, M., Winder, R., & Williams, J. M. G. (2009). Mindfulness-based cognitive therapy as a treatment for chronic depression: A preliminary study. *Behaviour Research and Therapy, 47*, 366–373.

Barraclough, B., Bunch, J., Nelson, B., & Sainsbury, P. (1974). A hundred cases of suicide: Clinical aspects. *British Journal of Psychiatry, 125*, 355.

Bauer, M. S., Wisniewski, S. R., Marangell, L. B., Chessick, C. A., Allen, M. H., Dennehy, E. B., et al. (2006). Are antidepressants associated with new-onset suicidality in bipolar disorder? A prospective study of participants in the systematic treatment enhancement program for bipolar disorder (STEP-BD). *Journal of Clinical Psychiatry, 67*, 48–55.

Bedford, J. J., Weggery, S., Ellis, G., McDonald, F. J., Joyce, P. R., Leader, J. P., et al. (2008). Lithium-induced nephrogenic diabetes insipidus: Renal effects of amiloride. *Clinical Journal of the American Society of Nephrology, 3*, 1324–1331.

Belmaker, R. H. (2004). Bipolar disorder. *New England Journal of Medicine, 351*, 476–486.

Bendz, H., & Aurell, M. (1999). Drug-induced diabetes insipidus: Incidence, prevention and management. [Review] [51 refs]. *Drug Safety, 21*, 449–456.

Black, D. W., Winokur, G., & Nasrallah, A. (1987). Suicide in subtypes of major affective disorder. A comparison with general population suicide mortality. *Archives of General Psychiatry, 44*, 878–880.

Blair-West, G. W., Cantor, C. H., Mellsop, G. W., & Eyeson-Annan, M. L. (1999). Lifetime suicide risk in major depression: Sex and age determinants. *Journal of Affective Disorders, 55*, 171–178.

Blair-West, G. W., Mellsop, G. W., & Eyeson-Annan, M. L. (1997). Down-rating lifetime suicide risk in major depression. *Acta Psychiatrica Scandinavica, 95*, 259–263.

Blanco, C., Laje, G., Olfson, M., Marcus, S. C., & Pincus, H. A. (2002). Trends in the treatment of bipolar disorder by outpatient psychiatrists. *American Journal of Psychiatry, 159*, 1005–1010.

Bostwick, J. M., & Pankratz, V. S. (2000). Affective disorders and suicide risk: A reexamination. *American Journal of Psychiatry, 157*, 1925–1932.

Bowden, C. L., Calabrese, J. R., Sachs, G., Yatham, L. N., Asghar, S. A., Hompland, M., et al. (2003). Placebo-controlled 18-month trial of lamotrigine and lithium maintenance treatment in recently manic or hypomanic patients with bipolar I disorder. *Archives of General Psychiatry, 60*, 392–400.

Brent, D. (2007). Antidepressants and suicidal behavior: Cause or cure? *American Journal of Psychiatry, 164*, 989–991.

Bridge, J. A., Birmaher, B., & Brent, D. A. (2007). Benefits and harms of pediatric antidepressant medications – Reply. *Journal of the American Medical Association, 298*, 627.

Bridge, J. A., Iyengar, S., Salary, C. B., Barbe, R. P., Birmaher, B., Pincus, H. A., et al. (2007). Clinical response and risk for reported suicidal ideation and suicide attempts in pediatric antidepressant treatment – A meta-analysis of randomized controlled trials. *Journal of the American Medical Association, 297*, 1683–1696.

Brown, E., Dunner, D. L., McElroy, S. L., Keck, P. E., Adams, D. H., Degenhardt, E., et al. (2009). Olanzapine/fluoxetine combination vs. lamotrigine in the 6-month treatment of bipolar I depression. *International Journal of Neuropsychopharmacology, 12*, 773–782.

Bruce, M. L., Ten Have, T. R., Reynolds, C. F., Katz, I. I., Schulberg, H. C., Mulsant, B. H., et al. (2004). Reducing suicidal ideation and depressive symptoms in depressed older primary care patients: A randomized controlled trial. *The Journal of the American Medical Association, 291*, 1081–1091.

Calabrese, J. R., Bowden, C. L., Sachs, G., Yatham, L. N., Behnke, K., Mehtonen, O.-P., et al. (2003). A placebo-controlled 18-month trial of lamotrigine and lithium maintenance treatment in recently depressed patients with bipolar I disorder. *Journal of Clinical Psychiatry, 64*, 1013–1024.

Carney, M. W. P., Roth, M., & Garside, R. F. (1965). The diagnosis of depressive syndromes and the prediction of ECT response. *British Journal of Psychiatry, 111*, 659–674.

Carney, S., Cowen, P., Dearness, K., Eastaugh, J., Freemantle, N. & UK ECT Review Group. (2003). Efficacy and safety of electroconvulsive therapy in depressive disorders: A systematic review and meta-analysis. *Lancet, 361*, 799–808.

Cavanagh, J. T. O., Carson, A. J., Sharpe, M., & Lawrie, S. M. (2003). Psychological autopsy studies of suicide: A systematic review. *Psychological Medicine, 33*, 395–405.

Chavez-Leon, E. (2004). Pharmacological treatment of the bipolar disorder, depressive phase (bipolar 33 depression). First part. *Salud Mental, 27*, 33–43.

Chynoweth, R., Tonge, J. I., & Armstrong, J. (1980). Suicide in Brisbane – A retrospective psychosocial study. *Australian and New Zealand Journal of Psychiatry, 14*, 37–45.

Ciapparelli, A., Dell'osso, L., Tundo, A., Pini, S., Chiavacci, M. C., Di Sacco, I., et al. (2001). Electroconvulsive therapy in medication-nonresponsive patients with mixed mania and bipolar depression. *Journal of Clinical Psychiatry, 62*, 552–555.

Cipriani, A., Geddes, J., Furukawa, T. A., & Barbui, C. (2007). Metareview on short-term effectiveness and safety of antidepressants for depression: An evidence-based approach to inform clinical practice. *Canadian Journal of Psychiatry, 53*, 553–562.

Cipriani, A., Pretty, H., Hawton, K., & Geddes, J. R. (2005). Lithium in the prevention of suicidal behavior and all-cause mortality in patients with mood disorders: A systematic review of randomized trials. *American Journal of Psychiatry, 162*, 1805–1819.

Claassen, C. A., Trivedi, M. H., Rush, A. J., Husain, M. M., Zisook, S., Young, E., et al. (2007). Clinical differences among depressed patients with and without a history of suicide attempts: Findings from the STAR*D trial. *Journal of Affective Disorders, 97*, 77–84.

Cohen, J. (1977). *Statistical power of analysis for the behavioral sciences*. New York: Academic Press.

Cohen, J. (1986). Statistical approaches to suicidal risk factor analysis. *Annals of the New York Academy of Sciences, 487*, 34–41.

Collins, J. C., & McFarland, B. H. (2008). Divalproex, lithium and suicide among Medicaid patients with bipolar disorder. *Journal of Affective Disorders, 107*, 23–28.

Colom, F., Vieta, E., Daban, C., Pacchiarotti, I., & Sanchez-Moreno, J. (2006). Clinical and therapeutic implications of predominant polarity in bipolar disorder. *Journal of Affective Disorders, 93*, 13–17.

Colom, F., Vieta, E., Martinez, A., Jorquera, A., Gasto, C., Colom, F., et al. (1998). What is the role of psychotherapy in the treatment of bipolar disorder? [Review] [65 refs]. *Psychotherapy and Psychosomatics, 67*, 3–9.

Cornelius, J. R., Salloum, I. M., Ehler, J. G., Jarrett, P. J., Cornelius, M. D., Perel, J. M., et al. (1997). Fluoxetine in depressed alcoholics. A double-blind, placebo-controlled trial. *Archives of General Psychiatry, 54*, 700–705.

Cornelius, J. R., Salloum, I. M., Lynch, K., Clark, D. B., & Mann, J. J. (2001). Treating the substance-abusing patient. *Annals of the New York Academy of Sciences, 932*, 78–90.

Cuijpers, P., & Schoevers, R. A. (2004). Increased mortality in depressive disorders: A review. *Current Psychiatry Reports, 6*, 430–437.

Daly, J. J., Prudic, J., Devanand, D. P., Nobler, M. S., Lisanby, S. H., Peyser, S., et al. (2001). ECT in bipolar and unipolar depression: Differences in speed of response. *Bipolar Disorders, 3*, 95–104.

Diagnostic and Statistical Manual of Mental Disorders (4th ed., Text Revision ed.). Washington, DC: American Psychiatric Association.

Dombrovski, A. Y., Cyranowski, J. M., Mulsant, B. H., Houck, P. R., Buysse, D. J., Andreescu, C., et al. (2008). Which symptoms predict recurrence of depression in women treated with maintenance interpersonal psychotherapy? *Depression and Anxiety, 25*, 1060–1066.

Dombrovski, A. Y., Mulsant, B. H., Houck, P. R., Mazumdar, S., Lenze, E. J., Andreescu, C., et al. (2007). Residual symptoms and recurrence during maintenance treatment of late-life depression. *Journal of Affective Disorders, 103*, 77–82.

Dube, S., Tollefson, G. D., Thase, M. E., Briggs, S. D., Van Campen, L. E., Case, M., et al. (2007). Onset of antidepressant effect of olanzapine and olanzapine/fluoxetine combination in bipolar depression. *Bipolar Disorders, 9*, 618–627.

Emslie, G. J., Ventura, D., Korotzer, A., & Tourkodimitris, S. (2009). Escitalopram in the treatment of adolescent depression: A randomized placebo-controlled multisite trial. *Journal of the American Academy of Child and Adolescent Psychiatry, 48*, 721–729.

Endicott, J., Rajagopalan, K., Minkwitz, M., Macfadden, W. & BOLDER Study Group. (2007). A randomized, double-blind, placebo-controlled study of quetiapine in the treatment of bipolar I and II depression: improvements in quality of life. *International Clinical Psychopharmacology, 22*, 29–37.

Fernandez, N., Grataloup, G., & Posner, K. (2008). Translation of the Columbia Suicide Severity Rating Scale (C-Ssrs) for use in 33 countries. *Value in Health, 11*, A340–A341.

Fountoulakis, K. N., Grunze, H., Panagiotidis, P., & Kaprinis, G. (2008). Treatment of bipolar depression: An update. *Journal of Affective Disorders, 109*, 21–34.

Gaudiano, B. A., Andover, M. S., & Miller, I. W. (2008). The emergence of suicidal ideation during the post-hospital treatment of depressed patients. *Suicide & Life Threatening Behavior, 38*, 539–551.

Geddes, J. R., Calabrese, J. R., & Goodwin, G. M. (2009). Lamotrigine for treatment of bipolar depression: Independent meta-analysis and meta-regression of individual patient data from five randomised trials. *British Journal of Psychiatry, 194*, 4–9.

Geddes, J. R., Carney, S. M., Davies, C., Furukawa, T. H., Kupfer, D. J., Frank, E., et al. (2003). Relapse prevention with antidepressant drug treatment in depressive disorders: A systematic review. *Lancet, 361*, 653–661.

Ghaemi, S. N., & Goodwin, F. K. (2005). Antidepressants for bipolar depression. *American Journal of Psychiatry, 162*, 1545–1546.

Gijsman, H. J., Geddes, J. R., Rendell, J. M., Goodwin, G. M., & Nolen, W. A. (2005). Antidepressants for bipolar depression. *American Journal of Psychiatry, 162*, 1547–1548.

Gijsman, H. J., Geddes, J. R., Rendell, J. M., Nolen, W. A., & Goodwin, G. M. (2004). Antidepressants for bipolar depression: A systematic review of randomised, controlled trials. *American Journal of Psychiatry, 161*, 1537–1547.

Gitlin, M. J. (1993). Lithium-induced renal insufficiency. *Journal of Clinical Psychopharmacology, 13*, 276–279.

Goldberg, J. F., Brooks, J. O., Kurita, K., Hoblyn, J. C., Ghaemi, N., Perlis, R. H., et al. (2009). Depressive illness burden associated with complex polypharmacy in patients with bipolar disorder: Findings from the STEP-BD. *Journal of Clinical Psychiatry, 70*, 155–162.

Goodwin, F. K., Fireman, B., Simon, G. E., Hunkeler, E. M., Lee, J., & Revicki, D. (2003). Suicide risk in bipolar disorder during treatment with lithium and divalproex. *Journal of the American Medical Association, 290*, 1467–1473.

Goodwin, F. K., & Jamison, K. R. (1990). *Manic-depressive illness* (pp. 228–230). New York: Oxford University Press.

Goodyer, I. M., Dubicka, B., Wilkinson, P., Kelvin, R., Roberts, C., Byford, S., et al. (2008). A randomised controlled trial of cognitive behavior therapy in adolescents with major depression treated by selective serotonin reuptake inhibitors. *The ADAPT trial. Health Technology Assessment, 12*, iii–60.

Grandjean, E. M., & Aubry, J. M. (2009a). Lithium: Updated human knowledge using an evidence-based approach: Part I: Clinical efficacy in bipolar disorder. *CNS Drugs, 23*, 225–240.

Grandjean, E. M., & Aubry, J. M. (2009b). Lithium: Updated human knowledge using an evidence-based approach: Part III: Clinical safety. *CNS Drugs, 23*, 225–240.

Greil, W., Ludwig-Mayerhofer, W., Erazo, N., Schocklin, C., Schmidt, S., Engel, R. R., et al. (1997). Lithium versus carbamazepine in the maintenance treatment of bipolar disorders – A randomised study. *Journal of Affective Disorders, 43*, 151–161.

Grof, P., & Muller-Oerlinghausen, B. (2009). A critical appraisal of lithium's efficacy and effectiveness: The last 60 years. *Bipolar Disorders, 11*, 10–19.

Grunze, H. C. R. (2008). Switching, induction of rapid cycling, and increased suicidality with antidepressants in bipolar patients: Fact or overinterpretation?. *CNS Spectrums, 13*, 790–795.

Gunnell, D., & Frankel, S. (1994). Prevention of suicide: Aspirations and evidence. *British Medical Journal, 308*, 1227–1233.

Guze, S. B., & Robins, E. (1970). Suicide and primary affective disorders. *British Journal of Psychiatry, 117*, 437–438.

Hagnell, O., & Rorsman, B. (1978). Suicide and endogenous depression with somatic symptoms in the Lundby study. *Neuropsychobiology, 4*, 180–187.

Harris, E. C., & Barraclough, B. M. (1997). Suicide as an outcome for mental disorders: A meta-analysis. *British Journal of Psychiatry, 170*, 205–228.

Harris, E. C., & Barraclough, B. M. (1998). Excess mortality of mental disorder. *British Journal of Psychiatry, 173*, 11–53.

Hawton, K., Sutton, L., Haw, C., Sinclair, J., & Harriss, L. (2005). Suicide and attempted suicide in bipolar disorder: A systematic review of risk factors. *Journal of Clinical Psychiatry, 66*, 693–704.

Healy, D. & Aldred, G. (2005). Antidepressant drug use & the risk of suicide. *International Review of Psychiatry, 17,* 163–172.

Hepburn, S. R., Crane, C., Barnhofer, T., Duggan, D. S., Fennell, M. J. V., & Williams, J. M. G. (2009). Mindfulness-based cognitive therapy may reduce thought suppression in previously suicidal participants: Findings from a preliminary study. *British Journal of Clinical Psychology, 48*, 209–215.

Hirschfeld, R., Fochtmann, L. J., & McIntyre, J. S. (2005). Antidepressants for bipolar depression. *American Journal of Psychiatry, 162*, 1547.

Hirschfeld, R. M., Keller, M. B., Panico, S., Arons, B. S., Barlow, D., Davidoff, F., et al. (1997). The National depressive and manic-depressive association consensus statement on the undertreatment of depression. [See comment]. [Review] [38 refs] *Journal of the American Medical Association, 277*, 333–340.

Hirschfeld, R. M. A., Bowden, C., Gitlin, M. J., Keck, P. E., Suppes, T., Thase, M. E., et al. (2002). *Practice guideline for the treatment of bipolar disorder* (2nd ed.). Washington, DC: American Psychiatric Association.

Hughes, C. W., Emslie, G. J., Crismon, M. L., Posner, K., Birmaher, B., Ryan, N. et al. (2007). Texas children's medication algorithm project: Update from Texas consensus conference panel on medication treatment of childhood major depressive disorder. *Journal of the American Academy of Child and Adolescent Psychiatry, 46,* 667–686.

Inskip, H. M., Harris, E. C., & Barraclough, B. (1998). Lifetime risk of suicide for affective disorder, alcoholism and schizophrenia. *British Journal of Psychiatry, 172*, 35–37.

Janicak, P. G., Dowd, D. M., Martis, B., Alam, D., Beedle, D., Krasuski, J., et al. (2002). Repetitive transcranial magnetic stimulation versus electroconvulsive therapy for major depression: Preliminary results of a randomized trial. *Biological Psychiatry, 51*, 659–667.

Johnson, F. N. (1999). The origins of lithium therapy. *Reviews in Contemporary Pharmacotherapy, 10*, 193–265.

Juurlink, D. N. (2006). Antidepressant-induced or clinician-induced suicidality in depression? Dr. Juurlink replies. *American Journal of Psychiatry, 163,* 1644–1645.

Juurlink, D. N., Mamdani, M. M., Kopp, A., & Redelmeier, D. A. (2006). The risk of suicide with selective serotonin reuptake inhibitors in the elderly. *American Journal of Psychiatry, 163,* 813–821.

Keck, J., McIntyre, R. S., & Shelton, R. C. (2007). Bipolar depression: Best practices for the outpatient. *CNS Spectrums, 12*(Suppl.), 1–15.

Keks, N. A., Hill, C., Sundram, S., Graham, A., Bellingham, K., Dean, B., et al. (2009). Evaluation of treatment in 35 cases of bipolar suicide. *Australian and New Zealand Journal of Psychiatry, 43*, 503–508.

Kellner, C. H., Fink, M., Knapp, R., Petrides, G., Husain, M., Rummans, T., et al. (2005). Relief of expressed suicidal intent by ECT: A consortium for research in ECT study. *American Journal of Psychiatry, 162*, 977–982.

Kemp, D. E., Muzina, D. J., McIntyre, R. S., & Calabrese, J. R. (2008). Bipolar depression: Trial-based insights to guide patient care. *Dialogues in Clinical Neuroscience, 10*, 181–192.

Kendell, R. E. (1968). *The classification of depressive illnesses*. London: Oxford University Press.

Kessing, L. V., Sondergard, L., Kvist, K., & Andersen, P. K. (2007). Adherence to lithium in naturalistic settings: Results from a nationwide pharmacoepidemiological study. *Bipolar Disorders, 9*, 730–736.

Kincaid-Smith, P., Burrows, G. D., Davies, B. M., Holwill, B., Walter, M., & Walker, R. G. (1979). Renal biopsy findings in lithium and prelithium patients. *Lancet, 1979*, 700–701.

Kirsch, I., Deacon, B. J., Huedo-Medina, T. B., Scoboria, A., Moore, T. J., & Johnson, B. T. (2008). Initial severity and antidepressant effects: A meta-analysis of data submitted to the Food and Drug Administration. *PLoS Medicine, 5*, e45.

Laje, G., Buervenich, S., Manji, H., Rush, A. J., Wilson, A., Charney, D. et al. (2006). Genetic markers of suicidal ideation emerging during antidepressant treatment. *American Journal of Medical Genetics Part B-Neuropsychiatric Genetics, 141B,* 724–725.

Laje, G., Paddock, S., Manji, H., Rush, A. J., Wilson, A. F., Charney, D. et al. (2007). Genetic markers of suicidal ideation emerging during citalopram treatment of major depression. *American Journal of Psychiatry, 164,* 1530–1538.

Lauterbach, E., Felber, W., Muller-Oerlinghausen, B., Ahrens, B., Bronisch, T., Meyer, T., et al. (2008). Adjunctive lithium treatment in the prevention of suicidal behaviour in depressive disorders: A randomised, placebo-controlled, 1-year trial. *Acta Psychiatrica Scandinavica, 118*, 469–479.

Lewis, A. J. (1979). 'Endogenous' and 'exogenous': A useful dichotomy? In *The later papers of Sir Aubrey Lewis* (pp. 173–178). Oxford University Press.

Maharaj, K., & Parasram, R. (1989). Characteristics of a rural area community mental health programme County Caroni. *International Journal of Social Psychiatry, 35*, 280–284.

Maltsberger, J. T. (1997). Ecstatic suicide. *Archives of Suicide Research, 3*, 283–301.

Mann, J. (2008). SSRIs have a specific risk among antidepressants to cause suicidality – Con debate. *International Journal of Neuropsychopharmacology, 11,* 4.

Mann, J.J., Brown, R. P., Halper, J. P., Sweeney, J. A., Kocsis, J. H., Stokes, P. E., et al. (1985). Reduced sensitivity of lymphocyte beta-adrenergic receptors in patients with endogenous depression and psychomotor agitation. *New England Journal of Medicine, 313*, 715–720.

Mann, J. J., Emslie, G., Baldessarini, R. J., Beardslee, W., Fawcett, J. A., Goodwin, F. K. et al. (2006). ACNP task force report on SSRIs and suicidal behavior in youth. *Neuropsychopharmacology, 31,* 473–492.

Mann, J. J., Goodwin, F. R., O'Brien, C. P., & Robinson, D. S. (1993). Suicidal behavior and psychotropic medication: Accepted as a consensus statement by the ACNP Council, March 2, 1992. *Neuropsychopharmacology, 8,* 177–183.

Marangell, L. B., Bauer, M. S., Dennehy, E. B., Wisniewski, S. R., Allen, M. H., Miklowitz, D. J., et al. (2006). Prospective predictors of suicide and suicide attempts in 1,556 patients with bipolar disorders followed for up to 2 years. *Bipolar Disorders, 8*, 566–575.

March, J. S., Klee, B. J., & Kremer, C. M. E. (2006). Treatment benefit and the risk of suicidality in multicenter, randomized, controlled trials of sertraline in children and adolescents. *Journal of Child & Adolescent Psychopharmacology, 16*, 91–102.

March, J., Silva, S., Petrycki, S., Curry, J., Wells, K., Fairbank, J., et al. (2004). Fluoxetine, cognitive-behavioral therapy, and their combination for adolescents with depression – Treatment for adolescents with depression study (TADS) randomized controlled trial. *Jama-Journal of The American Medical Association, 292*, 807–820.

March, J. S., Silva, S., Petrycki, S., Curry, J., Wells, K., Fairbank, J., et al. (2007). The Treatment for Adolescents With Depression Study (TADS): long-term effectiveness and safety outcomes. *Archives of General Psychiatry, 64*, 1132–1143.

Markowitz, G. S., Radhakrishnan, J., Kambham, N., Valeri, A. M., Hines, W. H., & D'Agati, V. D. (2000). Lithium nephrotoxicity: A progressive combined glomerular and tubulointerstitial nephropathy. *Journal of the American Society of Nephrology, 11*, 1439–1448.

Maruta, N. O., Yavdak, I. O., Denysenko, M. M., & Kharchenko, A. M. (2008). A suicidal risk in patients with neurotic and endogenous depressions. *European Psychiatry, 23*, S259.

Mayer-Gross, W., Slater, E., & Roth, M. (1960). *Clinical psychiatry.* London: Cassell.

McCann, S. M., Daly, J., & Kelly, C. B. (2008). The impact of long-term lithium treatment on renal function in an out-patient population. *Ulster Medical Journal, 77*, 102–105.

McElroy, S. L., Kotwal, R., Kaneria, R., & Keck, P. E. (2006). Antidepressants and suicidal behavior in bipolar disorder. *Bipolar Disorders, 8*, 596–617.

McGirr, A., Renaud, J., Seguin, M., Alda, M., & Turecki, G. (2008). Course of major depressive disorder and suicide outcome: A psychological autopsy study. *Journal of Clinical Psychiatry, 69*, 966–970.

McGrath, P. J., Khan, A. Y., Trivedi, M. H., Stewart, J. W., Morris, D. W., Wisniewski, S. R., et al. (2008). Response to a selective serotonin reuptake inhibitor (citalopram) in major depressive disorder with melancholic features: A STAR*D report. *The Journal of Clinical Psychiatry, 69*, 1847–1855.

Medda, P., Perugi, G., Zanello, S., Ciuffa, M., Rizzato, S., & Cassano, G. B. (2009). Comparative response to electroconvulsive therapy in medication-resistant bipolar I patients with depression and mixed state. *Journal of ECT,* doi: 10.1097/YCT.0b013e3181b00f1e.

Meltzer, H. Y., Alphs, L., Green, A. I., Altamura, A. C., Anand, R., Bertoldi, A., et al. (2003). Clozapine treatment for suicidality in schizophrenia: International suicide prevention trial (InterSePT). *Archives of General Psychiatry, 60*, 82–91.

Melvin, G. A., Tonge, B. J., King, N. J., Heyne, D., Gordon, M. S., & Klimkeit, E. (2006). A comparison of cognitive-behavioral therapy, sertraline, and their combination for adolescent depression. *Journal of the American Academy of Child and Adolescent Psychiatry, 45*, 1151–1161.

Miklowitz, D. J., Otto, M. W., Frank, E., Reilly-Harrington, N. A., Wisniewski, S. R., Kogan, J. N., et al. (2007). Psychosocial treatments for bipolar depression: A 1-year randomized trial from the systematic treatment enhancement program. [See comment]. *Archives of General Psychiatry, 64*, 419–426.

Miles, C. P. (1977). Conditions predisposing to suicide: A review [Review]. *Journal of Nervous and Mental Disease, 164*, 231–246.

Muller-Oerlinghausen, B., Ahrens, B., Grof, E., Grof, P., Lenz, G., Schou, M., et al. (1992). The effect of long-term lithium treatment on the mortality of patients with manic-depressive and schizoaffective illness. *Acta Psychiatrica Scandinavica, 86*, 218–222.

Muller-Oerlinghausen, B., Muser-Causemann, B., & Volk, J. (1992). Suicides and parasuicides in a high-risk patient group on and off lithium long-term medication. *Journal of Affective Disorders, 25*, 261–269.

Mulsant, B. H., Alexopoulos, G. S., Reynolds, C. F. III, Katz, I. R., Abrams, R., Oslin, D., et al. (2001). Pharmacological treatment of depression in older primary care patients: The PROSPECT algorithm. *International Journal of Geriatric Psychiatry, 16*, 585–592.

Murphy, J. M., Burke, J. D., Monson, R. R., Horton, N. J., Laird, N. M., Lesage, A., et al. (2008). Mortality associated with depression. A forty-year perspective from the Stirling County study. *Social Psychiatry and Psychiatric Epidemiology, 43*, 594–601.

Nakajima, S., Ishida, T., Akaishi, R., Takahata, K., Kitahata, R., Uchida, H., et al. (2009). Impacts of switching antidepressants after successful electroconvulsive therapy on the maintenance of clinical remission in patients with treatment-resistant depression: A chart review. *Journal of ECT, 25*, 178–181.

National Institute for Health and Clinical Excellence. (2006). Bipolar disorder: The management of bipolar disorder in adults, children, and adolescents, in primary and secondary care.

Nelson, J. C., Thase, M. E., Khan, A., Nelson, J. C., Nelson, J. C., Thase, M. E., et al. (2008). Are antidepressants effective? What's a clinician to think? *Journal of Clinical Psychiatry, 69*, 1014–1015.

Newman, S. C., & Bland, R. C. (1991). Suicide risk varies by subtype of affective disorder. *Acta Psychiatrica Scandinavica, 83*, 420–426.

O'Donovan, C., Garnham, J. S., Hajek, T., & Alda, M. (2008). Antidepressant monotherapy in pre-bipolar depression; predictive value and inherent risk. *Journal of Affective Disorders, 107*, 293–298.

Olfson, M. & Marcus, S. C. (2008). A case-control study of antidepressants and attempted suicide during early phase treatment of major depressive episodes. *Journal of Clinical Psychiatry, 69*, 425–432.

Olfson, M., Marcus, S. C., & Shaffer, D. (2006). Antidepressant drug therapy and suicide in severely depressed children and adults – A case-control study. *Archives of General Psychiatry, 63*, 865-872.

Oquendo, M. A. (2007). Lithium and divalproex in the treatment of bipolar suicide attempters. *Biological Psychiatry, 61*, 136S.

Oquendo, M. A. (2009). First RCT comparing lithium and divalproex in the prevention of suicidal behavior in bipolar suicide attempters. *Bipolar Disorders, 11*(Suppl. 1), 5–6.

Oquendo, M. A., Chaudhury, S. R., & Mann, J. J. (2005a). Pharmacotherapy of suicidal behaviour in bipolar disorder. *Archives of Suicide Research, 9*, 237–250.

Oquendo, M. A., Chaudhury, S. R., & Mann, J. J. (2005b). Pharmacotherapy of suicidal behavior in bipolar disorder. [Review] [124 refs]. *Archives of Suicide Research, 9*, 237–250.

Oquendo, M. A., Currier, D., & Mann, J. J. (2006). Prospective studies of suicidal behavior in major depressive and bipolar disorders: What is the evidence for predictive risk factors? *Acta Psychiatrica Scandinavica, 114*, 151–158.

Oquendo, M. A., & Mann, J. J. (2003). Intervention research for suicidal behaviour. *Lancet, 362*(9387), 844–845.

Orbach, I., Mikulincer, M., Gilboa-Schechtman, E., & Sirota, P. (2003). Mental pain and its relationship to suicidality and life meaning. *Suicide & Life-Threatening Behavior, 33*, 231–241.

Orbach, I., Mikulincer, M., Sirota, P., & Gilboa-Schechtman, E. (2003). Mental pain: A multidimensional operationalization and definition. *Suicide & Life-Threatening Behavior, 33*, 219–230.

Paddock, S., Laje, G., Charney, D., Rush, A. J., Wilson, A. F., Sorant, A. J. M. et al. (2007). Association of GRIK4 With Outcome of Antidepressant Treatment in the STAR*D Cohort. *American Journal of Psychiatry, 164*, 1181–1188.

Penland, H. R., & Ostroff, R. B. (2006). Combined use of lamotrigine and electroconvulsive therapy in bipolar depression: A case series. *Journal of ECT, 22*, 142–147.

Perlis, R. H. (2007). Treatment of bipolar disorder: The evolving role of atypical antipsychotics. [Erratum appears in Am J Manag Care 2008 Feb;14(2):76]. [Review] [82 refs]. *American Journal of Managed Care, 13*, S178–S188.

Perlis, R. H., Patrick, A., Smoller, J. W., & Wang, P. S. (2009). When is pharmacogenetic testing for antidepressant response ready for the clinic? A cost-effectiveness analysis based on data from the STAR*D study. *Neuropsychopharmacology, 34*, 2227–2236.

Pirkola, S. P., Suominen, K., & Isometsa, E. T. (2004). Suicide in alcohol-dependent individuals – Epidemiology and management. *CNS Drugs, 18*, 423–436.

Pompili, M., Lester, D., Leenaars, A. A., Tatarelli, R., & Girardi, P. (2008). Psychache and suicide: A preliminary investigation. *Suicide & Life-Threatening Behavior, 38*, 116–121.

Posner, K., Oquendo, M. A., Gould, M., Stanley, B., & Davies, M. (2007). Columbia Classification Algorithm of Suicide Assessment (C-CASA): Classification of suicidal events in the FDA's pediatric suicidal risk analysis of antidepressants. *American Journal of Psychiatry, 164*, 1035–1043.

Posner, K., Oquendo, M., Stanley, B., & Gould, M. (2004). *Suicidality classification project.* www.fda.gov/ohrms/dockets/ac/04/slides/2004–406551_06_FDA_Posnor_file/frame.htm#slide0088.htm.

Post, R. M. (2005). The impact of bipolar depression. *Journal of Clinical Psychiatry, 66*, 5–10.

Prien, R. F., Klett, C. J., & Caffey, E. M. Jr. (1973). Lithium carbonate and imipramine in prevention of affective episodes: A comparison in recurrent affective illness. *Archives of General Psychiatry, 29*, 420–425.

Reeves, H., Batra, S., May, R. S., Zhang, R., Dahl, D. C., & Li, X. H. (2008). Efficacy of risperidone augmentation to antidepressants in the management of suicidality in major depressive disorder: A randomized, double-blind, placebo-controlled pilot study. *Journal of Clinical Psychiatry, 69*, 1228–1236.

Rich, C. L., Young, D., & Fowler, R. C. (1986). San Diego suicide study. I. Young vs. old subjects. *Archives of General Psychiatry, 43*, 577–582.

Robins, E., Murphy, G. E., Wiltinson, R. H. Jr., Gassner, S., & Kayes, J. (1959). Some clinical considerations in the prevention of suicide based on a study of 134 successful suicides. *American Journal of Public Health, 49*, 888–899.

Rosa, A. R., Andreazza, A. C., Kunz, M., Gomes, F., Santin, A., Sanchez-Moreno, J., et al. (2008). Predominant polarity in bipolar disorder: Diagnostic implications. *Journal of Affective Disorders, 107*, 45–51.

Rucci, P., Frank, E., & Kostelnik, B. (2002). Suicide attempts in patients with bipolar I disorder during acute and maintenance phases of intensive treatment with pharmacotherapy and adjunctive psychotherapy. *American Journal of Psychiatry, 159*, 1160–1164.

Sachs, G. S., Nierenberg, A. A., Calabrese, J. R., Marangell, L. B., Wisniewski, S. R., Gyulai, L., et al. (2007). Effectiveness of adjunctive antidepressant treatment for bipolar depression. [See comment]. *New England Journal of Medicine, 356*, 1711–1722.

Sackeim, H. A., Haskett, R. F., Mulsant, B. H., Thase, M. E., Mann, J. J., Pettinati, H. M., et al. (2001). Continuation pharmacotherapy in the prevention of relapse following electroconvulsive therapy: A randomised controlled trial. *Journal of the American Medical Association, 285*, 1299–1307.

Sackeim, H. A., & Prudic, J. (2005). Length of the ECT course in bipolar and unipolar depression. *Journal of ECT, 21*, 195–197.

Sajatovic, M., Davies, M., & Hrouda, D. R. (2004). Enhancement of treatment adherence among patients with bipolar disorder. [Review] [50 refs]. *Psychiatric Services, 55*, 264–269.

Sakinofsky, I. (2005). Suicide and suicidality. In D. S. Goldbloom (Ed.), *Psychiatric clinical skills*. Burlington, MA: Elsevier.

Sakinofsky, I. (2007a). Treating suicidality in depressive illness. Part 1: Current controversies. *Canadian Journal of Psychiatry. Revue Canadienne De Psychiatrie, 52*, 71S–84S.

Sakinofsky, I. (2007b). Treating suicidality in depressive illness. Part 2: Does treatment cure or cause suicidality? *Canadian Journal of Psychiatry. Revue Canadienne De Psychiatrie, 52*, 85S–101S.

Sakinofsky, I., & Webster, G. (2010). The epidemiology of suicide in Canada. In J. Cairney & D. L. Streiner (Eds.), *Mental health in Canada: The epidemiologic perspective.* . University of Toronto Press.

Schaffer, A., Cairney, J., & Veldhuizen, S. (2006). Antidepressant use in a community sample of bipolar and unipolar subjects: Effect of diagnosis and comorbid anxiety. *Bipolar Disorders, 12*(Suppl.), 37.

Schaffer, A., Flint, A. J., Smith, E., Rothschild, A. J., Mulsant, B. H., Szanto, K., et al. (2008). Correlates of suicidality among patients with psychotic depression. *Suicide & Life Threatening Behavior, 38*, 403–414.

Schneider, B., Muller, M. J., & Philipp, M. (2001). Mortality in affective disorders. *Journal of Affective Disorders, 65*, 263–274.

Schou, M., & Schou, M. (1997). Forty years of lithium treatment. [See comment] [Review] [42 refs]. *Archives of General Psychiatry, 54*, 9–13.

Seemuller, F., Severus, E., Moller, H. J., & Riedel, M. (2009). Antidepressants and suicidality in younger adults – Is bipolar illness the missing link? *Acta Psychiatrica Scandinavica, 119*, 166.

Seguin, M., Lesage, A., Chawky, N., Guy, A., Daigle, F., Girard, G., et al. (2006). Suicide cases in New Brunswick from April 2002 to May 2003: The importance of better recognizing substance and mood disorder comorbidity. *Canadian Journal of Psychiatry – Revue Canadienne De Psychiatrie, 51*, 581–586.

Shelton, R. C., & Papakostas, G. I. (2008). Augmentation of antidepressants with atypical antipsychotics for treatment-resistant major depressive disorder. [Review] [51 refs]. *Acta Psychiatrica Scandinavica, 117*, 253–259.

Sher, L., Oquendo, M. A., & Mann, J. J. (2001). Risk of suicide in mood disorders. *Clinical Neuroscience Research, 1*, 337–344.

Shneidman, E. S. (1993). Commentary: Suicide as psychache. *Journal of Nervous and Mental Disease, 181*, 145–147.

Shneidman, E. S. (1998). Further reflections on suicide and psychache. *Suicide & Life-Threatening Behavior, 28*, 245–250.

Simon, G. (2008). Antidepressants and suicide – Treatment is probably too sporadic to affect overall suicide rates. *British Medical Journal, 336,* 515–516.

Simon, G. E., & Savarino, J. (2007). Suicide attempts among patients starting depression treatment with medications or psychotherapy. *American Journal of Psychiatry, 164*, 1029–1034.

Soares-Weiser, K., Bravo, V. Y., Beynon, S., Dunn, G., Barbieri, M., Duffy, S., et al. (2007). A systematic review and economic model of the clinical effectiveness and cost-effectiveness of interventions for preventing relapse in people with bipolar disorder. [Review] [122 refs]. *Health Technology Assessment (Winchester, England), 11*, iii–iiv.

Sondergard, L., Lopez, A. G., Andersen, P. K., & Kessing, L. V. (2008). Mood-stabilizing pharmacological treatment in bipolar disorders and risk of suicide. *Bipolar Disorders, 10*, 87–94.

Swannell, J. (Ed.). (1992). *The Oxford modern English Dictionary.* Oxford, Clarendon Press.

Stone, M., Laughren, T., Jones, M. L., Levenson, M., Holland, P. C., Hughes, A., et al. (2009). Risk of suicidality in clinical trials of antidepressants in adults: Analysis of proprietary data submitted to US Food and Drug Administration. *British Medical Journal, 339*, b2880, doi: 10.1136 BMJ.b2880.

Sturner, W. Q. (1986). Adolescent suicide fatalities. *Rhode Island Medical Journal, 69*, 471–474.

Suppes, T., Kelly, D. I., & Perla, J. M. (2005). Challenges in the management of bipolar depression. *Journal of Clinical Psychiatry, 66*, 11–16.

Szanto, K., Mulsant, B. H., Houck, P., Dew, M. A., & Reynolds, C. F. (2003). Occurrence and course of suicidality during short-term treatment of late-life depression. *Archives of General Psychiatry, 60*, 610–617.

Szanto, K., Mulsant, B. H., Houck, P. R., Dew, M. A., Dombrovski, A., Pollock, B. G., et al. (2007). Emergence, persistence, and resolution of suicidal ideation during treatment of depression in old age. *Journal of Affective Disorders, 98*, 153–161.

Szanto, K., Mulsant, B. H., Houck, P. R., Miller, M. D., Mazumdar, S., & Reynolds, C. F. III. (2001). Treatment outcome in suicidal vs. non-suicidal elderly patients. *American Journal of Geriatric Psychiatry, 9*, 261–268.

Teicher, M. H., Glod, C., & Cole, J. O. (1990). Emergence of intense suicidal preoccupation during fluoxetine treatment. *American Journal of Psychiatry, 147*, 207–210.

Teicher, M. H., Glod, C. A., & Cole, J. O. (1993). Antidepressant drugs and the emergence of suicidal tendencies. [Review]. *Drug Safety, 8*, 186–212.

Thase, M. E. (2005). Bipolar depression: Issues in diagnosis and treatment. *Harvard Review of Psychiatry, 13*, 257–271.

Thase, M. E. (2008). Do antidepressants really work? A clinicians' guide to evaluating the evidence. [Review] [23 refs]. *Current Psychiatry Reports, 10*, 487–494.

Thase, M. E., Corya, S. A., Osuntokun, O., Case, M., Henley, D. B., Sanger, T. M., et al. (2007). A randomized, double-blind comparison of olanzapine/fluoxetine combination, olanzapine, and fluoxetine in treatment-resistant major depressive disorder. *Journal of Clinical Psychiatry, 68*, 224–236.

Thase, M. E., Macfadden, W., Weisler, R. H., Chang, W., Paulsson, B., Khan, A., et al. (2006). Efficacy of quetiapine monotherapy in bipolar I and II depression: A double-blind, placebo-controlled study (the BOLDER II study). [See comment] [Erratum appears in J Clin Psychopharmacol. 2007 Feb;27(1):51]. *Journal of Clinical Psychopharmacology, 26*, 600–609.

Thies-Flechtner, K., Muller-Oerlinghausen, B., Seibert, W., Walther, A., & Greil, W. (1996). Effect of prophylactic treatment on suicide risk in patients with major affective disorders. Data from a randomized prospective trial. *Pharmacopsychiatry, 29*, 103–107.

Trivedi, M. H., Thase, M. E., Osuntokun, O., Henley, D. B., Case, M., Watson, S. B., et al. (2009). An integrated analysis of olanzapine/fluoxetine combination in clinical trials of treatment-resistant depression. *Journal of Clinical Psychiatry, 70*, 387–396.

Tuazon, J., Casalino, D., Syed, E., Batlle, D., Tuazon, J., Casalino, D., et al. (2008). Lithium-associated kidney microcysts. *The Scientific World Journal, 8*, 828–829.

Tundo, A., Marchetti, F., & Lega, I. (2006). Mood changes and suicidality in bipolar patients in maintenance treatment with mood stabilizers and antidepressants. A naturalistic study. *Bipolar Disorders, 8*, 40.

Turner, E. H., & Rosenthal, R. (2008). Efficacy of antidepressants. *British Medical Journal, 336*, 516–517.

Vaidya, N. A., Mahableshwarkar, A. R., & Shahid, R. (2003). Continuation and maintenance ECT in treatment-resistant bipolar disorder. *Journal of ECT, 19*, 10–16.

Valtonen, H. M., Suominen, K., Mantere, O., Leppamaki, S., Arvilommi, P., & Isometsa, E. T. (2006). Prospective study of risk factors for attempted suicide among patients with bipolar disorder. *Bipolar Disorders, 8*, 576–585.

Vitiello, B., Silva, S. G., Rohde, P., Kratochvil, C. J., Kennard, B. D., Reinecke, M. A., et al. (2009). Suicidal events in the treatment for adolescents with depression study (TADS). *Journal of Clinical Psychiatry, 70*, 741–747.

Wagner, K. D., Jonas, J., Findling, R. L., Ventura, D., & Saikali, K. (2006). A double-blind, randomized, placebo-controlled trial of escitalopram in the treatment of pediatric depression. *Journal of the American Academy of Child and Adolescent Psychiatry, 45*, 280–288.

Weisler, R. H., Calabrese, J. R., Thase, M. E., Arvekvist, R., Stening, G., Paulsson, B., et al. (2008). Efficacy of quetiapine monotherapy for the treatment of depressive episodes in bipolar I disorder: A post hoc analysis of combined results from 2 double-blind, randomized, placebo-controlled studies. *Journal of Clinical Psychiatry, 69*, 769–782.

Wheeler, B. W., Gunnell, D., Metcalfe, C., Stephens, P., & Martin, R. M. (2008). The population impact on incidence of suicide and non-fatal self harm of regulatory action against the use of selective serotonin reuptake inhibitors in under 18s in the United Kingdom: Ecological study. *BMJ*, doi:10.1136/bmj.39462.375613.BE.

Williams, J. M., Alatiq, Y., Crane, C., Barnhofer, T., Fennell, M. J., Duggan, D. S., et al. (2008). Mindfulness-based cognitive therapy (MBCT) in bipolar disorder: Preliminary evaluation of immediate effects on between-episode functioning. *Journal of Affective Disorders, 107*, 275–279.

Williams, J. M. G., Barnhofer, T., Crane, C., & Beck, A. T. (2005). Problem solving deteriorates following mood challenge in formerly depressed patients with a history of suicidal ideation. *Journal of Abnormal Psychology, 114*, 421–431.

Williams, J. M. G., Crane, C., Barnhofer, T., Van der Does, A. J. W., & Segal, Z. V. (2006). Recurrence of suicidal ideation across depressive episodes. *Journal of Affective Disorders, 91*, 189–194.

Williams, J. M. G., Duggan, D. S., Crane, C., & Fennell, M. J. V. (2006). Mindfulness-based cognitive therapy for prevention of recurrence of suicidal behavior. *Journal of Clinical Psychology, 62*, 201–210.

Williams, J. M. G., Van der Does, A. J. W., Barnhofer, T., Crane, C., & Segal, Z. S. (2008). Cognitive reactivity, suicidal ideation and future fluency: Preliminary investigation of a differential activation theory of hopelessness/suicidality. *Cognitive Therapy and Research, 32*, 83–104.

Wisniewski, S., Rush, A. J., Nierenberg, A. A., Gaynes, B. N., Warden, D., Luther, J. F., et al. (2009). Can phase III trial results of antidepressant medications be generalized to clinical practice? A STAR*D report. *American Journal of Psychiatry, 166*, 599–607.

Yatham, L. N., Kennedy, S. H., Schaffer, A., Parikh, S. V., Beaulieu, S., O'Donovan, C., et al. (2009). Canadian Network for Mood and Anxiety Treatments (CANMAT) and International Society for Bipolar Disorders (ISBD) collaborative update of CANMAT guidelines for the management of patients with bipolar disorder: Update 2009. *Bipolar Disorders, 11*, 225–255.

Yerevanian, B. I., Koek, R. J., & Mintz, J. (2003). Lithium, anticonvulsants and suicidal behavior in bipolar disorder. *Journal of Affective Disorders, 73*, 223–228.

Yerevanian, B. I., Koek, R. J., & Mintz, J. (2007). Bipolar pharmacotherapy and suicidal behavior. Part I: Lithium, divalproex and carbamazepine. *Journal of Affective Disorders, 103*, 5–11.

Yerevanian, B. I., Koek, R. J., Mintz, J., & Akiskal, H. S. (2007). Bipolar pharmacotherapy and suicidal behavior. Part 2: The impact of antidepressants. *Journal of Affective Disorders, 103*, 13–21.

About the Author

Isaac Sakinofsky, MB, ChB, MD, FRCPC, FRCPsych, is Professor Emeritus in psychiatry and public health sciences in the University of Toronto, Canada, and has worked with suicidal patients throughout his career. His doctoral thesis, about social and cultural determinants, contrasted prevalence rates and clinical pictures of nonfatal suicidality and mental illness in the racial groups of Cape Town, South Africa (where he grew up). He received his training in medicine, psychiatry, and neurology at the University of Cape Town and then completed a residency in psychiatry at the Institute of Psychiatry and the Maudsley Hospital, University of London, in the days when Sir Aubrey Lewis and

Professor Michael Shepherd taught their students rigorous critical analysis of the psychiatric literature. He emigrated to Canada in 1968 to join the faculty of the new McMaster University Medical School and later moved to the University of Toronto. He has researched, taught, and published on the epidemiology and clinical aspects of suicide and attempted suicide. He is a foundation member of the International Academy for Suicide Research.

Isaac Sakinofsky
University of Toronto
CAMH-Clarke site
250 College Street
Toronto ON M5T 1R8
Canada
Tel.: +1 416 979 4674
E-mail: isaac.sakinofsky@utoronto.ca

Evidence-Based Treatment for Reducing Suicide Risk in Schizophrenia

Herbert Y. Meltzer

Department of Psychiatry, Vanderbilt University School of Medicine, Nashville, TN, USA

Schizophrenia is a genetically determined syndrome that is caused by structural and functional brain abnormalities. Pre- and postnatal experience can influence the course and phenotype. This syndrome is characterized by positive symptoms (such as hallucinations and delusions), negative symptoms (such as withdrawal, anhedonia, flat affect, and loss of motivation), enduring multifaceted cognitive impairment (Freedman, 2003), and diverse mood symptoms that include depression. Schizophrenia affects about 1% of the adult population, but can occur in children and during early adolescence. It is most often initially diagnosed during late adolescence and early adulthood. Schizophrenia produces devastating effects on the functional outcome in many patients with schizophrenia, with the cognitive impairment considered to be the most important reason for this; but other domains of psychopathology listed above also contribute to poor outcome. As a result of this dysfunction, hopelessness can arise. This characteristic, along with command hallucinations and delusions, can bring individuals with schizophrenia to the point of deliberate self-harm.

The concept of "suicidality," as used herein, represents a spectrum of behaviors, to include suicidal thoughts or plans, suicide attempts, completed suicide, deliberate self-harm with no lethal intent, and passive thoughts of being "better off dead" when attempting to draw conclusions from studies with mixed samples. Suicide and suicidality, as indicated below, are exceptionally common among patients with schizophrenia, not just those with sufficient affective symptoms to be diagnosed as schizoaffective (Inskip, Harris, & Barra Clough, 1998). Earlier estimates suggested that between 9% and 13% of patients with schizophrenia completed suicide at some point in their lifetime, at an annual rate of 0.2–0.3% (Harris & Barraclough, 1997; Meltzer, 1998). A recent comprehensive review of the literature suggested that the lower end of this range, for example, 4.9%, is a more accurate figure (Palmer, Pakratz, & Bostwick, 2005). Most successful attempts appear to occur early in the disease process, especially within the first year and decade after the onset of illness (Palmer et al., 2005; Qin et al., 2006). However, the risk of suicide in schizophrenia persists throughout the patient's lifetime.

Compared with the general population, the rate of completed suicide among schizophrenic patients by earlier estimates was reported to be 25 times higher (Miles, 1977); however, more recent figures indicate that the rate of suicide in schizophrenia is approximately 90 per 100,000 or about 8–13 times greater than that of the general population in the US (Allebeck, 1989; Mortensen & Juel, 1993). The standardized mortality rate for schizophrenia worldwide is 8–9%, ranking third from among all mental disorders behind major depression (18–23%) and bipolar disorder (12–18%; Harris & Barraclough, 1997). These rates are likely an underestimate because of the reluctance to attribute death due to suicide in the official records, data from which most estimates of suicide frequency are derived.

The risk factors for suicide in patients with schizophrenia are well established. Thus, patients at greatest risk are those who have made a prior suicide attempt, who are in the second and third decades of life, first year of psychosis, male, Caucasian, unmarried, who have a relatively good premorbid level of social, school, or work function, who experience depression as their first or second episodes of psychotic symptoms subside, and who have a history of substance abuse (Bertelsen et al., 2007; Kohler & Lallart, 2002; Tapp, Kilzieh, Wood, Raskind, & Tandon, 2001). Hopelessness, social isolation, awareness of illness coupled with a dismal view of the prognosis, recent hospitalization due to any reason, recent loss of job, or forced withdrawal from formal education are also important risk factors in schizophrenic individuals who commit suicide (Kim, Jayathiake, & Meltzer, 2003; Siris, 2001). Rejection by their family members and the receipt of explicit messages sometimes that suicide might be a "way-out" are powerful but fortunately rare stimuli for the timing of a suicide attempt. Instability within the therapeutic relationship may also contribute to the risk for suicide. Acceptance of the diagnosis of schizophrenia and belief in poor prognosis regardless of the treatment, particularly if these include a sense that the desired level of recovery will never be attained, have been reported as risk factors in many studies (Amador et al., 1996; Kim et al., 2003). Many of these factors are present during the prodromal phase of schizophrenia. Thus, suicide is not uncommon in the prodrome of schizophrenia (Knittel et al., 2008).

Current Approaches to Treatment and Prevention

Current approaches to the prevention and treatment of schizophrenia rely heavily on early detection, protective care such as respite or hospitalization, appropriate pharmacotherapy, careful planning of discharge with the risk of suicide in mind, psychotherapy and psychosocial treatment, and possibly cognitive behavioral therapy. Early detection depends on awareness of the risk factors for suicide within schizophrenia mentioned above. However, identification of some individuals as suicidal who do not share any of these characteristics or who are unwilling or unable to make someone evaluating the risk of suicidality aware that these suicidal traits are present in them will be missed. Once identified, the most urgent decision to be reached is what level of care is appropriate: Send the patient back to their family or help the patient with some form of assisted living, stay overnight in the emergency ward, take respite, or undergo hospitalization. Restriction of access to means for committing suicide, for example, using guns, and a curb on methods used to commit suicide in a hospital, for example, by hanging or jumping from heights are useful in the short run. The most common approaches involve the application of those treatments that are most effective in treating schizophrenia per se. These approaches include the use of antipsychotic drugs, for which, as reviewed below, there is extremely robust evidence with regard to the efficacy of clozapine, the atypical antipsychotic drug. While there are some epidemiologic data supporting the use of antipsychotic drugs other than clozapine (Haukka, Tiihonen, Härkänen, & Lönnqvist, 2008; Tiihonen et al., 2006), there is little or no evidence supporting the use of mood stabilizers or antidepressant drugs. The reason for this factor may be because treatment of psychosis per se does not appear to affect the risk for suicide (Fialko et al., 2006). Psychotic symptoms that are not accompanied by depression and hopelessness do not increase the risk for suicide in schizophrenia. While there are no controlled studies on the role of ECT in treating patients with schizophrenia who are at risk for suicide, there is evidence to suggest that ECT is effective in reducing the risk for suicide in patients with severe depression (Greenhalgh, Knight, Hind, Beverley, & Walters, 2005) and ECT can potentiate the efficacy of clozapine (Masoudzadeh & Khalilian, 2007). However, there is no randomized evidence for the effectiveness of ECT in patients with schizophrenia (Greenhalgh et al., 2005). Using an economic model, these authors concluded that clozapine is a cost-effective treatment compared with ECT for suicidal patients with schizophrenia. For patients who fail to respond to clozapine, ECT treatment may be the preferred next step over switching medication.

Cognitive behavioral therapy in schizophrenia is a promising new endeavor that should be considered for treating those individuals with schizophrenia with insight into the effects of schizophrenia on their overall function, who had high function prior to the onset of illness, and who express concern over their perceived decline in function. However, the results from one open study of CBT in patients with schizophrenia who were considered to be at risk for suicide showed no beneficial effect (Tarrier et al., 2008).

Sources of Research Evidence

Evidence for Efficacy of Current Approaches

Systematic Reviews and Meta-Analyses

A random-effects meta-analysis of six studies compared the rates of suicides or suicide attempts by psychotic patients who were treated with clozapine versus other antipsychotics (Hennen & Baldessarini, 2005). There was a greater than threefold reduction in the risk of suicidal behaviors favoring clozapine, based on a calculated risk ratio of 3.3 (95% CI = 1.7–6.3, $p < .0001$). For completed suicides, the risk ratio was 2.9 (95% CI = 1.5–5.7, $p = .002$). They concluded that long-term treatment with clozapine was associated with a threefold overall reduction in the risk of suicidal behaviors. However, in this small number of studies, quantitative differences among the studies were noted; the only randomized trial, the International Suicide Prevention Trial (InterSePT) (Meltzer et al., 2003), did not find reduced risk of completed suicide.

Randomized Controlled Trials With Definitive Results

The InterSePT was a large-scale, multicenter, international, randomized, parallel-group study that compared the effects of clozapine (300–900 mg/day) versus those of olanzapine (10–20 mg/day) on suicidal events in 980 patients with schizophrenia or schizoaffective disorder who were at high risk for suicide. "High risk" was defined as having had a suicide attempt or hospitalization to prevent suicide within the 3 years prior to study entry, moderate-to-severe suicidal ideation at trial entry, and significant depressive symptoms or command hallucinations within one week of trial initiation. Olanzapine was chosen as the comparator agent because of its pharmacological similarity to clozapine and previously published evidence that it reduces depression and suicidality in patients with schizophrenia (Richelson, 1999; Tollefson, Sanger, Lu, & Thieme, 1998; Tran et al., 1997).

The monitoring of suicidal events was conducted by three blinded, independent raters. The patients were seen on a weekly basis for the first 6 months, then every other week thereafter. The clozapine-treated patients received hematological monitoring as required, while the patients who took olanzapine had their blood pressure taken as per the same schedule. All patients were questioned about suicidality at each visit. Steps taken for reducing suicidal risk included freedom to optimize the dose of each study drug to ensure adequate response and to use any medication deemed necessary to reduce the suicidal behavior (including additional antipsychotics, antidepressants, anxiolytics, and mood stabilizers). Prescribers could utilize the electroconvulsive therapy, request for hospitalization, or increase the surveillance as needed.

The primary endpoint of the study was the time for suicide attempts and hospitalizations to prevent the risk of imminent suicide (labeled as a Type 1 event). Compliance with all the study medications as assessed by the pill count was 99%. Thirty-nine percentage of the subjects dropped out of the study, reasons for which did not differ significantly between groups, except for an unsatisfactory effect on suicide risk for olanzapine ($p = .03$). The proportion of patients who experienced a Type 1 event was significantly less in the clozapine-treated group compared with the olanzapine-treated group ($p = .03$). Time elapsed before experiencing a Type 1 event, which was the primary endpoint, was also significantly longer for clozapine ($p = .03$). Over the 2-year study, the probability of a significant suicide attempt or hospitalization to prevent suicide was 24% for the clozapine-treated group and 32% for olanzapine-treated group.

The secondary endpoint of the study was the addition of antidepressant medication or a change in antipsychotic medication (defined as the switch to another drug or the addition of a second antipsychotic medication) as a "rescue" intervention. Significantly fewer clozapine-treated patients required a secondary endpoint intervention in comparison to olanzapine-treated patients (3.1% versus 6.7% for the addition of antidepressants, $p = .01$; 3.1% versus 5.9% for the use of adjunctive antipsychotics, $p = .04$). The number of patients needed to be treated to prevent a single suicide attempt or hospitalization to prevent suicide was 13. During the course of the study, three olanzapine-treated patients and five clozapine-treated patients committed suicide. The difference between the agents, however, was not statistically significant ($p = .73$). No other randomized controlled trial was conducted.

Cohort Studies

Clozapine was first reported to reduce the rate of suicidality in a mirror image study (Meltzer & Okayli, 1995). The rates of suicidality were examined among a cohort of 88 neuroleptic-resistant patients who were diagnosed with chronic schizophrenia ($N = 73$) or schizoaffective disorder ($N = 15$). The percentage of patients with no suicidality increased from 53% at baseline to 88% during clozapine treatment. During the 2 years prior to the initiation of clozapine therapy, 22 suicide attempts were reported in the total sample. During the 2-year study period in which clozapine was administered, there were only three such attempts, which translated to an 86% decrease in suicide attempts. A reduction in the lethal potential of these attempts was observed: The reported lethality of attempts before clozapine administration was minimal to mild in 11 instances and moderate to severe in another 11 cases. All three suicide attempts that occurred during clozapine treatment were considered to have no substantial potential for lethality. In this study, clozapine treatment was also associated with improvements in hopelessness and depressive symptoms that were indicated by improvements in the Hamilton Depression Scale total score at 6 weeks ($p = .002$) and at the end of the study ($p = .009$) relative to baseline in the 22 patients who had made previous suicide attempts. Hamilton suicide ratings were also significantly improved both at 6 weeks ($p = .03$) and at the end of the study ($p = .01$). It was not possible to determine if the observed effects on suicidality were the consequence of a specific antisuicidal effect of clozapine, nonspecific benefits from weekly clinical contact (owing to the need for frequent monitoring of the hematological status), poor psychopharmacological and psychosocial treatment prior to study entry, an interaction between clozapine and ongoing psychosocial treatment, or a cohort effect.

A reduction in suicide attempts ($p < .05$), impulsivity ($p < .05$), and aggressiveness ($p < .01$) was reported in a study of 30 neuroleptic-resistant patients with schizophrenia who were treated with clozapine for at least 1 year compared to 30 chronic schizophrenic patients treated with standard neuroleptics (Spivak, Mester, Wittenberg, Maman, & Weizman, 1997).

Modestin, Dal Pian, and Agarwalla (2005) conducted a retrospective comparison of the effects of continuous clozapine treatment (mean duration 15 months) and pre-clozapine treatment (for a similar time duration) using a mirror image design. The rates of suicidal behavior during the pre-clozapine and active clozapine periods were 28% and 3%, respectively. Odds ratios were 11.6 (95% CI = 3.4–39.9) for suicidal behavior and 12.3

(95% CI = 1.6–97.5) for severely suicidal behavior, both in favor of active clozapine treatment. These results were independent of cotreatment with antidepressants.

Haukka et al. (2008) studied the effect of medication on severe suicide attempts and completed suicide in a nationwide (Finland) cohort of suicidal schizophrenic individuals: The study population included all individuals in Finland who were hospitalized with a diagnosis of attempted suicide between January 1, 1997 and December 31, 2003, who also underwent at least one hospitalization due to the diagnosis of schizophrenia, and were at least 16 years old when the index hospitalization began. Cox's proportional hazards modeling and Bayesian intensity estimation were used in the analysis. There were 1,611 patients with a mean follow-up time of 4.3 years. Current use of antipsychotics was associated with decreased mortality due to suicide (HR 0.52, 95% CI = 0.34–0.81, $p = .004$), but no significant decrease in mortality was observed during current use of antidepressants (0.66, 0.41–1.08, $p = .099$), when compared to past use. In a more detailed analysis when current users were compared to nonusers, mixed use of antipsychotics was associated with reduced risk of suicide mortality. There were too few subjects treated with clozapine or other individual antipsychotic drugs to draw any firm conclusions about the use of these drugs. Current use of the antidepressant citalopram was associated with decreased mortality due to suicide as well.

In a subsequent epidemiologic follow-up study of all schizophrenic patients in Finland, covering the period of 1996–2006, Tiihonen et al. (2009) found that clozapine was associated with a substantially lower risk for suicide than any other medication. There were 19 deaths by suicide for clozapine treatment during 25,594 person-years. The adjusted hazard ratio was 0.30 (0.17–0.53). This compares with 44 deaths by suicide for olanzapine treatment during 19,629 person-years (0.95 (0.60–1.51)) and 37 deaths by suicide for risperidone treatment during 15,060 person-years (1.11 (0.69–1.80)). Similar advantages for clozapine were also observed with perphenazine.

Case-Control Study

All patients over a 4-year period who initiated treatment with clozapine while hospitalized within the Department of Veterans Affairs (VA) system ($N = 1,415$) were matched with a schizophrenic control group ($N = 2,830$) by propensity scoring. Centralized VA databases and a national death registry were used to identify all deaths within the two groups, along with listed causes, for the 3 years after discharge. Veterans exposed to clozapine as inpatients were significantly less likely to die during the follow-up period than those in the control group, but this was entirely attributable to the much lower rate of death due to respiratory disorders in the clozapine-treated group. There were no significant differences in the rates of suicide or accidental death. They concluded their results fail to support the hypothesis that clozapine treatment is associated with significantly fewer deaths due to suicide. A careful reading of this article indicates that the results do not lead to a rejection of the hypothesis that clozapine reduces the risk for suicide. Any conclusions from this article depend on the reliability of the propensity scoring to assemble the comparison group. It is likely that the efforts to identify an adequate control group with this method were inadequate. There are no other studies that have tried this approach.

Bateman, Hansen, Turkington, and Kingdon (2007) randomized 90 outpatients who were treatment-resistant schizophrenic patients treated with conventional antipsychotic medication to CBT or "befriending." The CBT-treated group showed significant reductions in suicidal ideation after 6 months of treatment, which persisted up to the time of a 9-month follow-up. As these patients were treatment resistant, and clozapine is the only treatment recognized to be efficacious for them, it is not clear why they chose not to use clozapine as the primary treatment and then add CBT or befriending. As it cannot be recommended that typical neuroleptic drugs be used to treat treatment-resistant schizophrenia, the utility of CBT treatment-resistant patients needs to be compared with a suitable comparator, for example, supportive psychotherapy, assisted work training, combination with clozapine. Similarly, CBT needs to be evaluated in randomized controlled trials in nontreatment-resistant patients as a means to prevent the emergence of suicidality in nontreatment-resistant patients. Current recommendations for treating the nontreatment-resistant suicidal patients with schizophrenia suggest clozapine as the treatment of choice (Meltzer et al., 2003; www.IPAP.org).

Registry Studies

In a retrospective analysis of morbidity and mortality, data from the Clozaril National Registry (April 1991 to December 1993) were cross-checked with the data from the national death Index and Social Security Administration for identifying the cause of death of 67,072 current and former users of clozapine; an 83% reduction in death by suicide was documented among current clozapine users compared with past users (Walker, Lanaza, Arellano, & Rothman, 1997). The results suggested that the risk of death by suicide had increased after the discontinuation of clozapine.

Meltzer and Okayli (1995), using the Clozaril National Registry data from 1990 to 1992, reported that the suicide rate in patients treated with clozapine was significantly lower than the expected rate. These results were supported by an additional analysis of Reid, Mason, and Hogan (1998), who examined the data from 1990 to 1996 and reported a 0.0157% per year incidence of completed suicide in patients treated with clozapine versus 0.4–0.8% per year reported in previous studies with typical neuroleptics (Allebeck, 1989; Caldwell & Gottesman, 1990). For first episode patients, the risk of suicide in those not taking any type of antipsychotic medication was 37-fold (5.1–276) greater than that in patients currently using any antipsychotic drug (Tiihonen et al., 2006).

Case Reports

Tarrier et al. (2006) reported the results of a trial of cognitive behavioral therapy, supportive counseling, and treatment as usual in recent onset schizophrenia on suicidal behavior.

Treatment was delivered over a 5-week period during hospitalization for an acute episode. The participants were assessed at baseline, 6 weeks, and 3 and 18 months. Over the 18 months of assessment, there were three definite suicides and two deaths by accidental causes. They concluded that there were no beneficial or adverse effects of this treatment regimen on suicide. None of the patients were treated with clozapine. This should not be considered an adequate trial of CBT. In particular, this might be tried as an adjunct with clozapine.

Improving and Optimizing Current Practice

Improving the current practice of treating patients with schizophrenia who have survived a serious suicide attempt or have been hospitalized to prevent a serious suicide attempt based upon evaluation of all information from multiple sources would appear to mandate initiation of treatment with clozapine. The body of information summarized here supports the conclusion that clozapine is superior to any other treatment for this purpose. The strongest evidence is the data obtained from the randomized controlled InterSePT (Meltzer et al., 2003). The data summarized in the meta-analysis of Hennen and Baldessarini (2005) support this conclusion. The recent epidemiologic data of Tiihonen et al. (2009) indicate that the effect of clozapine is manifest in routine clinical practice and can be life-saving. There is nothing other than clozapine for which there is substantial evidence of efficacy. As previously mentioned, the addition of ECT to clozapine might be considered in an individual who made an additional suicide attempt while taking an adequate dose of clozapine.

Potential Problems, Costs, and Resources

To minimize mortality from agranulocytosis, a patient treated with clozapine is required to have weekly monitoring of his or her white blood cell count when it is initiated, with the frequency of monitoring decreasing to monthly at differing rates in different countries. Clozapine also causes a number of other side effects: Hypersalivation, hypotension, drowsiness, weight gain, glucose dysregulation, lipid increases, myoclonus, major motor seizures, and myocarditis. These factors are not to be minimized but given the risk of suicide in patients who would meet the requirements for this indication, the potential benefit would be worth the additional risk to most individuals. It should be noted that after the first 6 and certainly 12 months of treatment with clozapine, the risk of agranulocytosis diminishes, whereas the risk of suicide does not, so the risk-benefit ratio becomes more favorable over time.

Acknowledgments

The author acknowledges the grant support received from Novartis during the period 1989–2001. He had served as their consultant for the period 2003–2009. He had also received grant support from or was a consultant for Eli Lilly, Janssen, Pfizer, Astra Zeneca, Roche, Wyeth, Organon, and Sanofi-Aventis. The author also wishes to thank Mr. and Mrs. Robert Paterson, and Mr. and Mrs. Edward Hintz for their financial support.

Further Reading

Meltzer, H. Y., Alphs, L., Green, A. I., Altamura, A. C., Anand, R., Bertoli, A., et al. (2003). Clozapine treatment for suicidality in schizophrenia: International Suicide Prevention Trial (InterSePT). *Archives of General Psychiatry, 60*, 82–91.

Fialko, L., Freeman, D., Bebbington, P. E., Kuipers, E., Garety, P. A., Dunn, G., & Fowler, D. (2006). Understanding suicidal ideation in psychosis: Findings from the Psychological Prevention of Relapse in Psychosis (PRP) trial. *Acta Psychiatr Scandinavica, 114*(3), 177–178.

Haukka, J., Tiihonen, J., Härkänen, T., & Lönnqvist, J. (2008). Association between medication and risk of suicide, attempted suicide and death in nationwide cohort of suicidal patients with schizophrenia. *Pharmacoepidemiol Drug Safety, 17*(7), 686–696.

References

Allebeck, P. (1989). Schizophrenia: A life-shortening disease. *Schizophrenia Bulletin, 15*, 81–89.

Amador, X. F., Friedman, J. H., Kasapis, C., Yale, S. A., Flaum, M., & Gorman, J. M. (1996). Suicidal behavior in schizophrenia and its relationship to awareness of illness. *American Journal of Psychiatry, 153*(9), 1185–1188.

Bateman, K., Hansen, L., Turkington, D., & Kingdon, D. (2007). Cognitive behavioral therapy reduces suicidal ideation in schizophrenia: Results from a randomized controlled trial. *Suicide & Life-Threatening Behavior, 37*(3), 284–290.

Bertelsen, M., Jeppesen, P., Petersen, L., Thorup, A., Øhlenschlaeger, J., le Quach, P., et al. (2007). Suicidal behaviour and mortality in first-episode psychosis: The OPUS trial. *British Journal of Psychiatry, 51*(Suppl.), 140–146.

Caldwell, C. B., & Gottesman, I. I. (1990). Schizophrenics kill themselves too: A review of risk factors for suicide. *Schizophrenic Bulletin, 16*, 571–589.

Fialko, L., Freeman, D., Bebbington, P. E., Kuipers, E., Garety, P. A., Dunn, G., et al. (2006). Understanding suicidal ideation in psychosis: Findings from the Psychological Prevention of Relapse in Psychosis (PRP) trial. *Acta Psychiatrica Scandinavica, 114*(3), 177–178.

Freedman, R. (2003). Schizophrenia. *The New England Journal of Medicine, 349*, 1738–1749.

Greenhalgh, J., Knight, C., Hind, D., Beverley, C., & Walters, S. (2005). Clinical and cost-effectiveness of electroconvulsive therapy for depressive illness, schizophrenia, catatonia and mania: Systematic reviews and economic modelling studies. *Health Technology Assessment, 9*, 1–156.

Harris, B. C., & Barraclough, B. (1997). Suicide as an outcome for mental disorders: A meta-analysis. *British Journal of Psychiatry, 170*, 205–228.

Haukka, J., Tiihonen, J., Härkänen, T., & Lönnqvist, J. (2008). Association between medication and risk of suicide, attempted suicide and death in nationwide cohort of suicidal patients with schizophrenia. *Pharmacoepidemiology and Drug Safety, 17*(7), 686–696.

Hennen, J., & Baldessarini, R. J. (2005). Suicidal risk during treatment with clozapine: A meta-analysis. *Schizophrenia Research, 73*, 139–145.

Inskip, H. M., Harris, E. C., & Barraclough, B. (1998). Lifetime risk of suicide for affective disorder, alcoholism and schizophrenia. *British Journal of Psychiatry, 172*, 35–37.

Kim, C. H., Jayathiake, K., & Meltzer, H. Y. (2003). Hopelessness, neurocognitive function, and insight in schizophrenia: Relationship to suicidal behavior. *Schizophrenia Research, 60*, 71–80.

Knittel, D., Munn, G., & Simmer, E. (2008). Prodromal psychosis as an etiology of suicide: A case report and review of the literature. *American Journal of Forensic Medicine and Pathology, 29*(3), 238–241.

Kohler, C. G., & Lallart, E. A. (2002). Postpsychotic depression in schizophrenia patients. *Current Psychiatry Reports, 4*, 273–278.

Masoudzadeh, A., & Khalilian, A. R. (2007). Comparative study of clozapine, electroshock and the combination of ECT with clozapine in treatment-resistant schizophrenic patients. *Pakistan Journal of Biological Science, 10*(23), 4287–4290.

Meltzer, H. Y. (1998). Suicide in schizophrenia: Risk factors and clozapine treatment. *Journal of Clinical Psychiatry, 59*(Suppl. 3), 15–20.

Meltzer, H. Y., Alphs, L., Green, A. I., Altamura, A. C., Anand, R., Bertoli, A., et al. (2003). Clozapine treatment for suicidality in schizophrenia: International Suicide Prevention Trial (InterSePT). *Archives of General Psychiatry, 60*, 82–91.

Meltzer, H. Y., & Okayli, G. (1995). Reduction of suicidality during clozapine treatment of neuroleptic-resistant schizophrenia: Impact on risk-benefit assessment. *American Journal of Psychiatry, 152*, 183–190.

Miles, C. P. (1977). Conditions predisposing to suicide: A review. *Journal of Nervous and Mental Disease, 164*, 246–321.

Modestin, J., Dal Pian, D., & Agarwalla, P. (2005). Clozapine diminishes suicidal behavior; a retrospective evaluation of clinical records. *Journal of Clinical Psychiatry, 66*(4), 534–538.

Mortensen, P. B., & Juel, K. (1993). Mortality and causes of death in first admitted schizophrenic patients. *British Journal of Psychiatry, 163*, 183–189.

Palmer, B. A., Pankratz, V. S., & Bostwick, J. M. (2005). The lifetime risk of suicide in schizophrenia: A re-examination of the evidence. *Archives of General Psychiatry, 62*, 247–253.

Qin, P., Nordentoft, M., Høyer, E. H., Agerbo, E., Laursen, T. M., & Mortensen, P. B. (2006). Trends in suicide risk associated with hospitalized psychiatric illness: A case-control study based on Danish longitudinal registers. *Journal of Clinical Psychiatry, 67*(12), 1936–1941.

Reid, W. H., Mason, M., & Hogan, T. (1998). Suicide prevention effects associated with clozapine therapy in schizophrenia and schizoaffective disorder. *Psychiatric Services, 49*, 1029–1033.

Richelson, E. (1999). Receptor pharmacology of neuroleptics: Relation to clinical effects. *Journal of Clinical Psychiatry, 60*(Suppl. 10), 5–14.

Sernyak, M. J., Hoff, R., & Rosenheck, R. (1999). Clozapine and suicide. *Psychiatric Services, 50*(1), 116–117.

Siris, S. (2001). Suicide and schizophrenia. *Journal of Psychopharmacology, 15*, 127–135.

Spivak, B., Mester, R., Wittenberg, N., Maman, Z., & Weizman, A. (1997). Reduction of aggressiveness and impulsiveness during clozapine treatment in chronic neuroleptic-resistant schizophrenic patients. *Clinical Neuropharmacology, 20*, 442–446.

Tapp, A., Kilzieh, N., Wood, A. E., Raskind, M., & Tandon, R. (2001). Depression in patients with schizophrenia during an acute psychotic episode. *Comprehensive Psychiatry, 42*, 314–318.

Tarrier, N., Haddock, G., Lewis, S., Drake, R., & Gregg, L. (2006). SoCRATES Trial Group. Suicide behaviour over 18 months in recent onset schizophrenic patients: The effects of CBT. *Schizophrenia Research, 83*(1), 15–27.

Tarrier, N., Taylor, K., & Gooding, P. (2008). Cognitive-behavioral interventions to reduce suicide behavior: A systematic review and meta-analysis. *Behavior Modification, 32*(1), 77–108.

Tiihonen, J., Lönnqvist, J., Wahlbeck, K., Klaukka, T., Niskanen, L., Tanskanen, A., et al. (2009). Mortality in schizophrenia: An 11-year follow-up study of the total Finnish population (FIN11 Study). *The Lancet, 374*, 620–627.

Tiihonen, J., Wahlbeck, K., Lönnqvist, J., Klaukka, T., Ioannidis, J. P., Volavka, J., et al. (2006). Effectiveness of antipsychotic treatments in a nationwide cohort of patients in community care after first hospitalisation due to schizophrenia and schizoaffective disorder: Observational follow-up study. *British Medical Journal, 333*(7561), 224–229.

Tollefson, G. S., Sanger, T. M., Lu, Y., & Thieme, M. E. (1998). Depressive signs and symptoms in schizophrenia: A prospective blinded trial of olanzapine and haloperidol. *Archives of General Psychiatry, 55*, 250–258.

Tran, P. V., Hamilton, S. H., Kuntz, A. J., Potvin, J. H., Andersen, S. W., Beasley, C., et al. (1997). Double-blind comparison of olanzapine versus risperidone in the treatment of schizophrenia and other psychotic disorders. *Journal of Clinical Psychopharmacology, 17*, 407–418.

Walker, A. M., Lanaza, L. L., Arellano, F., & Rothman, K. J. (1997). Mortality in current and former users of clozapine. *Epidemiology, 8*, 671–677.

About the Author

Herbert Y. Meltzer, MD, is Bixler/May/Johnson Professor of Psychiatry and Pharmacology and Director of the Psychobiology Program for Translational Research at the Vanderbilt University School of Medicine, in Nashville, TN. He is also Director of the Schizophrenia Program of Centerstone Mental Health System in Nashville and Chair of the Young Investigator Grant Review Committee for NARSAD. He is Chairman of the International Psychopharmacology Algorithm Project (www.IPAP.org). Dr. Meltzer is the recipient of the Efron and Paul Hoch Awards of the ACNP, the Noyes Prize of the Commonwealth of Pennsylvania, the Edward J. Sachar Award from Columbia University, the Lieber Prize for Schizophrenia Research from NARSAD, the Stanley Dean Award for Research in Schizophrenia of the American College of Psychiatry, the Gold Medal Award of the Society of Biological Psychiatry, the Earl Sutherland Prize for Achievement in Research of Vanderbilt University (2004), the Research Prize of the American Psychiatric Association (2005), and the Grant Liddle Award for Clinical Research from Vanderbilt University (2008). His research interests include clinical and basic psychopharmacology, with an emphasis on antipsychotic drug efficacy, safety, and tolerability, the mechanism of action of antipsychotic drugs, genetic factors in schizophrenia and pharmacogenomics, prevention of suicide in schizophrenia, and cognitive impairment in schizophrenia.

Herbert Y. Meltzer
Department of Psychiatry
Vanderbilt University School of Medicine
Nashville
TN 37215
USA
E-mail: herbert.meltzer@Vanderbilt.Edu

Evidence-Based Approach to Suicide Risk in First-Episode Psychosis

Merete Nordentoft

Faculty of Health Sciences, Psychiatric Centre Bispebjerg, Copenhagen University, Copenhagen NV, Denmark

Much attention has been paid to the risk of suicide in schizophrenia and early psychosis, and suicide risk in psychosis is a serious public health problem. Based on Danish register-based research, it can be estimated that in Denmark and probably in other Western European societies, approximately 7% of all deaths from suicide is attributed to suicides among patients who have been diagnosed with schizophrenia during their inpatient stay (Qin & Nordentoft, 2005).

The American epidemiologist Ezra Susser pinpointed the risk of suicide and other unwanted outcomes during the early phases of psychosis with this sentence: "At first admission, half the story is told," thereby referring to the well-known fact that many patients attempted suicide before first admission, and that some had even died from suicide before they managed to get into contact with psychiatric services.

Suicidal behavior and suicidal ideation is much more common than suicides. A total of 28% of patients included in the OPUS trial had had at least one suicide attempt before first contact with psychiatric services (Bertelsen et al., 2007), and the same percentage with suicide attempt before first contact was found in the LEO trial (Craig et al., 2004). In the TIPS project, Melle et al. found lower figures: 16% of first-episode psychotic patients from the nonearly detection areas attempted suicide before first contact with psychiatric services, and 5% in the early detection areas had done so previously in their lifetime (Melle et al., 2006). A recent Australian study showed that violent suicide attempts were more frequent among patients with first-episode psychosis than in later psychotic episodes.

The suicide risk was analyzed using data extracted from register-based studies, especially studies from Denmark, Sweden, and Finland. Some of these analyses revealed that the greatest risk of suicide occurred just after admission to a psychiatric department or just after discharge (Qin & Nordentoft, 2005), and that for patients with disorders in schizophrenia spectrum, the first year of treatment was associated with approximately 60% increased risk of suicide compared to the whole group of patients who had been admitted because of these disorders (Nordentoft et al., 2004). As in the general population, the absolute risk of suicide is higher among male patients than among female patients, but the *excess* risk compared to the general population is equal for the two genders. As in the general population, the suicide risk among patients with psychosis increases with increasing age, but the *excess* risk compared to the general population was highest in the young age groups (Nordentoft et al., 2004; Qin & Nordentoft, 2005). As the analyses are based on psychiatric case registers, these analyses could only indicate the risk of suicide after contact with secondary mental health services. However, there are some indications that suicide risk for patients in the early phases of psychosis is also high before first contact, but for obvious reasons we cannot get a direct measure of that aspect, as these persons are not identified with a diagnosed disease, registered in a register. However, several studies of patients who for the first time came into contact with mental health services with a psychotic condition, showed that almost one third have attempted suicide before first contact. A more indirect measure of the suicide risk during untreated psychosis can be extracted from studies evaluating the risk of suicide in the offspring of parents with psychiatric disorders. A recent study showed that children aged 10–21 years had an almost twofold risk of suicide if their parent had a history of psychiatric illness. This fact was also seen in cases where the children had had no psychiatric treatment. This might indicate suicide during untreated phases of a psychotic disorder or it could reflect the strain of living in a family with a mentally ill parent.

Since Miles (1977) in a review estimated that the risk of suicide in schizophrenia was 10%, this figure had been repeated many times in reviews and comments, and even in the latest version of the so-called NICE guidelines on schizophrenia from the National Institute for Health and Clinical Excellence (National Collaborating Center for Mental Health, 2009). However, it is likely that this estimate could be too high. Most likely, it is not 10% who eventually die from suicide. In a recent review, Palmer, Pankratz, and Bostwick (2005) identified all first-episode studies and estimated the lifetime risk to be 5.6%. Both antipsychotic treatment and the organization of psychiatric treatment have undergone changes; therefore, only studies published after 1965 were included. Their meta-analysis was split into an evaluation of mixed samples and an evaluation of first-episode studies. In the latter analysis, two large studies estimated a case fatality rate of 6% and 5% after a follow-up period of 9 and 14 years, respectively (Mortensen & Juel, 1993; Osby, Correia, Brandt, Ekbom, & Sparen, 2000). High case fatality rates due to zsuicide were mostly found in smaller studies (Carone, Harrow, & Westermeyer, 1991; Finnerty, Keogh, O'Grady-Walsh, & Walsh, 2002; Krausz, Muller-Thomsen, & Haasen, 1995; Tsoi & Wong, 1991; Wiersma, Nienhuis, Slooff, & Giel, 1998). Thus, it seems reasonable to conclude that case fatality rate due to suicide will not reach figures as high as 10%, because suicide risk is highest in the first few years after first admission. It is more likely that the true case fatality rate is between 5% and 6%. However, estimating lifetime suicide risk is very much complicated and is also susceptible to change along with changes in the treatment support offered to the patient group and in the general features of society. It is likely that large prospective studies of first-onset cases with a long follow-up period would provide a better estimate of the suicide risk; but an inherent problem with these studies is that by the time the results of these studies become available, the risk for new first-episode patients may have changed because of the changes in treatment and other factors. Studies should also be reviewed with regard to the age of onset, because cases with early onset have worse outcomes than cases with later onset pertaining to other outcome measures. Likewise, in their estimation of lifetime risk of suicide in various disorders, Inskip, Harris, and Baraclough (1998) estimated the lifetime risk in schizophrenia to be 4%.

To give a true estimate of suicide risk in schizophrenia, it is necessary to base the estimates on the follow-up of first-episode schizophrenia patients. If the patient group followed is not a consecutive or a representative sample of first-episode patients, as is the case in most studies, the estimates of the suicide risk might be inflated, because the mixed sample consists of the most severe cases; or these estimates might be underestimated, because those patients represent the positively selected survivors of the initial high-risk suicide period after first admission. Also, varying duration of follow-up or difficulties in following the patients over longer periods may make studies difficult to compare and interpret. A statement such as "10% die from suicide" is sometimes based on the calculation of the proportion of suicides in relation to all deaths; but since follow-up periods are not lifelong, there is an obvious risk of overestimating the suicide risk, since suicides often occur early in the course of schizophrenia, natural deaths occur later in life (Inskip et al., 1998). Or the suicide rate can be underestimated because of the survival bias as mentioned above. Another way of expressing suicide risk is to estimate suicide rate as the number of suicides per 100,000 person-years. This measure does take into account the fact that follow-up periods are different in different studies; but just as the case fatality rate, the suicide mortality rate does not take into account the fact that suicide rates are higher during the first few years after first admission. Estimating the suicide risk in first-episode schizophrenia also depends on diagnostic criteria, setting, and age limits in the sampling. Gender distribution in the sample could also play an important role.

Even with a lifetime risk of approximately 4–6%, the suicide risk is much higher among these patients compared to the general population. Comprehensive analyses of suicides have shown that people with severe mental illness form a particularly high-risk group, with only small variation between diagnostic groups (Mortensen, Agerbo, Erikson, Qin, & Westergaard-Nielsen, 2000). Though both Danish studies and a recent Finnish study have shown decreasing suicide rates among patients with schizophrenia during the last decades (Melle et al., 2006; Pirkola, Sohlman, Heila, & Wahlbeck, 2007), the risk of suicide in patients with disorders in schizophrenia spectrum is still approximately 20-fold higher than in the general population. Three large Danish register-based studies of suicide risk in patients with schizophrenia indicate that male gender, young age, short duration of illness, many admissions during last year, current inpatient, short time since discharge, and comorbid depression were independent risk factors (Melle et al., 2006; Mortensen & Juel, 1993; Rossau & Mortensen, 1997).

Some of the clinical studies have small sample size; therefore, some risk factors might not be identified due to lack of power. Previous suicide attempt is taken into consideration in almost all clinical studies. Apart from that, since different studies evaluate different risk factors, we cannot conclude that not mentioning a risk factor in a specific study excludes this risk factor from being a significant predictor of suicide. The information extracted from clinical studies supplies the register-based studies with the following risk factors as the most important and frequently observed predictors: previous suicide attempt, comorbid depression, drug abuse, poor compliance with medication, poor adherence to treatment, high IQ, and suicidal ideations. The results of the analyses of psychotic symptoms as risk factors for suicide are contradictory and are reported in different categories. Hawton et al. conducted a review of the risk factors for suicide in schizophrenia and found that hopelessness and depressive symptoms, suicidal thinking and suicidal attempts, agitation and motor restlessness, fear of mental disintegration, poor adherence to treatment, and recent loss were the strongest risk factors, as was drug (but not alcohol) abuse (Hawton, Sutton, Haw, Sinclair, & Deeks, 2005). In the meta-analysis of risk factors for suicide in schizophrenia, Hawton concluded that pooled odds ratio for suicide for positive symptoms was not significantly different from 1.0. However when the symptoms were divided into hallucinations and delusions, both hallucinations and delusions seemed to be protective (delusions: OR = 0.53 (95% CI 0.28–1.01) and hallucinations: OR = 0.5 (95% CI 0.35–0.71)); but there was a nonsignificant tendency that command hallucinations were associated with higher suicide risk (Hawton et al., 2005). One study identified high dose of antipsychotic medication as a predictor (Cheng, Leung, Lo, & Lam, 1990), while another found low dose of antipsychotic medication as a risk factor (Taiminen & Kujari, 1994). We could interpret this factor as a proxy variable for positive psychotic symptoms, but it could also reflect the lack of compliance with medication, mirrored in lower prescribed doses. Several studies reported that negative symptoms were protective, but in the meta-analysis by Hawton it turned out to be insignificant (Hawton et al., 2005).

A review of risk factors for suicide attempt in schizophrenia identified past or recent suicidal ideation, previous deliberate self-harm, past depressive episode, drug abuse or dependence, and higher mean number of psychiatric admissions as predictors (Haw, Hawton, Sutton, Sinclair, & Deeks, 2005). Depression, previous suicidal plans, and suicidal thoughts were also the strongest predictors of suicide attempt in the OPUS trial (Bertelsen et al., 2007). These results clearly indicate that to prevent suicidal behavior among first-episode psychotic patients, we have to necessarily focus on the group of patients with depressive symptoms and suicidal behavior and ideation.

Current Approaches to Treatment and Prevention

Due to poor evidence basis, there are no international guidelines for treating suicide risk in the early phases of schizophrenia (National Collaborating Center for Mental Health, 2009). However, many secondary care programs have developed guidelines for assessing the risk of suicide, safety procedures during inpatient stay, such as limiting access to potential dangerous means for suicide, and taking the risk of suicide into consideration, when deciding on the level of observation. There is no international agreement on these procedures; but for obvious reasons, these procedures have been implemented in different health services all over the world (see Table 1). As with other patients at increased risk of suicide, outpatient treatment services have worked with crisis plans.

Table 1. Screening of suicide risk in all psychiatric patients coming into contact with psychiatric services in the Capitol Region, Denmark

1. Has the patient previously attempted suicide?
2. Has the patient current suicidal ideation?
3. Has the patient current suicidal plans?
4. Is the patient impulsive?
5. Can the patient convincingly state that he or she will refrain from suicidal acts?
6. Is the patient characterized by suffering, hopelessness, pessimism, and is he or she unable to state the reasons for living?
7. Has there been an important negative life event or has the patient's mental state deteriorated?
8. Have the relatives been concerned that the patient will harm him- or herself?

Sources of Research Evidence

Few randomized controlled trials have been conducted with the aim of reducing the suicidal behavior in schizophrenia, and there is hardly any evidence to prove the effect of interventions on suicidal behavior and mortality. This problem had arisen partly due to studies needing very high numbers of participants to show a significant, clinically relevant difference between two or more treatment groups. There is very little evidence about the effectiveness of treatment on suicidal behavior in schizophrenia. In the InterSePT study, Meltzer et al. found that clozapine treatment showed superiority to olanzapine therapy in preventing suicide attempts in patients with schizophrenia and schizoaffective disorder who are at high risk for suicide (Meltzer et al., 2003). Apart from this trial, the evidence base is weak.

The OPUS trial revealed differences in overall mortality and in suicide mortality in favor of the experimental intensive treatment. Even though this study has been, until now, the largest randomized clinical trial in early psychosis with 547 patients randomized, the sample size is far too small to allow firm conclusions about the effect on completed suicide (Bertelsen et al., 2007) (see Figure 1). Despite lacking evidence, we must also anticipate that interventions with documented effect on schizophrenia symptoms might also be effective in preventing suicide; consequently, it is natural to recommend evidence based on psychiatric treatment for schizophrenia (American Psychiatric Association, 2004; National Institute for Clinical Excellence, 2006; Sekretariatet for referenceprogrammer, 2004).

The randomized clinical trial is the gold standard when evaluating the possible effects of an intervention. Because large randomized studies with suicide as outcome measure are almost practically impossible, we have to consider whether other study designs could provide evidence about any possible treatment effect. The nested case-control study is an effective tool to examine the influence of risk factors for which information is available in the Danish registers. In the nested case-control design, we could control some social and psychiatric confounders. Prospective cohort studies could also be used for assessing

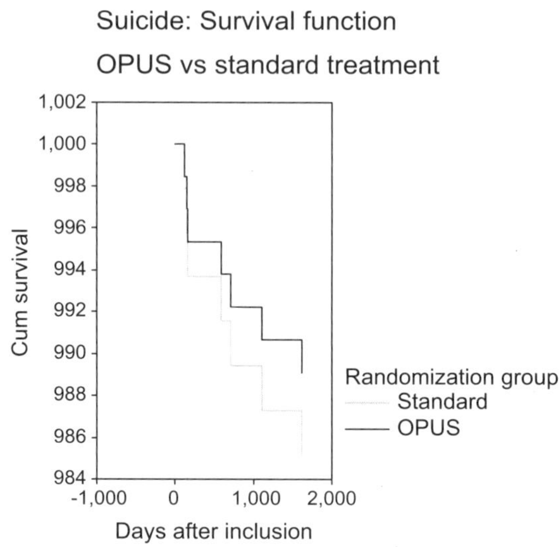

Figure 1. Suicide in the OPUS trial during a 5-year follow-up.

the influence of risk factors; but even with the most meticulous confounder control, all kinds of nonexperimental studies must be interpreted with caution. This is because the subjects who receive specific treatment and follow treatment recommendations constitute a select group. This group is characterized by positive (or negative) prognostic factors that increase (or decrease) the likelihood that the patients would benefit from this specific treatment, from other types of treatment, or even without treatment.

Evidence for the Efficacy of Current Approaches

There is a large evidence basis for restrictions in means for suicide in general (Hawton et al., 2004; Nordentoft, 2007; Nordentoft, Qin, Helweg-Larsen, & Juel, 2007), and this approach is also relevant for patients in the early phases of psychosis. Apart from that, the current approaches are based on a limited evidence basis, mainly based on expert's opinion.

Improving and Optimizing Current Practice

In daily clinical work, it seems sound to consider cognitive behavioral therapy, the concept of crisis plans, and green cards. Early intervention teams should in collaboration

Crisis plan

- Try to distract myself
  - TV, draw, paint, surf internet,messenger
- Think: "I have tried this before – it will end soon"
- Run in the park
- Write my thoughts down in my diary
- Take Truxal 25 mg
- Repeat: "I have promised not to hurt myself"
- Call Lis from OPUS 20607556
- Call my parents 33316274
- Call Lene 28763268
- Call Jacob 25245576
- Call Life line 70210210 (all days 11-23)
- Call psychiatric outreach via doctor on call 70130041
- Take a taxi to psychiatric emergency room, Bispebjerg Bakke 23, 35312300

Figure 2. Example of a crisis plan with actions, identified by the patient, likely to reduce suicide risk.

with the patients with suicidal thought and plans develop and rehearse crisis plans. The patient can contribute to these plans by identifying helpful thoughts and actions that to them have proven to be effective such as to call relatives or professionals, helplines, medication that can reduce anxiety and emotional pain, or actions that can distract unpleasant thoughts. The identified thoughts and actions should be written down, scheduled, prioritized, and rehearsed to make them an active resource in a critical situation (see Figure 2).

In a randomized clinical trial, Brown et al. found that cognitive therapy (mean 9 sessions) for adults who attempted suicide ($N = 120$) reduced the repetition rate and increased the repetition-free period (Brown et al., 2005). Part of this approach consisted of problem solving, identifying reasons for living, constructing a "hope box" or "survivor kit" with items such as pictures, letters, poetry, and coping cards. "Survivor kits" could easily be implemented in Early Intervention Services. Another promising tool is green cards (Morgan, Jones, & Owen, 1993) with instructions about how to access psychiatric emergency rooms or other interventions available in critical situations.

Randomized clinical trials with these interventions should be carried out to improve our knowledge basis. Most likely, due to small sample size, the outcome measure will have to be attempted suicide rather than suicide. Suicidal behavior is an important challenge for psychiatric services, and particularly so for services involved in treatment in the early phases of psychosis. Taking the challenge of suicidal behavior seriously involves development and evaluation of new methods for coping with suicidal crisis.

Further Reading

1. Nordentoft, M., Melau, M., Iversen, T., & Kjær S. (2009). *Psykose hos unge – symptomer, behandling og fremtid. Erfaringer fra OPUS*. København: Psykiatrifonden (Nordentoft, Melau, Iversen, & Kjær, 2009). Danish book about rationale, approach, and elements in the OPUS treatment. There are, for example, chapters about barriers to seek treatment, family work, and social skills training.
2. Jackson, H. J., & McGorry, P. D. (2009). The recognition and management of early psychosis. A preventive approach (2nd ed.). Cambridge: Cambridge University Press (Jackson & McGorry, 2009). This book describes stage-specific model highlighting the clinical and biological factors present during the development of the illness and the best treatment available for each of these stages. The book is highly recommendable for those involved in the care of people with early psychotic illness.
3. McFarlane W. R. (2002). Multifamilygroups in the treatment of severe psychiatric disorders. New York and London: Guilford Press (McFarlane, 2002). In this book, the rationale, the theoretical, and empirical foundation, for involving families are presented together with an extraordinarily clear explanation of how to work with psychoeducative multifamily groups. It is a manual in which the reader can find answers to almost all questions in relation to the practical therapeutic work.
4. Compton, M. T., & Broussard, B. (2009). The first episode of psychosis. A guide for patients and their families (1st ed.). New York: Oxford University Press (Compton & Broussard, 2009). The First Episode of Psychosis is the ideal book for patients experiencing the frightening and confusing initial episode of psychosis. The book can help patients and relatives to take an active and informed role in their care to ensure the best possible prognosis.

References

American Psychiatric Association. (2004). *Practice guideline for the treatment of patients with schizophrenia* (2nd ed.). Arlington: American Psychiatric Association.

Bertelsen, M., Jeppesen, P., Petersen, L., Thorup, A., Øhlenschlæger, J., le Quack, P., et al. (2007). Suicidal behaviour and mortality in first-episode psychosis: The OPUS trial. *British Journal of Psychiatry, 191*, 140–146.

Brown, G. K., Ten, H. T., Henriques, G. R., Xie, S. X., Hollander, J. E., & Beck, A. T. (2005). Cognitive therapy for the prevention of suicide attempts: A randomized controlled trial. *Journal of the American Medical Association, 294*, 563–570.

Carone, B. J., Harrow, M., & Westermeyer, J. F. (1991). Posthospital course and outcome in schizophrenia. *Archives of General Psychiatry, 48*, 247–253.

Cheng, K. K., Leung, C. M., Lo, W. H., & Lam, T. H. (1990). Risk factors of suicide among schizophrenics. *Acta Psychiatrica Scandinavica, 81*, 220–224.

Compton, M. T., & Broussard, B. (2009). *The first episode of psychosis. A guide for patients and their families*. New York, NY: Oxford University Press.

Craig, T. K., Garety, P., Power, P., Rahaman, N., Colbert, S., Fornells-Ambrojo, M., et al. (2004). The Lambeth Early Onset (LEO) Team: Randomised controlled trial of the effectiveness of specialised care for early psychosis. *British Medical Journal, 329*(7474), 1067.

Finnerty, A., Keogh, F., O'Grady-Walsh, A., & Walsh, D. (2002). A 15-year follow-up of schizophrenia in Ireland. *Irish Journal of Psychological Medicine, 19*(4), 108–114.

Haw, C., Hawton, K., Sutton, L., Sinclair, J., & Deeks, J. (2005). Schizophrenia and deliberate self-harm: A systematic review of risk factors. *Suicide & Life-Threatening Behavior, 35*, 50–62.

Hawton, K., Simkin, S., Deeks, J., Cooper, J., Johnston, A., Waters, K., et al. (2004). UK legislation on analgesic packs: Before and after study of long term effect on poisonings. *British Medical Journal, 329*(7474), 1076.

Hawton, K., Sutton, L., Haw, C., Sinclair, J., & Deeks, J. J. (2005). Schizophrenia and suicide: Systematic review of risk factors. *British Journal of Psychiatry, 187*, 9–20.

Inskip, H. M., Harris, E. C., & Barraclough, B. (1998). Lifetime risk of suicide for affective disorder, alcoholism and schizophrenia. *British Journal of Psychiatry, 172*, 35–37.

Jackson, H. J., & McGorry, P. D. (2009). *The recognition and management of early psychosis. A preventive approach* (2nd ed.). Cambridge: Cambridge University Press.

Krausz, M., Muller-Thomsen, T., & Haasen, C. (1995). Suicide among schizophrenic adolescents in the long-term course of illness. *Psychopathology, 28*(2), 95–103.

McFarlane, W. R. (2002). *Multifamily groups in the treatment of severe psychiatric disorders*. New York, London: Guilford Press.

Melle, I., Johannesen, J. O., Friis, S., Haahr, U., Joa, I., Larsen, T. K., et al. (2006). Early detection of the first episode of schizophrenia and suicidal behavior. *American Journal of Psychiatry, 163*, 800–804.

Meltzer, H. Y., Alphs, L., Green, A. I., Altamura, A. C., Anand, R., Bertoldi, A., et al. (2003). Clozapine treatment for suicidality in schizophrenia: International suicide prevention trial (InterSePT). *Archives of General Psychiatry, 60*, 82–91.

Miles, C. P. (1977). Conditions predisposing to suicide: A review. *Journal of Nervous and Mental Disease, 164*, 231–246.

Morgan, H. G., Jones, E. M., & Owen, J. H. (1993). Secondary prevention of non-fatal deliberate self-harm. The green card study. *British Journal of Psychiatry, 163*, 111–112.

Mortensen, P. B., Agerbo, E., Erikson, T., Qin, P., & Westergaard-Nielsen, N. (2000). Psychiatric illness and risk factors for suicide in Denmark. *Lancet, 355*(9197), 9–12.

Mortensen, P. B., & Juel, K. (1993). Mortality and causes of death in first admitted schizophrenic patients. *British Journal of Psychiatry, 163*, 183–189.

National Collaborating Center for Mental Health. (2009). *Schizophrenia. Core interventions in the treatment and management of schizophrenia in primary and secondary care*. National Clinical Practice Guideline number 82. London: National Institute for Health and Clinical Excellence.

National Institute for Clinical Excellence. (2006). *Schizophrenia. Full national clinical guideline for interventions in primary and secondary care*. London: Royal College of Psychiatrist and British Psychological Society.

Nordentoft, M. (2007). Prevention of suicide and attempted suicide in Denmark. Epidemiological studies of suicide and intervention studies in selected risk groups. *Danish Medical Bulletin, 54*, 306–369.

Nordentoft, M., Laursen, T. M., Agerbo, E., Qin, P., Hoyer, E. H., & Mortensen, P. B. (2004). Change in suicide rates for patients with schizophrenia in Denmark, 1981–97: Nested case-control study. *British Medical Journal, 329*, 261–266.

Nordentoft, M., Melau, M., Iversen, T., & Kjær, S. (2009). *Psykose hos unge – symptomer, behandling og fremtid. Erfaringer fra OPUS* [Psychosis in young people – symptoms, treatment, future. Experiences from OPUS]. København: Psykiatrifonden.

Nordentoft, M., Qin, P., Helweg-Larsen, K., & Juel, K. (2007). Restrictions in means for suicide: An effective tool in preventing suicide: The Danish experience. *Suicide & Life-Threatening Behavior, 37*, 688–697.

Osby, U., Correia, N., Brandt, L., Ekbom, A., & Sparen, P. (2000). Mortality and causes of death in schizophrenia in Stockholm county, Sweden. *Schizophrenac Research, 45*, 21–28.

Palmer, B. A., Pankratz, V. S., & Bostwick, J. M. (2005). The lifetime risk of suicide in schizophrenia: A reexamination. *Archives of General Psychiatry, 62*, 247–253.
Pirkola, S., Sohlman, B., Heila, H., & Wahlbeck, K. (2007). Reductions in postdischarge suicide after deinstitutionalization and decentralization: A nationwide register study in Finland. *Psychiatric Services, 58*, 221–226.
Qin, P., & Nordentoft, M. (2005). Suicide risk in relation to psychiatric hospitalization: Evidence based on longitudinal registers. *Archives of General Psychiatry, 62*, 427–432.
Rossau, C. D., & Mortensen, P. B. (1997). Risk factors for suicide in patients with schizophrenia: Nested case-control study. *British Journal of Psychiatry, 171*, 355–359.
Sekretariatet for referenceprogrammer. (2004). *Referenceprogram for udredning og behandling af skizofreni* [Guidelines for diagnosis and treatment of schizophrenia]. København: Sundhedsstyrelsen.
Taiminen, T. J., & Kujari, H. (1994). Antipsychotic medication and suicide risk among schizophrenic and paranoid inpatients. A controlled retrospective study 1. *Acta Psychiatrica Scandinavica, 90*, 247–251.
Tsoi, W. F., & Wong, K. E. (1991). A 15-year follow-up study of Chinese schizophrenic patients. *Acta Psychiatrica Scandinavica, 84*, 217–220.
Wiersma, D., Nienhuis, F. J., Slooff, C. J., & Giel, R. (1998). Natural course of schizophrenic disorders: A 15-year followup of a Dutch incidence cohort. *Schizophrenia Bulletin, 24*, 75–85.

About the Author

Merete Nordentoft, MD, PhD, is Professor and Chief Psychiatrist at the Psychiatric Center Copenhagen, University of Copenhagen. She was PI for several large randomized clinical trials, the OPUS trial (specialized assertive intervention in first episode psychosis) being the most well known. She was the leader of the intervention in Copenhagen during the process of transforming the project into a permanent part of psychiatric services. Her fields of expertise include psychiatric epidemiology, suicidal behavior, and psychopathology. Among others, she was Chairman of the Danish Psychiatric Association (2000–2002), the Nordic Joint Psychiatric Committee (2003–2006), the Danish National Board of Health, Danish National Action Plan for Prevention of Suicidal Behaviour Committee (1997–1998), and the Copenhagen Medical Society (2003–2005). She is a member of the Danish Medical Research Council since 2005.

Merete Nordentoft
Faculty of Health Sciences
Copenhagen University
Psychiatric Centre Bispebjerg
2400 Copenhagen NV
Denmark
Tel.: +45 206 075 52
E-mail: mn@dadlnet.dk

Reducing Suicide Risk in Personality Disorders

The State of Current Evidence

Joel Paris

Professor of Psychiatry, McGill University, Institute of Community and Family Psychiatry, Quebec, Canada

Personality disorders (PDs) are a diagnostic group characterized by abnormal patterns of inner experience and behavior that affect cognition, emotion interpersonal functioning, and impulse control, are inflexible and pervasive, lead to clinically significant distress or impairment, are stable and of long duration, and have an onset in adolescence or early adulthood (American Psychiatric Association, 2000). In clinical settings, PDs can be identified in about 45% of all patients (Zimmerman, Rothschild, & Chelminski, 2005). Borderline personality disorder (BPD), while not the most frequent of these diagnoses, is of particular importance because it is associated with a wide range of severe psychopathology (Paris, 2008a). This condition is characterized by unstable mood, a wide range of impulsive behaviors, as well as unstable interpersonal relationships. It is very rare to find BPD patients who have never shown any suicidal behavior; Soloff, Lynch, Kelly, Malone, and Mann (2000) reported a mean of three lifetime attempts. In fact, suicidality is one of the defining features of the disorder in DSM-IV-TR (American Psychiatric Association, 2000).

While BPD is only one of 10 categories of PD, along with antisocial personality disorder (ASPD), it has been the subject of a large body of research. The only other PD to be examined for suicide as an outcome is ASPD (Links, Gould, & Ratnayake, 2003; Martin, Cloninger, Guze, & Clayton, 1985; Robins, 1966), in which the rate of completion is around 5%.

The rest of the published literature on suicide and PD concerns BPD. Several types of suicidal behaviors could be observed in this condition. Self-harm, usually involving superficial cuts to the wrists and arms, is very common, but is not suicidal in intent; patients report that they cut to relieve emotional tension and have no intention to die (Brown, Comtois, & Linehan, 2002). This supports the theory that BPD patients have problems with emotion regulation, and that they cut themselves addictively in order to reduce painful inner states (Linehan, 1993).

Overdoses of pills can sometimes be truly suicidal in intent, and they are sometimes life-threatening. Nonetheless, these behaviors vary greatly in their nature and their intent (Soloff et al., 2000). Overdoses tend to occur following stressful live events, and patients describe this behavior as motivated by a wish to escape (Brown et al., 2002). However, most overdoses are marked by ambivalent motivation. Clinicians often see patients who take small quantities of medication and then call significant others for help. Even when potentially fatal overdoses are taken, it is not unusual for rescuers to be contacted.

Suicidal attempts, although often repetitive, tend to decrease as patients age: The pattern is one of the recurrent attempts in the 20s, requiring medical treatment, followed by a tapering off over time (Maris, 1981). These findings are consistent with the observation that overdoses are most common in younger BPD patients (Soloff et al., 2000), and with the well-known observation that attempters and completers are separate but overlapping populations (Beautrais, 2001). Hawton, Zahl, and Weatherall (2003), in a large-scale follow-up of attempters seen in an emergency room, found that only about 3% eventually died by suicide.

This is not to say that patients with BPD never kill themselves. Several studies using psychological autopsy methods have examined the frequency of PD diagnoses in patients who have died by suicide (Hunt et al., 2006; Lesage et al., 1994, 2008; Tidemalm, Elofsson, Stefansson, Waern, & Runeson, 2005). These data suggest that PDs are present in about half of cases under the age of 35 and that BPD is the most common Axis II diagnosis. Several follow-back studies have been conducted in which patients diagnosed with BPD were followed over time. These data generally show that suicide occurs in about 10% of the cases (Paris & Zweig-Frank, 2001; Stone, 1990). Lower rates (3–4%) have been reported in one retrospective study (McGlashan, 1986) as well as in a prospectively followed cohort (Zanarini, Frankenburg, Hennen, & Silk, 2003). But patients who agree to be followed over time may be less likely to die by suicide.

By and large, suicides occur late in the course of illness and are often associated with long courses of unsuccessful treatment (Paris, 2003). One study found the mean age at suicide to be 30 (Stone, 1990). In the longest follow-up, the mean age was 37, with a standard deviation of 10 years (Paris & Zweig-Frank, 2001). Thus, patients are not at highest risk when they are young and are frequent visitors to ER, but later in the course of their illness. Since a great majority of BPD patients improve over time (Paris, 2003), those who eventually end their lives may belong to a subgroup that fail to recover.

Most clinical cases of BPD are female (Zimmerman et al., 2005) and highly treatment-seeking. However, epidemiological studies suggest that males in the community may have this disorder in equal numbers, even if they do not present clinically (Coid, Yang, Tyrer, Roberts, & Ullrich, 2006; Lenzenweger, Lane, Loranger, & Kessler, 2007). Males with BPD have a different pattern of suicidality from females. Nearly a third of youth suicides (most are men) can be diagnosed by psychological autopsy with BPD (Lesage et al., 1994). Autopsy studies of BPD patients who died by suicide also show a preponderance of males (McGirr, Paris, Lesage, Renaud, & Turecki, 2007). But few of these cases were under treatment at the time of their death.

Current Approaches to the Treatment of BPD

Patients with BPD have to undergo complex courses of treatment, with multiple attempts at psychotherapy, repeated emergency room visits and hospitalizations, and multiple prescriptions in a polypharmacy "cocktail" (Zanarini, Frankenburg, Khera, & Bleichmar, 2001). In the context of their tumultuous course, BPD patients often threaten to (or attempt to) kill themselves. Thus, much effort goes in trying to prevent them from doing so (Hull, Yeomans, Clarkin, Li, & Goodman, 1996).

One of the most frequent interventions is hospitalization, and this procedure was recommended by the American Psychiatric Association guidelines for the treatment of suicidal threats in BPD (Oldham et al., 2001). However, the guidelines did not present any evidence that hospital admission is efficacious for this purpose nor any data showing that doing so has any preventive effect against suicide (Paris, 2008a). Moreover, repeated hospitalization tends to be counterproductive, as it interferes with the outpatient treatment and makes it impossible for patients to stay in the workplace. In addition, hospital admission often leads to "regression," with an increase of symptoms (Linehan, 1993). It may make more sense to carry out evidence-based treatment of the disorder.

Sources of Research Evidence

A search of Medline from 1950 to 2008 with the keywords "personality disorder and suicide or suicidality" yielded 2,642 references. However, the vast majority of these were either clinical reports or studies in which the assessment of PD was not a primary aim. No study has directly tested the efficacy of any intervention for the prevention of suicide in this population. The references used for this review were therefore chosen by the author of this chapter as most relevant to the subject.

A Medline search over the same period using the keywords "personality disorder and suicide prevention" yielded 18 references. However, none of these studies actually measured suicide prevention. Three studies that looked at the frequency of PD diagnoses among people who committed suicide were also included.

Evidence for Efficacy of Current Approaches

The treatment methods with the strongest evidence for efficacy in BPD are psychotherapies specifically designed for patients with this disorder (Paris, 2008b). The most extensively investigated method is dialectical behavior therapy (DBT; Linehan, 1993). The efficacy of DBT has been confirmed in multiple RCTs (Linehan, Armstrong, Suarez, Allmon, & Heard, 1991; Linehan et al., 2006) as well as in replications outside the clinic where it was developed (Paris, 2008b). Reductions in overdoses, and in emergency room visits for suicidality, as well as reduced frequency of self-harm, were some of the main outcomes of the two large clinical trials of DBT (Linehan et al., 1991, 2006). However, there was only one death by suicide in the first trial and none in the second. Since patients who die by suicide are probably not to be found in clinical trials, there is no evidence that DBT prevents suicide.

Other psychotherapy methods have also been developed for BPD, and several of them have been tested in single clinical trials. The list includes mentalization-based therapy (Bateman & Fonagy, 1999), transference-focused psychotherapy (Clarkin, Levy, Lenzenweger, & Kernberg, 2007), schema therapy (Giesen-Bloo et al., 2006), and standard cognitive therapy (Davidson et al., 2006). All of them showed some degree of success, suggesting that psychological treatments that are well structured and specifically designed for this population could be superior to standard clinical management. However, much more research is needed to determine how generalizable these findings are and to establish which patients benefit from what kind of psychotherapy. A Cochrane report (Binks et al., 2006a) concluded, rather conservatively, that cognitive therapy for BPD has "promise," but it also noted that the subject needs much more systematic investigation. (In view of the spurt of recent research, a second Cochrane report is forthcoming.)

The efficacy of pharmacological agents in BPD is less firmly established. Although most patients are on medication – antidepressants, mood stabilizers, and/or neuroleptics (Zanarini et al., 2001), this practice is only supported by single trials in small samples. A Cochrane report (Binks et al., 2006b) concluded that there is insufficient evidence, on the basis of existing clinical trials, to prescribe *any* drug for patients with BPD. A review of all clinical trials concluded that the effects of the drugs that have been tested are, at best, modest (Paris, 2008b). However, most of the patients with BPD receive polypharmacy (Zanarini et al., 2001). Although this practice is encouraged by the current APA guidelines (Oldham et al., 2001), it is in no way an evidence-based one.

The pharmacological treatment of BPD has also been influenced by the proposal that this diagnosis should be considered a bipolar variant (Akiskal, Chen, Davis, & Puzantian, 2001). Those who accept that point of view reject the BPD construct and focus on treating mood instability. However, there is little evidence to support the use of mood-stabilizing drugs in BPD (Paris, 2008b; Paris, Gunderson, & Weinberg, 2007). There is also no evidence that psychopharmacological interventions reduce suicidal behavior. Again, the problem that afflicts these clinical trials is generalizability (Westen & Morrison, 2001). Patients who enter RCTs may not be representative of the populations seen in clinical practice. In BPD, patients who end up dying by suicide may be much less compliant with treatment.

Improving and Optimizing Current Practice

What differentiates the suicidality in BPD from patterns seen in other mental disorders is the chronicity of suicidal ideation (Paris, 2008a). Patients with mood disorders may be suicidal when depressed, but usually put these ideas aside when they go into remission. In contrast, BPD patients can consider suicide on a daily basis for months to years.

These symptoms vary in intensity over time, waxing when life events are stressful and waning when they are not (Paris, 2006a). On the other hand, if suicidal behaviors usually remit over time, treatment may find ways to make naturalistic recovery go faster.

The traits that underlie BPD can help us to treat the disorder. Affective instability (AI) is a characteristic feature of BPD (Russell et al., 2007) that differentiates it from other PDs (Siever & Davis, 1991) and is the least likely aspect of BPD to remit on long-term follow-up (Paris, 2003). DBT refers to this trait as emotion dysregulation and specifically aims to modify it (Linehan, 1993). The method involves teaching patients how to regulate negative emotions in ways that do not involve cutting or overdoses. However, while AI is linked to self-harm, it does not have such a direct link to other forms of suicidal behavior.

The other trait that characterizes BPD is impulsivity (Links, Heslegrave, & van Reekum, 1999). Patients who are emotionally dysregulated are more likely to turn to suicidal actions if they are also impulsive (Siever & Davis, 1991). The frequency of suicide attempts tends to be strongly related to levels of impulsivity (Soloff et al., 2000). Moreover in follow-up studies, declines in impulsivity are strongly associated with reductions in suicidal behaviors (Paris, 2003).

While any patient with suicidal behaviors is at higher risk of completion, research has not been able to identify in advance which patients are most likely to die by suicide. Completions are rare events relative to the frequency of attempts, and large-scale studies of patients hospitalized for depression have found it impossible to predict who will commit suicide (Goldstein, Black, Nasrallah, & Winokur, 1991; Pokorny, 1982). There are too many false positives (patients who fit the profile of a completer, but never actually kill themselves).

While there is no evidence that any specific intervention prevents suicide in BPD, it is reassuring that most clinical patients with BPD, despite of having suicidal thoughts for long periods of time, and multiple suicide attempts, never kill themselves. Thus, the level of alarm created by young women with BPD who present in clinics and ERs with suicidal threats is not necessarily justified. Clinicians can therefore concentrate on treating the problems they see and not be distracted by chronic suicidality.

However, chronic suicidality can be draining for psychotherapists (Maltsberger & Buie, 1974). But once one embarks on the treatment of a patient with BPD, suicidality "goes with the territory" (Schwartz, Flinn, & Slawson, 1974). It has been suggested that these patients cannot be treated without accepting the risk (Maltsberger, 1994). Moreover, applying management strategies designed for acute suicidality to chronic suicidality may be counterproductive, particularly if they reinforce the very behaviors they are designed to treat (Linehan, 1993; Paris, 2006b).

By and large, hospitalization, while recommended by APA guidelines (Oldham et al., 2001), is an ineffective and counterproductive strategy for suicide prevention in BPD. It has never been supported by evidence (Paris, 2008a). When suicidality is chronic, admission to hospital provides only temporary relief, and most patients continue to have suicidal ideas after discharge. Moreover, hospitalization can also do harm when admissions are repetitive and regressive. In contrast, clinical trials suggest that day treatment can be helpful for BPD patients (Bateman & Fonagy, 1999). Day hospitals have the advantages of wards (intensive treatment by an experienced team) without their disadvantages.

Potential Problems, Costs, and Resources

Clinical decisions in chronically suicidal patients with BPD are problematic. Hospitalization is expensive and of unproven value. However, these patients continue to be held over in ERs or admitted to wards when they threaten suicide. These options are determined in part by a fear of litigation. However, there are ways to minimize the risk of lawsuits, including careful record keeping, frequent consultation, and involvement with families (Gutheil, 1992; Gutheil & Brodsky, 2008).

The most conservative recommendation based on current evidence is to treat suicidal patients with BPD on an outpatient basis with evidence-based psychological treatments designed for this group. Psychopharmacology has to be seen as adjunctive and optional. Hospital admission should be rare and could only be justified either by a near-fatal attempt or by a micropsychotic episode (Paris, 2008a). While some of these patients may commit suicide, one cannot conduct therapy in a state of fear and chaos. Effective treatment of this population requires the acceptance of some degree of calculated risk (Maltsberger, 1994), while proceeding with a therapeutic plan.

Further Reading

Gunderson, J. G. (2008). *Borderline personality disorder: A clinical guide* (2nd ed.). Washington, DC: American Psychiatric Press (this clinical guide is research-based and highly practical, including many recommendations for managing suicidality).

Gutheil, T. A., Brodsky, A. (2008). *Preventing boundary violations in clinical practice*. New York: Guilford Press (a practical and up-to-date book showing how to stay out of legal trouble with suicidal patients).

Links, P. S., Gould, B., & Ratnayake, R. (2003). Assessing suicidal youth with antisocial, borderline, or narcissistic personality disorder. *Canadian Journal of Psychiatry, 48*, 301–310 (a review of suicidality in young patients with PDs, identifying some of the most important risk factors).

Paris, J. (2006). *Half in love with death: Managing the chronically suicidal patient*. Florence, KY: Erlbaum (this book-length essay on chronic suicidality examines the problem in the context of broader issues of suicide prediction).

Paris, J. (2008). *Treatment of borderline personality disorder: A guide to evidence-based practice*. New York: Guilford Press (this recently published book by the author of this chapter covers all aspects of BPD research and makes detailed recommendations for integrating these data into clinical practice).

Pokorny, A. D. (1982). Prediction of suicide in psychiatric patients: Report of a prospective study. *Archives of general psychiatry, 40*, 249–257 (this classic study shows how difficult it is to predict death by suicide).

References

Akiskal, H., Chen, S., Davis, G., & Puzantian, V. (2001). Do patients with borderline personality disorder belong to the bipolar spectrum? *Journal of Affective Disorders, 67*, 221–228.

American Psychiatric Association. (2000). *Diagnostic and statistical manual of mental disorders* (4th ed., Text Revision). Washington, DC: American Psychiatric Press.

Bateman, A., & Fonagy, P. (1999). Effectiveness of partial hospitalization in the treatment of borderline personality disorder: A randomized controlled trial. *American Journal of Psychiatry, 156*, 1563–1569.

Beautrais, A. L. (2001). Suicides and serious suicide attempts: Two populations or one? *Psychological Medicine, 31*, 837–845.

Binks, C. A., Fenton, M., McCarthy, L., Lee, T., Adams, C. E., & Duggan, C. (2006a). Psychological therapies for people with borderline personality disorder. *Cochrane Database of Systematic Reviews* (1), CD005652.

Binks, C. A., Fenton, M., McCarthy, L., Lee, T., Adams, C. E., & Duggan, C. (2006b). Pharmacological interventions for people with borderline personality disorder. *Cochrane Database of Systematic Reviews* (1), CD005653.

Brown, M. Z., Comtois, K. A., & Linehan, M. M. (2002). Reasons for suicide attempts and nonsuicidal self-injury in women with borderline personality disorder. *Journal of Abnormal Psychology, 111*, 198–202.

Clarkin, J. F., Levy, K. N., Lenzenweger, M. F., & Kernberg, O. F. (2007). Evaluating three treatments for borderline personality disorder: A multiwave study. *American Journal of Psychiatry, 164*, 1–8.

Coid, J., Yang, M., Tyrer, P., Roberts, A., & Ullrich, S. (2006). Prevalence and correlates of personality disorder in Great Britain. *British Journal of Psychiatry, 188*, 423–431.

Davidson, K., Norrie, J., Tyrer, P., Gumley, A., Tata, P., & Murray, H. (2006). The effectiveness of cognitive behavior therapy for borderline personality disorder: Results from the borderline personality disorder study of cognitive therapy (BOSCOT) trial. *Journal of Personality Disorders, 20*, 450–465.

Giesen-Bloo, J., van Dyck, R., Spinhoven, P., van Tilburg, W., Dirksen, C., van Asselt, T., et al. (2006). Outpatient psychotherapy for borderline personality disorder: Randomized trial of schema-focused therapy vs transference-focused psychotherapy. *Archives of General Psychiatry, 63*, 649–658.

Goldstein, R. B., Black, D. W., Nasrallah, A., & Winokur, G. (1991). The prediction of suicide. *Archives of General Psychiatry, 48*, 418–422.

Gutheil, T. G. (1992). Suicide and suit: Liability after self-destruction. In D. Jacobs (Ed.), *Suicide and clinical practice* (pp. 147–167). Washington, DC: American Psychiatric Press.

Gutheil, T. A., & Brodsky, A. (2008). *Preventing boundary violations in clinical practice*. New York: Guilford Press.

Hawton, K., Zahl, D., & Weatherall, R. (2003). Suicide following deliberate self-harm: Long-term follow-up of patients who presented to a general hospital. *British Journal of Psychiatry, 182*, 537–542.

Hull, J. W., Yeomans, F., Clarkin, J., Li, C., & Goodman, G. (1996). Factors associated with multiple hospitalizations of patients with borderline personality disorder. *Psychiatric Services, 47*, 638–641.

Hunt, I. M., Kapur, N., Robinson, J., Shaw, J., Flynn, S., Bailey, H., et al. (2006). Suicide within 12 months of mental health service contact in different age and diagnostic groups: National clinical survey. *British Journal of Psychiatry, 188*, 135–142.

Lenzenweger, M. F., Lane, M. C., Loranger, A. W., & Kessler, R. C. (2007). DSM-IV personality disorders in the national comorbidity survey replication. *Biological Psychiatry, 62*, 553–556.

Lesage, A. D., Boyer, R., Grunberg, F., Morisette, R., Vanier, C., Morrisette, R., et al. (1994). Suicide and mental disorders: A case control study of young men. *American Journal of Psychiatry, 151*, 1063–1068.

Lesage, Al., Seguin, M., Guy, A., Daigle, F., Bayle, M.-N., Chawky, N., et al. (2008). Systematic services audit of consecutive suicides in New Brunswick: The case for coordinating specialist mental health and addiction services. *Canadian Journal of Psychiatry, 53*, 671–678.

Linehan, M. M. (1993). *Cognitive behavioral therapy of borderline personality disorder.* New York: Guilford.

Linehan, M. M., Armstrong, H. E., Suarez, A., Allmon, D., & Heard, H. (1991). Cognitive behavioral treatment of chronically parasuicidal borderline patients. *Archives of General Psychiatry, 48*, 1060–1064.

Linehan, M. M., Comtois, K. A., Murray, A. M., Brown, M. Z., Gallop, R. J., Heard, H. L., et al. (2006). Two-year randomized controlled trial and follow-up of dialectical behavior therapy vs therapy by experts for suicidal behaviors and borderline personality disorder. *Archives of General Psychiatry, 63*, 757–766.

Links, P. S., Gould, B., & Ratnayake, R. (2003). Assessing suicidal youth with antisocial, borderline, or narcissistic personality disorder. *Canadian Journal of Psychiatry, 48*, 301–310.

Links, P. S., Heslegrave, R., & van Reekum, R. (1999). Impulsivity: Core aspect of borderline personality disorder. *Journal of Personality Disorders,* 131–139.

Maltsberger, J. T. (1994). Calculated risk taking in the treatment of suicidal patients: Ethical and legal problems. *Death Studies, 18*, 439–452.

Maltsberger, J. T., & Buie, D. H. (1974). Countertransference hate in the treatment of suicidal patients. *Archives of General Psychiatry, 30*, 625–633.

Maris, R. (1981). *Pathways to suicide.* Baltimore: Johns Hopkins Press.

Martin, R. L., Cloninger, C. R., Guze, S. B., & Clayton, P. J. (1985). Mortality in a follow-up of 500 psychiatric outpatients. II. Cause-specific mortality. *Archives of General Psychiatry, 42*, 58–66.

McGirr, A., Paris, J., Lesage, A., Renaud, J., & Turecki, G. (2007). Risk factors for suicide completion in borderline personality disorder: A case-control study of cluster B comorbidity and impulsive aggression. *Journal of Clinical Psychiatry, 68*, 721–729.

McGlashan, T. H. (1986). The Chestnut Lodge follow-up study. III: Long-term outcome of borderline personalities. *Archives of General Psychiatry, 43*, 2–30.

Oldham, J. M., Gabbard, G. O., Goin, M. K., Gunderson, J., Soloff, P., Spiegel, D., et al. (2001). Practice guideline for the treatment of borderline personality disorder. *American Journal of Psychiatry, 158*(Suppl.), 1–52.

Paris, J. (2003). *Personality disorders over time.* Washington, DC: American Psychiatric Press.

Paris, J. (2006a). *Half in love with easeful death: The meaning of chronic suicidality.* Mahwah, NJ: Erlbaum.

Paris, J. (2006b). Predicting and preventing suicide: Do we know enough to do either? *Harvard Review of Psychiatry, 14*, 233–240.

Paris, J. (2008a). *Treatment of borderline personality disorder: A guide to evidence-based practice.* New York: Guilford Press.

Paris, J. (2008b). Clinical trials in personality disorders. *Psychiatric Clinics of North America, 31*, 517–526.

Paris, J., Gunderson, J. G., & Weinberg, I. (2007). The interface between borderline personality disorder and bipolar spectrum disorder. *Comprehensive Psychiatry, 48*, 145–154.

Paris, J., & Zweig-Frank, H. (2001). A twenty-seven year follow-up of borderline patients. *Comprehensive Psychiatry, 42*, 482–487.

Pokorny, A. D. (1982). Prediction of suicide in psychiatric patients: Report of a prospective study. *Archives of General Psychiatry, 40*, 249–257.

Robins, L. (1966). *Deviant children grown up.* Baltimore: Williams and Wilkins.

Russell, J., Moskowitz, D., Sookman, D., Zuroff, D. C., & Paris, J. (2007). Affective instability in patients with borderline personality disorder. *Journal of Abnormal Psychology, 116*, 578–588.

Schwartz, D. A., Flinn, D. E., & Slawson, P. F. (1974). Treatment of the suicidal character. *American Journal of Psychotherapy, 28*, 194–207.

Siever, L. J., & Davis, K. L. (1991). A psychobiological perspective on the personality disorders. *American Journal of Psychiatry, 148*, 1647–1658.

Soloff, P. H., Lynch, K. G., Kelly, T. M., Malone, K. M., & Mann, J. J. (2000). Characteristics of suicide attempts of patients with major depressive episode and borderline personality disorder: A comparative study. *American Journal of Psychiatry, 157*, 601–608.

Stone, M. H. (1990). *The fate of borderline patients*. New York: Guilford.

Tidemalm, D., Elofsson, S., Stefansson, C.-G., Waern, M., & Runeson, B. (2005). Predictors of suicide in a community-based cohort of individuals with severe mental disorder. *Social Psychiatry and Psychiatric Epidemiology, 40*, 595–600.

Westen, D., & Morrison, K. (2001). A multidimensional meta-analysis of treatments for depression, panic, and generalized anxiety disorder: An empirical examination of the status of empirically supported therapies. *Journal of Consulting and Clinical Psychology, 69*, 875–899.

Zanarini, M. C., Frankenburg, F. R., Hennen, J., & Silk, K. R. (2003). The longitudinal course of borderline psychopathology: 6-year prospective follow-up of the phenomenology of borderline personality disorder. *American Journal of Psychiatry, 160*, 274–283.

Zanarini, M. C., Frankenburg, F. R., Khera, G. S., & Bleichmar, J. (2001). Treatment histories of borderline inpatients. *Comprehensive Psychiatry, 42*, 144–150.

Zimmerman, M., Rothschild, L., & Chelminski, I. (2005). The prevalence of DSM-IV personality disorders in psychiatric outpatients. *American Journal of Psychiatry, 162*, 1911–1918.

About the Author

Joel Paris was born in New York City, but has spent most of his life in Canada. He obtained an MD from McGill University in 1964, where he also trained in psychiatry. Dr. Paris has been a member of the McGill psychiatry department since 1972. Since 1994, he has been a full Professor and served as Department Chair from 1997 to 2007. Dr. Paris is currently a Research Associate at the SMBD-Jewish General Hospital and heads personality clinics at two hospitals. He is also Editor-in-Chief of the *Canadian Journal of Psychiatry*. Dr. Paris' research interest is in borderline personality disorder, and he is a Past President of the Association for Research on Personality Disorders. Over the last 20 years, Dr. Paris has been conducting research on the biological and psychosocial causes and the long-term outcome of BPD. Dr. Paris has 153 peer-reviewed articles and is the author of 12 books and 36 book chapters. He is an educator who has supervised psychiatric evaluation with residents for over 30 years and who has won awards for his teaching.

Joel Paris
McGill University
Institute of Community and Family Psychiatry
4333 chemin de la cote ste. Catherine
Montreal, Quebec H3T1E4
Canada
Tel.: +1 514 340 8210
E-mail: joel.paris@mcgill.ca

Where Do We Go From Here?

Perspectives in Suicide Research and Prevention*

A Commentary

Alan L. Berman

American Association of Suicidology, Washington, DC, USA

A Look Back

In 1965, the Center for Studies of Suicide Prevention (CSSP) was established, under the direction of Dr. Edwin Shneidman, at the National Institutes of Mental Health in Washington, DC. One of the first acts of the CSSP was the appointment of some 50 leaders and students in the field of suicide prevention, self-destructive behaviors, and dying and bereavement to a Task Force charged with establishing directions and priorities for the field for the decade ahead. The Task Force assembled in Phoenix in January, 1970 and published its reports and recommendations 3 years later (Resnik & Hathorne, 1973).

Elsewhere (Berman, 2006a), I have reviewed the recommendations of this historic report measured from the perspective of 35 years of hindsight. Notably, in spite of considerable growth and evidence of much greater research sophistication in the field of Suicidology, it is painfully apparent that there remain significant gaps in the state of our knowledge and, consequently, in our efforts to translate that knowledge into practical clinical and public health applications. This perspective documents the fact that we have yet much work ahead of us to improve Suicidology as a scientific discipline and to use that science to inform clinical practice and public health approaches to prevent suicide.

To wit, let me illustrate with a few examples:

- The Task Force's Committee on Classification and Nomenclature recommended establishing a universally accepted nomenclature and disseminating a training manual to support it. As of 2007, we are still in process toward this goal both in the United States (Silverman, Berman, Sanddal, O'Carroll, & Joiner, 2007a,

* Reprinted by permission from: Tatarelli, R., Pompili, M., & Girardi, P. (Eds.). (2007). Suicide in psychiatric disorders (pp. 215–221). New York: Nova Science.

2007b) and internationally (De Leo, Burgis, Bertolote, Kerkhof, & Bille-Brahe, 2006). The Committee further recommended the establishment of nationally standardized case finding forms and training coroners and medical examiners to study these forms, a recommendation far from being fulfilled. Both within the United States and internationally, the lack of standardization in certifying suicides continues to plague our ability to meaningfully identify cases and to reliably establish and compare the rates across jurisdictions, states, provinces, and countries. Would it not be terrific to be able to look at five countries with high suicide rates versus five countries with low suicide rates, knowing that these rates were, indeed, based on reasonably reliable and valid data collection and certification systems, to be able to identify cultural, ecological, and sociological level data to put forth research hypotheses about the risk for and protection from suicide?

- The Committee on Research recommended both conducting longitudinal studies to chart the developmental course of suicidal behavior and improving methodologies for, thus conducting evaluation studies of, suicide prevention programs. To this day, we have few significant longitudinal studies (of presuicidal pathways) in the literature, and those very few program evaluation studies (with any degree of methodological sophistication) on the effectiveness of suicide prevention programs have found only a handful of programs to be either effective or even "promising" (see www.sprc.org). Pena and Caine's recent (2006) review of screening programs (a "promising" strategy) and their relative lack of evidence for effectiveness well illustrates the work ahead of us.
- The Committee on Treatment urged a focus on *acute* risk, aggressive outreach programs, and a fostering of continuity of care. Only recently has attention begun to be applied to the question of acute risk for suicide (Rudd et al., 2006), and, at that, our best research to date defines acute risk as risk found to be associated with the *last 12 months* of a decedent's life. Aggressive outreach programs are few and far between; and issues of continuity of care continue to plague our systems of care for the at-risk patient with consequent high rates of suicide even after hospitalization (Beautrais, 2006).

There are a host of other unfulfilled hopes from the early 1970s – to increase the proportion of deaths receiving physical autopsies (and toxicology studies), to more widely employ and improve methodologies for psychological autopsies of suicides, to create a large database of cases for research, to improve our treatments, to upgrade our training of clinicians, etc. – that remain before us as yet-unfulfilled challenges for decades to come.

As the present volume has, as its particular focus, suicide in psychiatric disorders, this brief commentary necessarily focuses on some of the more salient, yet-unanswered questions within the frame of this theme. What follows is a decidedly idiosyncratic (in part even iconoclastic) perspective, but one that hopefully helps to shape an applied research agenda for the next several decades.

Toward the Future

Near-Term Suicide Risk

As noted above, we have yet to define sensitive markers to describe the acute risk for suicide or suicidal behaviors, in any time frame more proximate to the suicide than 12 months. The clinical demand is to better observe and judge the risk in the very short term, that is, hours to days, as this judgment must inform triage and the need for close monitoring or hospitalization. Simon (2006) has appropriately noted that the notion of *imminent* risk is illusory, a construction of our attorney friends, without any tie to empirical validity or reliability. Thus, there is a siren call to intensively study a large number of completed suicides and suicide attempts of various lethalities relative to both observed and observable signs and symptoms in the very near term (e.g., last 24 hours or last week of life) through psychological autopsies or standardized chart review studies and, then, to validate any derived acute risk factors through case-control research with high-risk subjects. Further, the potential to link near-term clinical manifestations of heightened risk to a biologic marker to predict these, no less to pharmacologic interventions to inhibit these, presents an exciting collaboration between the psychosocial and neurobiological research communities.

Psychiatric Disorders

This volume focuses on a wide range of psychiatric disorders and their relationship to suicide. The role of comorbidity in increasing suicide risk appears undisputed, but our understanding of the variations of comorbidities (e.g., two or more Axis I disorders versus an Axis I and an Axis II disorder) and their relationship to increased suicide risk begs further research. Similarly, there is a dearth of literature on subclinical syndromes, singly or comorbid, and their relationship to suicidality. As psychological autopsies have well documented the fact that ~ 90% of completed suicides may be retrospectively diagnosed with at least one mental disorder, our understanding of "the other 10%" (Berman, 2006b) remains hypothetical and understudied. As well, there is great need to go beyond the medical model and explore and explicate the impact and role of specific affects and cognitions common to suicide; the role of shame and humiliation, for example, as they interact with particular aspects of character and coping ability.

Cause Versus Association

Tanney (1992) appropriately noted that mental disorders have clearly been found to be associated with suicide, yet cautioned and reminded us that association does not equate to causation. He proposed a number of direct, indirect, interactive, and co-occurring mechanisms to explain the observed association. There remains a compelling need to better understand and explore these underlying mechanisms and, in particular, the multiple driving forces that lead one severely pathological person to suicide and an equally pathological person to sustaining life in spite of the impact of their mental disorder. In the same vein, we have insufficient knowledge to differentiate what turns one person's psychological despair into suicide ideation and another's into suicidal impulse, and yet a third's into suicidal behavior; no less to describe the pathway from despair to ideation to impulse to behavior when all occur in the same individual.

Similarly, although an association has been found between selective serotonin reuptake inhibitors (SSRIs) and suicide ideation and nonfatal suicide attempts in children, adolescents, and young adults, leading to an FDA-mandated black box warning in the US, this does not mean that SSRIs cause increased suicidality among those under 25. A more sophisticated study of those suffering adverse events such as increased suicidality has yet to be reported.

Where Goes Theory?

The development of a comprehensive theory of suicide, a recommendation from the CSSP Task Force almost four decades ago, remains elusive. Those few newer theoretical positions that have been put forth have yet to stimulate significant research interest to advance the field. For example, Shneidman (1996) has forcefully argued that there can be no suicide without psychological pain (*psychache*) stemming from thwarted, frustrated, or distorted psychological needs. His theoretical postulates present a goldmine of research hypotheses in need of testing. More recently, Joiner (2006) has articulated a theory that adds considerably to our need to better understand concepts such as thwarted belongingness and burdensomeness which he argues are central to the suicidal process.

Strategies for Risk Formulation

Ultimately, the significance of our better understanding of the risk factors for suicide and suicidal behaviors lies in the translation of research into practice. Models and strategies for making judgments of levels of risk, for example, have been proposed (see American Association of Suicidology Behavioral Skills Competency Training Program: www.suicidology.org; Berman, Jobes, & Silverman, 2006; Joiner et al., 2007; Rudd et al., 2006); however, there is no research, to my knowledge, that has specifically examined the relative validity of any of these proposed schemas, no less the process and outcome of clinical decision-making that is intended to result. As an example of the latter issue, given the observed odds ratios for suicide consequent to discharge from psychiatric hospitalization (Qin & Nordentoft, 2005), the effectiveness of hospitalization as a treatment intervention and questions regarding discharge planning and continuity of care procedures and implementation (Beautrais, 2006) all call for investigation and answer.

Interventions and Treatments

The relative scarcity of randomized clinical trials has been well documented elsewhere (Hawton et al., 2000; Linehan, 1997; Rudd, 2000). Research in this area remains hampered by the relative exclusion from the study of high-risk patients; relatively short follow-up durations, necessarily limited by available funding, but therefore maximizing focus on brief cognitive-behavioral and other structured interventions and relatively short-term outcomes (long-term treatment follow-up studies appear to be bounded at only 24 months); a lack of differentiation among those studied into groups judged to be at acute versus chronic risk; a lack of precision, consequent to our continuing muddled nomenclature, in defining homogeneous groups (ideators, attempters, repetitive attempters, etc.) for research study; a lack of differentiation, thereby, among patient-subjects with regard to their relative lethality and intent; and our reliance, consequent to the relatively short-term duration of study, on indirect markers, for example, symptom reduction or one-time measures of suicide ideation, for treatment outcomes, versus direct markers, for example, no suicidal behavior, sustained over longer periods of follow-up.

Similarly, the available research on psychopharmacologic interventions is plagued by problems of classification and a lack of standardized data collection by pharmaceutical houses during clinical trials; relatively brief durations of study; overreliance on single question markers of treatment response, for example, responses to a single scale (e.g., HAM-D) or even one item (HAM-D, item 3) on a rating scale to measure suicidality; the lack of dechallenge-rechallenge studies; better understanding of why nonresponders are nonresponders; and, with regard to the SSRIs in particular, an understandable lack of interest in exploring the relatively high rate of placebo response, which may account for as much as 80% of observed benefit from active medications.

Adherence

Crucial to effective treatment interventions is a patient who adheres to a prescribed treatment regimen; yet, adherence remains more theoretical than empirically studied. We have reason to presume that nonadherent patients are compromised by a number of factors ranging from gender role socialization (males are more nonadherent than females) to influences stemming from their psychopathology and character that compromise trust, willingness to be in a dependent position to a caregiver, etc. It is noteworthy, for example, that two recent studies (Leon et al., 2006; Moskos, Olson, Halbern, Keller, & Gray, 2005) of adolescent suicides found that only 1 patient of 72 (combined samples) prescribed an antidepressant had evidence of that medication in their blood upon toxicological analysis at the time of autopsy! In this regard, issues of help-seeking and help-receiving, particularly among males at risk for suicide, are crucial to better develop methods to enhance these behaviors, thus engagement in caregiving and adherence to recommended treatments (Berman, 2005; Stanley, 2006).

In the US, *The Surgeon General's National Strategy for Suicide Prevention* (USDHHS, 2001) established 5-year objectives to develop a national research agenda, and to increase public and private funding for suicide prevention research and for translating scientific knowledge into practice, among other notable goals. As of this date, we remain without a national agenda and, where funding has increased, significantly as a consequence of one US Senator's tragic loss of a son to suicide, it has not been for research and prevention programs directed toward those at higher risk for suicide. As but one example, one third of all suicides in the States involve alcohol or substance use disorder, yet less than 10% of federally funded suicide studies involve even a mention of interest in these disorders (Berman, 2006a).

Similarly, the Institute of Medicine's report *Reducing Suicide*: *A National Imperative* (Goldsmith, Pellmar, Kleinman, & Bunney, 2002) set out an ambitious research and prevention agenda for years to come that has yet to be translated into significant action steps. We must hope that when we look back 35 years from now, we will have made significantly greater progress in accomplishing these objectives and fulfilling these recommendations and, thereby, saving lives.

References

Beautrais, A. (2006). *Is suicidal behavior a chronic condition?* Presented at the 39th Annual Conference of the American Association of Suicidology, Seattle.

Berman, A. L. (2005). Help-seeking among men: Implications for suicide prevention. *Acta Suicidologica Slovenica, III*(1–2), 36–51.

Berman, A. L. (2006a). "*The Time Has Come,*" *the Walrus said,* "*To Talk of Many Things.*" Dublin Award presentation to the 39th Annual Conference of the American Association of Suicidology, Seattle.

Berman, A. L. (2006b). The other ten percent. *Newslink* (American Association of Suicidology), *33*(3), 3.

Berman, A. L., Jobes, D. A., & Silverman, M. M. (2006). *Adolescent suicide: Assessment and intervention* (2nd ed.). Washington, DC: American Psychological Association.

De Leo, D., Burgis, S., Bertolote, J. M., Kerkhof, A. J. F., & Bille-Brahe, U. (2006). Definitions of suicidal behavior: Lessons learned from the WHO/EURO Multicentre Study. *Crisis, 27*(1), 4–15.

Goldsmith, S. K., Pellmar, T. C., Kleinman, A. M., & Bunney, W. E. (2002). *Reducing suicide: A national imperative*. Washington, DC: The National Academies Press.

Hawton, K., Townsend, E., Arensman, E., Gunnel, D., Hazell, P., House, A., et al. (2000). Psychosocial versus pharmacological treatments for deliberate self harm. *Cochrane Database System Review.* (2), CD001764.

Joiner, T. (2006). *Why people die by suicide*. Cambridge, MW: Harvard University Press.

Joiner, T., Kalafat, J., Draper, J., Stokes, H., Knudson, M., Berman, A. L., et al. (2007). Establishing standards for the assessment of suicide risk among callers to the National Suicide Prevention Lifeline. *Suicide & Life-Threatening Behavior, 37*, 353–365.

Leon, A. C., Marzuk, P. M., Tardiff, K., Bucciarelli, A., Markham Piper, T., & Galea, S. (2006). Antidepressants and youth suicide in New York City, 1999–2002. *Journal of the American Academy of Child and Adolescent Psychiatry, 45*(9), 1054–1058.

Linehan, M. M. (1997). Behavioral treatments of suicidal behaviors. In D. M. Stoff & J. J. Mann (Eds.), *The neurobiology of suicide: From the bench to the clinic. Annals of the New York Academy of Sciences, 836*, 302–328.

Moskos, M., Olson, L., Halbern, S., Keller, T., & Gray, D. (2005). Utah youth suicide study: Psychological autopsy. *Suicide & Life-Threatening Behavior, 35*(5), 536–546.

Pena, J. B., & Caine, E. D. (2006). Screening as an approach for adolescent suicide prevention. *Suicide & Life-Threatening Behavior, 36*(6), 614–637.

Qin, P., & Nordentoft, M. (2005). Suicide risk in relation to psychiatric hospitalization: Evidence based in longitudinal registers. *Archives of General Psychiatry, 62*(4), 427–432.

Resnik, H. L. P., & Hathorne, B. C. (1973). Suicide prevention in the 70's (CHEW Publication No. (HSM) 72-9054). Washington, DC: US Government Printing Office.

Rudd, M. D. (2000). Integrating science into the practice of clinical suicidology: A review of the psychotherapy literature and a research agenda for the future. In R. W. Maris, S. S. Canetto, J. L. McIntosh, & M. M. Silverman (Eds.), *Review of suicidology* (pp. 47–83). NY: Guilford Press.

Rudd, M. D., Berman, L., Joiner, T., Nock, M., Silverman, M. M., Mandrusiak, M., et al. (2006). Warning signs for suicide: Theory, research, and clinical application. *Suicide & Life-Threatening Behavior, 36*(3), 255–262.

Shneidman, E. S. (1996). *The suicidal mind*. NY: Oxford University Press.

Silverman, M. M., Berman, A. L., Sanddal, N. D., O'Carroll, P. W., & Joiner, T. E. (2007a). Rebuilding the Tower of Babel: A revised nomenclature for the study of suicide and suicidal behaviors. Part I. Background, rationale, and methodology. *Suicide & Life-Threatening Behavior, 37*(3), 248–263.

Silverman, M. M., Berman, A. L., Sanddal, N. D., O'Carroll, P. W., & Joiner, T. E. (2007b). Rebuilding the Tower of Babel: A revised nomenclature for the study of suicide and suicidal behaviors. Part II. Suicide-related ideations, communications, and behaviors. *Suicide & Life-Threatening Behavior, 37*(3), 264–277.

Simon, R. I. (2006). Imminent suicide: The illusion of short-term prediction. *Suicide & Life-Threatening Behavior, 36*(3), 296–301.

Stanley, B. (2006). Psychological interventions for people at risk for suicide: What works and what does not? Slovenia: Potoroz, Presented at 11th European Symposium on Suicide and Suicidal Behaviours.

Tanney, B. L. (1992). Mental disorders, psychiatric patients, and suicide. In R. W. Maris, A. L. Berman, J. T. Maltsberger, & R. I. Yufit (Eds.), *Assessment and prediction of suicide* (pp. 277–320). NY: Guilford Press.

USDHHS. (2001). *National strategy for suicide prevention: Goals and objectives for action*. Rockville, MD: Public Health Service.

About the Author

Alan L. (Lanny) Berman, PhD, is Executive Director of the American Association of Suicidology and former Director of the National Center for the Study and Prevention of Suicide at the Washington School of Psychiatry. He is a recipient of both the Shneidman and the Dublin Awards for outstanding contributions to suicidology and the field of suicide prevention and is the author/editor of seven books and more than 100 peer-reviewed articles, and book chapters in the field. He is a Fellow of both the International Academy of Suicide Research and the American Psychological Association.

Alan (Lanny) Berman
5221 Wisconsin Ave.
NW
Washington, DC 20015
USA
Tel.: +1 202 237 2280
E-mail: berman@suicidology.org

Where Is More Evidence Needed?

Research Priorities in Suicidology

David Lester

Department of Psychology, The Richard Stockton College of New Jersey, Pomona, NJ, USA

In a number of articles, Lester has severely criticized research as well as organizations for the poor quality of the output (Lester, 2000a, 2000b). For example, with regard to epidemiology, the World Health Organization (WHO) maintains a database on mortality, but the rates have not been kept up-to-date; there are few reports from the nations in Africa, the Middle East, and Central and South America. National data on the marital status of completed suicides, or the month of occurrence, method used, and motive, are rarely produced by any nation. Many nations, such as England and Wales, consistently undercount completed suicides (by as much as 40%), making the evaluation of suicide prevention efforts impossible (Lester, 2002). Although WHO/EURO study on attempted suicide has produced the relevant data in some cities around the world (De Leo, Burgis, Bertolote, Kerkhof, & Bille-Brahe, 2006), there is no nation that counts attempted suicides comprehensively at a national level.

Recommendation 1: Comprehensive efforts must be made to count accurately completed suicides and attempted suicides in nations around the world, to report these rates broken down by demographic variables and by the circumstances of the suicidal acts.

Lester (2000a) has also criticized the research into and theorizing about suicide.[1] A brief summary of some of his comments on psychiatric, psychological, and anthropological research follows.

---

[1] See also Rogers and Lester (2010) for a critique of suicidology and a series of recommendations for future research.

Psychiatric Research

The sample sizes used in physiological research into suicidal behavior are typically quite small or much too small to control for extraneous variables (e.g., in brain studies, the time of storage of the tissue samples, age, sex, and medication status). There have been few meta-analyses of the research findings, and there has often been a failure to control for depression. Indeed, many of the physiological studies on suicidal individuals are but a side effect of the physiological studies of affective disorders, schizophrenia, etc.

Lester has also criticized the psychiatric diagnostic system for being based on symptom clusters rather than causes. For example, diagnosable depression could have been caused by neurotransmitter defects, psychodynamic forces (such as suppressed and repressed anger), learning experiences (such as learned helplessness and a deficit of positive reinforcers), and labeling (where ordinary sadness and melancholy are now "labeled" as depression).[2]

Recommendation 2: Psychiatric research into suicide should move toward an etiologically based diagnostic system rather than relying on a symptom-cluster diagnostic system.

Recommendation 3: Psychiatric research into suicidal behavior needs to improve its methodological rigor, using larger sample sizes and controlling for extraneous variables.

Psychological Research

Lester has criticized psychological research into suicidal behavior for its lack of theoretical grounding. Few proponents of the major theories of personality or systems of psychotherapy have addressed how suicidal behavior fits into their theory or system. Psychological research tends to be driven by multiple regression techniques of analysis, wherein a series of variables (such as hopelessness, impulsivity, problem-solving skills, and perfectionism) are entered into a multiple regression for predicting suicidality. Suicidality is viewed, therefore, as a simple weighted sum of the predictor variables. In contrast, the natural sciences propose much more complex relationships. For example, in Einstein's theory of relativity, the relationship between the speed of an object relative to an observer (*V*) and the mass of an object (*M*) is as follows (Smith, 1960):

$$M = M_o/\text{sqrt}(1 - V^2/C^2),$$

where C is the speed of light and M_o is the mass of the object at rest relative to the observer. Multiple regression techniques cannot test this type of relationship between variables.

2 See Wilson (2008) for this theory of depression.

Recommendation 4: Psychological research into suicidal behavior needs to be grounded in theory and to explore more complex relationships than simple additive models.

Anthropological Research

An anthropological perspective suggests that suicidologists have typically ignored many cultures in their study of suicide. For example, most developed nations have minority ethnic groups, but suicidal behavior is rarely studied in these groups – such as the Basques in France and Spain or the Cornish in England. In some countries where there is a clear ethnic division, such as the Flemings and Walloons in Belgium, suicide is not studied in these groups individually, but rather for the nation as a whole. Indeed, Lester had an article on suicide in Wales (Lester, 1994) rejected by a British psychiatric journal as "being of no interest."

The situation is more complex in many other nations (particularly in Central and South America, and Asia) where almost all of them have indigenous groups whose behavior is rarely studied. An exception is the research by Cheng (1995) on the indigenous groups in Taiwan. In Africa, most of the nations were established by the colonial powers who grouped together many ethnic groups into single nations, a disastrous policy that has resulted in many civil conflicts and wars in African nations.
Recommendation 5: Studies of suicidal behavior should take into account the ethnicities of the individuals, especially in nations that are multiethnic in composition.

Evaluation of Suicide Prevention Programs

Several tactics have been proposed for preventing suicide, but only a few have received adequate evaluation.

School Suicide Prevention Programs

Many different programs have been tried out in schools to inform the students about suicide and suicide prevention, tell them about the resources in the school and community for suicidal youths, and, in some programs, improve the students' coping skills (with the aim of preventing suicidal crises from occurring). Leenaars, Lester, and Wenckstern (2002) reviewed the research evaluating these programs and found evidence that they could improve the help-seeking responses of students and increase their knowledge about suicide. Only two studies that dealt with the impact of the programs on suicidal ideation were identified, of which one found an impact on suicidal ideation but not on hopelessness, whereas the other found no impact on either measure. However, no study was located that investigated the impact of the programs on attempted or completed suicide.

Recommendation 6: More research needs to be conducted on whether school suicide prevention programs have a detectable impact on attempted and completed suicide.

Educating Physicians

In Gotland, Sweden, the general practitioners in the community were educated on depression and suicide, and informed on ways of treating these problems. The initial results indicated that the program led to a reduction in suicides in the community, at least among women, for the next few years (Rutz et al., 1989).[3] A replication of this study in Hungary by Zonda and Lester (2006–2007), however, failed to find any beneficial impact on the suicide rate from the training of general practitioners.
Recommendation 7: The impact of training physicians on the recognition and appropriate treatment of depression and suicide in the patients that they encounter needs to be studied further.

Suicide Prevention Centers

Lester (1997) conducted a meta-analysis of all the studies that had explored whether the establishment of suicide prevention centers had an impact on the suicide rate of the communities or regions that the centers served. Lester identified 14 studies, and the meta-analysis found an average effect size (using a Pearson's product-moment correlation) of −0.16, a significant preventive effect. Most suicide prevention centers have a telephone crisis counseling service, and some provide other services such as walk-in clinics and outreach services to attempted suicides. It is interesting to note that no studies on evaluating the impact of suicide prevention centers, or the various components, have appeared in the last 10 years.[4]

An excellent example of program evaluation was published by De Leo, Carollo, and Della Buono (1995). They investigated the impact of a Tele-Help/Tele-Check system for 12,135 elderly people in a region of Italy over a period of 4 years. Staff at the service contacted the users at least twice a week, and the users could call the center for assistance at anytime of the day or week. They found one suicide in this group as compared to an expected number of 7.4.
Recommendation 8: More research needs to be conducted on whether suicide prevention centers have an impact on suicide in the communities they serve. This research should explore whether the impact, if any, is found in all subgroups of the population (by age, sex, social class, and ethnicity) or only in some subgroups.

3 See MacDonald (1995) for some criticisms of the study.
4 Lester (1970a, 1970b, 1970c, 1970d) suggested ways for evaluating suicide prevention centers that did not rely on their impact on completed suicide.

Restricting Access to Lethal Methods for Suicide

Restricting access to lethal methods for suicide is the best evaluated technique for suicide prevention. Clarke and Lester (1989) reviewed the research on this topic, and Lester (2009) has updated that earlier review. It is quite clear that preventing access to a lethal method for suicide eliminates its use for suicide. Fencing in a particular bridge or high place from which suicides jump eliminates the use of that venue for suicide. A similar impact is found for detoxifying domestic gas (changing from coal gas with highly toxic carbon monoxide to less toxic natural gas) and for enclosing the stations in subway systems (so that doors in the walls enclosing the platforms match the doors in the subway train when it stops in the station).

What is less clear, however, is whether people switch to other venues for suicide or to other methods. The research on this aspect has produced contradictory conclusions, with some studies finding no substitution of the method, while other studies did find substitution of the method. For example, while suicide using domestic gas was eliminated in England, suicide using car exhaust rose in popularity. The result is that sometimes this tactic for preventing suicide reduces the overall suicide rate in the country, but sometimes it does not.

Recommendation 9: More research needs to be conducted on whether and the extent to which people do substitute other methods for suicide when access to one method is restricted. This research should take into account whether the answer to the question depends on the particular method and the subgroup of the population (by age, sex, social class, and ethnicity).

Helping Survivors

Survivors are those who have lost a significant other to suicide. There has been much discussion of how psychotherapy may help survivors deal with this trauma (see Maris, Berman, & Silverman, 2000), and there are many popular books on this topic (Lukas & Seiden, 1990). In addition, many self-help groups have been established for survivors across the United States and in other countries. However, Berman (2008) asked the pointed question of whether there was any evidence "that cathartic treatments (support groups or therapeutic interventions designed to facilitate emotion and talk about the decedent) are more helpful to the long-term recovery of survivors than either no support group or no therapy . . .?" (p. 3). Berman also asked whether there was any evidence that surviving the suicide of a significant other requires catharsis rather than a simple decision by survivors to move on with their lives?

Recommendation 10: Careful controlled studies are needed to determine whether self-help groups for survivors reduce their distress and prevent their own suicidal behavior as compared to no treatment.

Public Health Programs

There are many public health-related activities that are now spreading nationwide and worldwide, but there has been no evidence of their effectiveness. These include programs like a day for depression awareness and screening. In 2008, the 18th such day was held on October 10. Individuals could go to a local site for taking a self-report depression inventory and for obtaining information on treatment and resources. Steps taken toward suicide prevention include public service announcements made about the prevention of such an act, dissemination of brochures on suicide awareness and prevention, and listings of suicide prevention hotline numbers in newspapers, telephone books, and online.

The International Association for Suicide Prevention (IASP) sponsors an annual World Suicide Prevention Day, cosponsored by WHO. In 2008, this day was September 10 and had the theme "Think globally, plan nationally, act locally" (Beautrais & Mishara, 2008). The information that was disseminated encouraged international collaboration on suicide research and prevention, formulation of national plans, and local activities. The local activities include holding conferences and educational seminars, writing articles for newspapers and magazines, holding press conferences, placing information on websites, organizing memorial services for those who died from suicide, organizing walks to highlight suicide prevention, and distributing leaflets, posters, and other written information.

Berman (2008) asked the question of whether these activities save lives, but there is no research that evaluates these activities. For most of these activities, the common measure of success is volume. This many people attended a meeting or a walk; this many came for depression screening; this amount of money was raised. Indeed, the volume of activity is the primary measure that suicide prevention services (whether telephone hotlines or walk-in clinics) use to measure their success – not how many lives they saved. The early suicide prevention services often changed their name to crisis intervention services to reflect their activity more accurately.

Berman asked, more pointedly, if there are no data to support the effectiveness of these public health programs, then why do organizations continue to spend limited available monies on them? Perhaps, a cynical answer is that these activities draw attention to the sponsoring organizations (e.g., IASP and WHO for World Suicide Prevention Day), hopefully increasing their membership and revenue.

In other areas, the evidence for the effectiveness of such campaigns has been questioned. For example, Hornik, Jacobson, Orwin, Piesse, and Kalton (2008) examined the impact of an antidrug media campaign on youths aged 12–18 years. In samples ranging from 5,126 to 8,117, Hornik and his associates observed that most of the analyses found no impact of the campaign on marijuana use. There was evidence in some samples that exposure to the campaign predicted *weaker* antidrug social norms and *increased* the likelihood of initiating marijuana use. The campaign, in fact, appeared to have the opposite impact of what was desired.

Recommendation 11: It is important that evaluation research be built into the design and planning of public awareness programs for suicide prevention.

Psychotherapy

There has been a major effort made for evaluating the effectiveness of psychotherapy in helping suicidal clients, and much of the research has been supportive of the cognitive therapies and related therapies such as dialectic behavior therapy. However, Larzelere, Kuhn, and Johnson (2004) noted that many of these studies have a selection bias in which those clients with the more severe presenting problems are more likely to be assigned to the treatment group, probably, out of ethical concerns. (It is viewed as unethical to deprive such clients of immediate help.) However, if the assignment of clients to the treatment and placebo groups were not completely random, then no valid cause-and-effect conclusions could be drawn. In the six studies that they identified on the effectiveness of psychotherapy for suicidal adolescents, treatment predicted subsequent suicidal behavior. This may mean that psychotherapy is detrimental to suicidal adolescents or it may mean that the more severely suicidal clients were assigned to the treatment group.
Recommendation 12: Studies of the effectiveness of psychotherapy for suicidal clients must be methodologically rigorous, especially with regard to random assignment of clients to the treatment and placebo groups.

Suicide Prevention Organizations

It is not surprising to note that people's desires for power and self-aggrandizement intrude into the scholarly world for, after all, those desires pervade human behavior in general. Nevertheless, the manifestation of these desires in scholars is disappointing because scholars, of all groups, might be expected to be above such concerns. How do these desires manifest themselves in suicidology?

The People and the Organizations

The first way is in the fragmentation of groups concerned with suicide prevention. One organization is formed and then, apparently, some who feel that their importance is not recognized by the organization form their own organization. Everyone wants his or her own little kingdom, and the idea of working together in harmony is rarely contemplated.

There are three international organizations that organize telephone crisis intervention centers – Befrienders International, IFOTES, and Life Line International. The IASP was followed by the European Symposium[5] and then the International Academy for Suicide Research (IASR).[6] In the United States, the first national organization developed

[5] The European Symposium initially limited the number of Americans permitted to attend. Eventually this restriction was removed, most likely to increase attendance and revenues.

[6] The IASR was suggested by a member of IASP who wanted his own organization. IASP attempted to keep IASR under its umbrella, but eventually IASR became independent.

to advance the cause of suicide prevention, the American Association of Suicidology (AAS), was followed by the American Suicide Foundation (now renamed as AFSP[7]) and then the Suicide Prevention Awareness Network (SPAN).[8]

Each of these groups has its own leaders, and it seems that each leader desires the spotlight. To be sure, the cause is of some importance to these leaders, but the attention and trappings of power appear to be equally seductive. After all, if the cause were really important, more could be achieved by one large organization than by many smaller ones fighting for attention.

AAS has been a fine organization. It has been active, fair, and inclusive – embracing scholars, crisis centers, and survivors. Founded by Edwin Shneidman and now admirably run by Alan Berman, it has proven itself to be an effective organization. I see no need for rival organizations, and I distrust the motives of the founders and directors of AFSP and SPAN. They could have easily worked with the AAS if they truly valued the cause and if they had been able to subjugate their desires for recognition. AAS currently encourages other groups (such as Contact and AFSP) to participate in its annual meeting and also other activities.

How might such organizations be evaluated? Initially, the organizations need to specify their goals and missions, both at an abstract level of discourse and at a more pragmatic level. For example, do they expect to prevent suicide? If so, how might this be assessed? *Recommendation 13: All suicidology organizations should have clearly stated missions and goals and, in addition, specify exactly what they hope to accomplish at a pragmatic level so that their impact can be assessed.*

The Money

There were two major disappointments with regard to the funding of suicidology in the 1990s. First, the widow of Arthur Sommer Rotenberg helped raise enough money to endow a chair in suicidology at the University of Toronto. Here was a chance to appoint a leading suicidologist to organize a center for the study of suicide, and Canada had several fine scholars who merited the position. Instead, the university chose to appoint a psychiatrist who was a researcher in borderline personality. Perhaps, funding for his position had run out?

Senators and congressmen in the United States often appropriate money simply to provide funds for their constituents. It is called "pork," and it is, in my opinion, unethical behavior on the part of these individuals since it is not part of rational and planned expenditures for government functions. As an example, recently a congressman in Pennsylvania removed the tolls for trucks from one exit of the Pennsylvania Turnpike, so that truck drivers would exit there and use the restaurants and gas stations in his district.

---

7 The AFSP has recently experienced a conflict and a group has broken off to compete with AFSP.

8 For essays written by the leaders of some of these organizations, see Lester (2001).

Recently, Senator Harry Reid obtained $1.5 million for a suicide center and, since he was the Senator from Nevada, the center was of course established at a university in Nevada, unfortunately one with no history of suicide research. There are many fine young suicidologists across the United States who could have formed the nucleus for a center. Some institutions already have a couple of suicidologists on the staff, and AAS would have been able to make fine use of the funds. But the Senator was from Nevada, and so the money had to go to Nevada.

When these events happen, we are supposed to cheer and be enthusiastic. Isn't this great for suicidology? No. Both these events were tragic because they were missed opportunities. Furthermore, there has been no evaluation of the impact of these expenditures. Was anything worthwhile achieved?

Recommendation 14: All funding should have an evaluative component built into the program so that the activity which has been funded can be evaluated.

Conclusion

It has been argued in this chapter that the evaluation of tactics for prevention was neglected in the past. Many of the programs established have not incorporated an evaluation component for examining whether they have met their goals or not. All too often, the volume of activity has been used as a measure of success rather than the direct impact on suicidal behavior. The recent research by Hornik et al. (2008), which suggested that antidrug public education may have increased drug use, is a warning that evaluation is critical if we are to promote successful suicide prevention programs and cease the promotion of ineffective or detrimental suicide prevention programs.

References

Beautrais, A. L., & Mishara, B. L. (2008). World Suicide Prevention Day. *Crisis, 29*, 59–63.

Berman, L. (2008). Twenty questions, maybe more. *Newslink (American Association of Suicidology), 35*(3), 3–6.

Cheng, A. T. A. (1995). Mental illness and suicide. *Archives of General Psychiatry, 52*, 594–603.

Clarke, R. V., & Lester, D. (1989). *Suicide: Closing the exits*. New York: Springer-Verlag.

De Leo, D., Burgis, S., Bertolote, J. M., Kerkhof, A. J. F. M., & Bille-Brahe, U. (2006). Definitions of suicidal behavior. *Crisis, 27*, 4–15.

De Leo, D., Carollo, G., & Della Buono, M. (1995). Lower suicide rates associated with a Tele-Help/Tele-Check service for the elderly at home. *American Journal of Psychiatry, 152*, 632–634.

Hornik, R., Jacobson, L., Orwin, R., Piesse, A., & Kalton, G. (2008). Effects of the National Youth Anti-Drug Media Campaign on youths. *American Journal of Public Health, 98*, 2229–2236.

Larzelere, R. E., Kuhn, B. R., & Johnson, B. (2004). The intervention selection bias. *Psychological Bulletin, 130*, 289–303.

Leenaars, A. A., Lester, D., & Wenckstern, S. (2002). Social support in suicide prevention. In J. D. Morgan (Ed.), *Social support* (pp. 99–111). Amityville, NY: Baywood.
Lester, D. (1970a). Steps toward the evaluation of a suicide prevention center: Part one. *Crisis Intervention, 2*(Suppl. #2), 42–45.
Lester, D. (1970b). Steps toward the evaluation of a suicide prevention center: Part two. *Crisis Intervention, 2*(Suppl. #1), 12–18.
Lester, D. (1970c). Steps toward the evaluation of a suicide prevention center: Part three. *Crisis Intervention, 2*(Suppl. #1), 19–21.
Lester, D. (1970d). Steps toward the evaluation of a suicide prevention center: Part four. *Crisis Intervention, 2*(Suppl. #4), 20–22.
Lester, D. (1994). Predicting the suicide rate in Wales. *Psychological Reports, 75*, 1054.
Lester, D. (1997). The effectiveness of suicide prevention centers. *Suicide & Life-Threatening Behavior, 27*, 304–310.
Lester, D. (2000a). Decades of suicide research: Wherefrom and whereto? In T. Joiner & M. D. Rudd (Eds.), *Suicide science* (pp. 9–16). Boston: Kluwer Academic.
Lester, D. (2000b). The end of suicidology. *Crisis, 21*, 158–159.
Lester, D. (Ed.). (2001). *Suicide prevention: Resources for the Millennium*. Philadelphia: Brunner-Routledge.
Lester, D. (2002). The scientific study of suicide requires accurate data. *Crisis, 23*, 133–134.
Lester, D. (2009). *Preventing suicide: Closing the exits revisited.* Hauppauge, NY: Nova Science.
Lukas, C., & Seiden, H. M. (1990). *Silent grief.* New York: Bantam.
MacDonald, A. J. D. (1995). Suicide prevention in Gotland. *British Journal of Psychiatry, 166*, 402.
Maris, R. W., Berman, A. L., & Silverman, M. M. (2000). *Comprehensive textbook of suicidology.* New York: Guilford.
Rogers, J. R., & Lester, D. (2010). *Understanding suicide: Why we don't and how we might.* Cambridge, MA, Göttingen, Germany: Hogrefe Publishing.
Rutz, W., Walinder, J., Eberhard, G., Holmberg, G., von Knorring, A. L., von Knorring, L., Wistedt, B., & Aberg-Wistedt, A. (1989). An educational program on depressive disorders for general practitioners on Gotland. *Acta Psychiatrica Scandinavica, 79*, 19–26.
Smith, M. S. (1960). *Modern physics.* London, UK: Longmans.
Wilson, E. G. (2008). *Against happiness: In praise of melancholy.* New York: Farrar, Straus, & Giroux.
Zonda, T., & Lester, D. (2006–2007). Preventing suicide by educating general practitioners. *Omega, 54*, 53–57.

About the Author

David Lester has doctoral degrees from Cambridge University (UK) in social and political science and Brandeis University (USA) in psychology. He is Distinguished Professor of Psychology at the Richard Stockton College of New Jersey. He has been President of the International Association for Suicide Prevention, and he has published extensively on suicide, murder, and other issues in thanatology. His recent books include *Katie's Diary: Unlocking the Mystery of a Suicide* (2004), *Suicide and the Holocaust* (2005), *Is there Life after Death?* (2005), *Preventing Suicide: Closing the Exits Revisited* (2009), and *Understanding Suicide: Why We Don't and How We Might* (2010).

David Lester
The Richard Stockton College of New Jersey
PO Box 195
Jimmie Leeds Road
Pomona, NJ 08240-0195
USA
Tel.: +1 609 652 4512
E-mail: lesterd@stockton.edu

Index